The Fountain of the Love of Wisdom

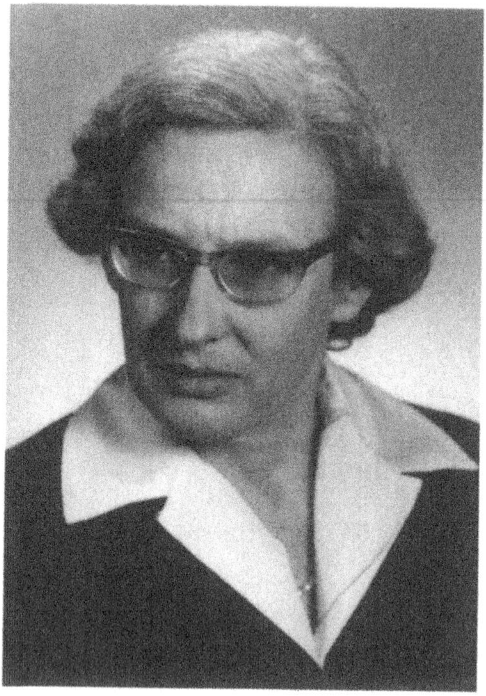

Marie-Louise von Franz

The Fountain of the Love of Wisdom

AN HOMAGE TO

MARIE-LOUISE VON FRANZ

Edited by Emmanuel Kennedy-Xypolitas

CHIRON PUBLICATIONS
Asheville, North Carolina

Book and cover design by Greta Polo.
Printed in the United States of America.

Library of Congress Cataloging-in-Publication Data

The fountain of the love of wisdom : an homage to Marie-Louise von Franz / edited by Emmanuel Kennedy-Xypolitas.

p. cm.

ISBN 978-1-63051-525-6 (alk. paper)

1. Franz, Marie-Louise von, 1915– 2. Jungian psychology. 3. Psychoanalysis. I. Franz, Marie-Louise von, 1915– II. Kennedy-Xypolitas, Emmanuel.

BF109.F72F68 2006

150.19'54092—dc22

[B]

2006010410

When a man holds a high position
and is nevertheless modest,
he shines with the light of wisdom.

I Ching, hexagram 15, "Modesty"

Contents

A gallery of color photographs follows page 68.

A gallery of black and white photographs follows page 132.

. . . the manifestations of the spirit are truly wondrous, and as varied as Creation itself.

The living spirit grows and even outgrows its earlier forms of expression; it freely chooses the men who proclaim it and in whom it lives. This living spirit is eternally renewed and pursues its goal in manifold and inconceivable ways throughout the history of mankind. Measured against it, the names and forms which men have given it mean very little; they are only the changing leaves and blossoms on the stem of the eternal tree.

—CARL GUSTAV JUNG, "PSYCHOTHERAPISTS OR THE CLERGY"

Acknowledgments

My cordial and sincere thanks for their help with this work go to Marie-Anne von Franz, the Psychological Club of Zürich, the Stiftung für Jung'sche Psychologie, and the Marie-Louise von Franz Stiftung. Due to their encouragement and generous support, this commemorative Festschrift was made possible.

—EMMANUEL KENNEDY-XYPOLITAS

Foreword

It is a great pleasure that Manolis Kennedy has taken the initiative to put together a commemorative Festschrift for Marie-Louise von Franz. The students and acquaintances of Marie-Louise are getting older and passing on, and the time will soon come when there will be but few witnesses who can report of her from firsthand experience.

Marie-Louise was a very complex personality—as are all genius personalities. She had so many facets, twists and turns, of her personality that all of her students and acquaintances had a different picture of her. Therefore, a simple presentation of the personality of Marie-Louise cannot be expected to follow, but rather a colorful and at times even contradictory image. The contributions will all agree on one point, and that is that Marie-Louise was a unique, great, and, at times, paradoxical personality. With diverse facets of her personality she was able to address the most varied types of people who, in turn, had a wide range of personalities and sundry expectations of her. Thanks to the broad spectrum of this woman's personality, along with her most comprehensive knowledge, she was able to give something to many people, and highly diverging types of characters felt addressed in many different ways. The common denominator was an immense, far-reaching, and often nondiscriminating eros that accepted everyone seeking help and answered their distress with a depth of feeling. It is not the intention of this commemorative Festschrift to sing praises to Marie-Louise von Franz, but rather to render this woman in all her contradictions, with both her light and shadow sides, and to preserve these for following generations who did not have the luck to have come into direct contact with her. If primarily the light and more beautiful and charismatic sides of her personality find expression in the following contributions, this has to do with the fact that in the face of the magnitude of her comprehensive and many faceted personality, one is hesitant to speak of her shadow side where she may, for example, have failed to fulfill the expectations that one had of her. This does not mean that such sides were not present but that it lies not with us to judge. I hope that one important side of her personality will be clear in the contributions that follow and that is her immense sense of humor with her insight into the ridiculous sides of human beings who feel lofty and sublime and whose fate then took care that their inflation was reduced to a tolerable measure. Marie-Louise von Franz had the sensitivity to detect these synchronicities and to mirror them back to the person concerned always in a benevolent manner.

With this Festschrift for Marie-Louise von Franz something essential for the future of the research of the history of depth psychology will be retained and this is that, in my opinion, she was the student of Jung who most clearly understood his thoughts and rendered them in her own books in such a personal manner. We were all fortunate to have received the spirit of Jung from her hands, we who did not have the luck of personally meeting Jung himself.

It remains to be hoped that through this Festschrift the spirit of Jung—which was rendered in such an original manner by Marie-Louise von Franz—will be passed on by her students and acquaintances. We also hope that this Festschrift will contribute to a concord among the conflicting Jungians, who will have the opportunity once again to reflect on the original meaning and spirit of C. G. Jung. And finally, with this Festschrift, we hope to have made a permanent contribution to the prosperousness and continuance of Jungian psychology. The life of Marie-Louise von Franz was an exemplary contribution toward this goal.

—ALFRED RIBI, M.D.

Introduction

"It is the quiet ones who sow seeds."
MARIE-LOUISE VON FRANZ

Marie-Louise von Franz was a unique individual human being, a woman who became a true embodiment of the "living spirit." All who knew her were touched by that greater spirit of openness and devotion toward the unconscious as envisioned by Carl Gustav Jung toward the end of his life.[1] The contributions in this commemorative publication have been gathered to honor this spirit and this devotion to the unconscious, the very essence of the woman herself.

Editors of a book are generally known to the reader. As this may not be the case here, it seems proper that I briefly introduce myself. I am a Greek national, born on a small island in the Aegean sea. I was adopted by William H. Kennedy—who personally knew both C. G. Jung and Marie-Louise von Franz—and came to Switzerland in 1973. That was a fateful year for me as it was the year I first met Marie-Louise von Franz. As the years passed and I established myself as a Jungian analyst, a valuable friendship developed between the two of us which lasted until her death in 1998.

The idea of a commemorative publication for Marie-Louise von Franz spontaneously arose during a stay in the vicinity of her "tower" where I sought retreat in the summer of 2001, two and a half years after her death. I let the idea sink within and dwell quietly for several weeks. Prompted by relevant signs from the unconscious, I discussed the idea first with Dr. Marie-Anne von Franz, the sister of Marie-Louise von Franz, and then with Dr. Alfred Ribi. Both of them welcomed the idea and encouraged me to proceed with the project. For their continuous moral support throughout the subsequent years of this project, I wish to express my heartfelt gratitude.

But mostly it was out of the deep bond of friendship with Marie-Louise von Franz that I—along with the President of the Psychological Club of Zürich, Dr. Alfred Ribi—addressed her friends and colleagues with the following letter.[2]

Psychological Club of Zurich
Gemeindestrasse 27
Zürich 8032
February 2002

Commemorative Publication ("Festschrift")
honoring Dr. Marie-Louise von Franz

Dear Friends and Colleagues,

We are sending this letter to people who knew Dr. von Franz or were related to her in one way or the other. Our purpose is to collect written "dedications" as contributions for a Festschrift, i.e., a commemorative publication honoring Marie-Louise von Franz.

The form of your donated contributions is left to your own judgment. For example, it can be any of the following:

- An account of an encounter (analytical or personal) with Dr. von Franz
- Memories or recollections of her
- Personal experiences of her
- Synchronistic events or any other relevant unconscious constellations related to her
- Impressions of her and/or her work

In addition, you might indicate what fateful impetus or

strong influence Dr. von Franz and/or her written work had on your life. Especially valuable contributions for this Festschrift could also be dreams of yours and/or your analysands about Marie-Louise von Franz. Even though such dreams have a personal aspect, they may still show *how the unconscious perceives her.*

Heartily welcomed are also "dedications" of a creative nature; for example, an essay or short paper of *general psychological interest,* an interpretation of a dream, myth, fairy tale, vision, spontaneous picture or fantasy, and so on. However, this creative work should *not* be an old work of yours—a "frozen fish" as it were—which was lying in the deep freezer and was simply taken out for this Festschrift. Rather, it should be a new work, a "fresh fish," written especially for the commemorative publication *in honor of Marie-Louise von Franz.* In the latter case, one has a better chance for the creative spirit of the unconscious to meaningfully express itself through *Eros:* a feeling-relatedness to inner values and love for the genuine spirit of truth. Please feel free to express your feeling and emotion for the late Dr. von Franz, even at the cost of being accused of writing something hagiographical. In other words, *your* heart knows, not the others. Everyone who felt close to Dr. von Franz knows that she was a *Mana-Personality.*

It is important to mention here that there is no obligation from our part to publish all the contributions for the Festschrift. Your contribution should not exceed 8–9 typed double-spaced pages. The typed text should be free of mistakes and ready for publication. Let us add that the author is completely responsible for the text. The deadline for your submission is the end of December 2002. Any contributions may be written in English or German.

Hoping for a positive echo, we remain sincerely yours,

President	Member of the Board
Alfred Ribi, M.D.	Emmanuel Kennedy, Ph.D.

Marie-Anne von Franz (known as "Mandi" among her friends) accompanied me faithfully throughout the preparation of this volume and advised me on various matters.[3] She presented me with highly valuable material regarding her sister. I would like to express here my deepest thanks to Mandi. Her inestimable contribution immensely enriched this commemorative volume for her sister, Marlus. This Festschrift owes a great deal to her commitment and most generous gesture.

When Marie-Anne von Franz and I decided to proceed with this project, the first question that arose was, naturally, who do we ask for contributions? Marie-Louise von Franz knew a great number of people, and we wanted to avoid leaving anyone out. We solved the problem by simply sending the letter to *all* the people whose names were in M.-L. von Franz's address book: acquaintances, relatives, friends, colleagues, analysands, doctors, lawyers, assistants, secretaries, nurses, publishers and professional associates, workmen and craftsmen, the hairdresser, the postwoman, the taxi chauffeur, and finally to people she did not know personally but with whom she had corresponded.[4] We sent out a total of 372 letters and received 75 responses, the majority of which were accompanied by a contribution. Happily enough, we were able to use all contributions. A couple of the essays needed some editing, which we were glad to do. The rest were left more or less as we received them, requiring only minor corrections and alterations. We felt it was important to retain the individual manner of expression of the authors, so although the text has been edited, there remain certain inconsistencies with regard to style, references, and notes.

As English is neither Dr. Marie-Anne von Franz's nor my mother tongue, we entrusted the editing to Chiron Publications and to my colleague Dr. David Eldred. He also translated the German contributions into English. We would like to express our gratitude to him as well as to Dr. Robert Mercurio, an American analyst living in Italy who translated two essays from Italian into English. He also offered to do editorial or any other work and thus assist in the realization of this project. His generosity is an expression of his true devotion to von Franz which stems from the depths of the heart. This is also evident in his contribution.

Some relatives of deceased addressees were kind enough to respond to our circular letter. In one such case we received the following note: "Mrs. N passed away just before your letter arrived. It's a pity, for Mrs. N had great respect for von Franz. Be that as it may, she will certainly tell her this herself 'there' on the other side."

We would like to express our deepest gratitude to those individuals who responded with a written contribution; without their heartfelt reaction, this publication would not have been possible. We are aware of the fact that it was not an easy task for many to write something about Marie-Louise von Franz, especially if one happened to have had a close relationship to her. This is partly due to the fact that there are encounters, feelings, and experiences—also dreams—which one cannot and need not reveal; they are part of the mystery of eros.

Our sincere thanks also goes out to those who did not wish to make a contribution but responded to our letter with encouraging words for the project, wishing it success. We are grateful for their sincerity and solidarity toward our efforts but even more toward the person and spirit of Marie-Louise von Franz, who untiringly and selflessly devoted her life—and whole being—to helping friends, analysands, colleagues, and many others in need. As we will see in the contributions which follow, in serving others Marie-Louise von Franz played an instrumental role in the lives of many people, thus gaining their everlasting devotion and love.

After receiving our call for contributions, a loyal friend of von Franz called me and asked, "Manolis, what shall I contribute? Marlus saved my life. I owe my life to her." This kind of gesture—in this case, an expression of introverted feeling—is in its essence worth a hundred pages of contribution. We would like to express our sincere thanks to this person as well.

When we examined the various contributions more closely, we made some interesting observations. First, the greater part of the contributions were of a personal nature, an expression of eros, of feeling relatedness, something for which von Franz was known. Even the contributions that were of a nonpersonal creative nature (an interpretation of a myth, a fairy tale, dreams, and so forth) were still related to von Franz, for these are fields in which she herself worked her entire life. There is also a considerable heterogeneity of the contributions, an element we hope will appeal to the general public. The multifacetedness of the responses was a major reason that prompted us to undertake this venture and make this present volume available to a wider readership.

We were very pleased to receive a considerable number of contributions from laypersons and simple people: a barber, a young female truck driver, a veterinary surgeon, a doctor's secretary, a schoolteacher, a bank employee, an elderly Swiss peasant woman who shared her love of nature with von Franz, an elderly Italian amateur painter who expressed her admiration by painting pictures of von Franz's tower and of a frog (plates 3 and 4 in the color gallery following page 68).[5]

The simple individuals, so it seems, are the true and living paradigms of love, the true recipients of gratitude which, in the opinion of Marie-Louise von Franz, transgresses conscious earthly borders and extends even into the beyond. According to Jung, it is the simple, poor people who are the real carriers of the spirit of analytical psychology. There is a story about Jung who was purportedly celebrating his birthday one evening when someone knocked at his door. It was an unknown and simple woman with a book of Jung's in her hands. She was kindly asked what she wanted, and she replied that she had come to congratulate the man who had written this valuable book. Jung's reaction was: "It is in the hearts of such inconspicuous simple people—and not of highbrow scholars, academic people, professors and the like—that my work will live on."[6]

Marie-Louise von Franz expressed a similar idea when I told her once that in a small village in a rural area of Switzerland a simple Catholic priest was giving seminars to laypersons on dreams and the Bible, incorporating Jung's ideas. She remarked: "It is the quiet ones who sow seeds." And in an interview with Gordon Young, Jung said:

> Most of [the highbrows] haven't the remotest idea what I am talking about. Trouble is, they don't bother to read my books because they're too high hat. I'm not a bit taken in by intellectuals. . . . Do you know who reads my books? Not the academic people, oh no, they think they know everything already. It's the ordinary people, often quite poor people and

> why do they do it? Because there's a need in the world just now for spiritual guidance . . . almost any sort of spiritual guidance.[7]

In our letter, we encouraged people to contribute a new work of their own, a "fresh fish" as we called it. By this we meant—and hoped—that people would actually sit down and write something exclusively for this commemorative publication honoring von Franz. As far as we are able to judge and know, apart from a very few exceptions, the majority of the contributions are indeed "fresh fish": personal creative dedications, genuine expressions of the unified chthonic spirit in struggle for differentiation and realization.

We were especially happy to receive contributions that included dreams about Marie-Louise von Franz, for the unconscious is the more "objective" and reliable source of information about the true being of an individual whose essence and fate is a mystery to man. At bottom, we never really know what the life of the individual human being is.[8]

We feel we owe an explanation to the reader as to the form of this rather unorthodox commemorative publication. The deadline for submission of contributions was the end of 2002. By then, we had received the greater part of the contributions. Nevertheless we were still uncertain whether or not the project should be realized. We left the question open and were waiting for some clear sign. Furthermore, were the project to be realized, we were uncertain about the form of the publication. One possibility was to have a file of all the contributions kept at the library of the Psychological Club of Zürich, available for internal use. Another possibility was to bind all the contributions in a single volume and give personal copies solely to each contributor. A third possibility was to publish the contributions in book form, a meal of "fresh fish," so to speak, without entrée, side dish, or dessert. Still a fourth possibility was a more elaborate and illustrated volume including not only the contributions but also additional material: paintings, photographs, various documents, and the like. These questions were still unanswered when, on January 10, 2003, we received a most valuable response from Mrs. Françoise Selhofer. Her contribution included a profound archetypal dream. This product of the unconscious seemed to contain an answer to our question of whether or not a more elaborate commemorative publication should be realized. We took it as a sign from the unconscious.

Geneva
January 8, 2003

Dear Dr. Kennedy,

Since I received your letter regarding the Festschrift—a letter that I would like to thank you for—I have been waiting for a dream, a sign, a "north-sea fish." Yesterday evening I set your letter to the side, the deadline is now past, and this morning I awoke having had this impressive dream:

I pick up a book by C. G. Jung in my library and am astounded that I have never seen the pictures in it before. One sees a mountain with a tower perched on a precipice. It is supposed to be the north tower of Jung (possibly in Bollingen?). Yet when I approach this tower (I am now in this landscape), I see that it is a part of an immense church buried in the mountain. As I climb upwards (half mountain, half tower) the entire building slowly appears: it is an old cathedral. The round tower that I am climbing looks now like the top of a bell tower although the bell is missing. When I look down I can see many people down in the nave of the church working to dig it out and restore it. Then I am down below. A young worker says to me that we should go no further as one should not trample the earth with ones feet. The bottom of the nave is still covered in a beautiful brown earth much like a large bed in a garden. The young worker smiles at me and I feel very comfortable with him. Later I see young students and children that are preparing themselves for a production. A banquet is also being prepared. Then Dr. von Franz arrives. I can only greet her briefly as many people are accompanying her into the cathedral which is now fully lit up. I remain outside and feel very sad. I know that it is now too late to contribute to the Festschrift, the book must have already gone to press.

Sincerely yours,
Françoise Selhofer

The dream seems to me to move on different levels. Besides its personal meaning or personal message to the dreamer, it seems to have a transpersonal quality, a quality characteristic of big dreams. The newly discovered book from C. G. Jung in the exposition of the dream—along with the allusion to Jung's tower—would seem to imply that the dream is revealing something about the nature of analytical psychology. Like several other people, Marie-Louise von Franz was, as it were, the very embodiment of Jungian psychology. The symbols of the earth and the cathedral point to the collective archetypal dimension of the whole inner-psychic experience.

Taking into account the outer context, as well as the end of the dream, I had the feeling that through this dream the unconscious tried to say something not only about the realization but also about the form of this present volume. The dream helped us decide what kind of Festschrift was suitable to honor Marie-Louise von Franz, namely, a banquetlike commemorative volume, a feast of spiritual nourishment, so to speak, a task to which Marie-Louise von Franz herself devoted her entire life. For as Jung once said: "There is a terrible spiritual famine in our world."[9]

In their contributions people expressed their intimate feelings, many exposed their innermost being and even shared their dreams. Due to the highly personal nature of the writings, we would like to set forth that no material in this volume can be quoted or reproduced without the written permission of the editor.

In Part One of this Festschrift—Reflections on the Death of Marie-Louise von Franz—one will find a selection of death announcements, obituaries, and responses to her death shared on the Internet.

Part Two—Eulogies—includes three eulogies delivered at the memorial service for Marie-Louise von Franz at the Reformed Church in

Küsnacht, Switzerland, on February 26, 1998. We would like to express our deep gratitude to Dr. Gotthilf Isler, Dr. Anne Maguire, and Dr. Nora Mindell for offering to include their valedictions in this present volume.[10]

Several speeches and comments given, for instance, at her birthday dinners constitute Part Three—Birthday Addresses.

In Part Four—Personal Impressions—one will find numerous shorter reflections and comments about Marie-Louise von Franz. The remarks come from various people and concern the woman Marie-Louise von Franz as well as M.-L. von Franz the analyst, the lecturer, the scholar, and the author.

Comments and reflections on her books published in English can be found in Part Five—Book Reviews and Publishers' Comments.

Part Six—Some Biographic Data on Marie-Louise von Franz— is reserved for the short but most valuable and revealing contribution from Marie-Anne von Franz in honor of her sister. She chose to write about "things and incidents which nobody else knows about." I am especially grateful to Mandi for her Herculean labor: she is now ninety-three years old.

The main body of this volume, Part Seven—Contributions—is devoted to the texts and essays submitted by the contributors themselves. They are presented alphabetically by the authors' names. In all of the contributions the emphasis is on personal, not scientific, work. References have been transcribed as the authors have given them to us. Some are incomplete, others in simplified forms. We have left them in the format that the author chose, making only minor adjustments. We have not checked the accuracy of citations or bibliographical references, and we have relied on the authors to have checked the spelling of words in languages other than English and German.

The final section—Part Eight—contains a list of Marie-Louise von Franz's writings in English, including books, articles, and her work on film.

In reading the various and most valuable contributions in this volume, it strikes one that the authors stress the *light* side of Marie-Louise von Franz and avoid speaking about the dark aspect of her being. I had explicitly asked and even urged some individuals—who I knew had occasionally experienced the less agreeable, fiery side of von Franz—to relate such encounters in their contributions. For reasons unknown, these people did not mention the shadowy aspect of von Franz's personality or wrote nothing at all.

It is not easy to speak about the shadow of someone who had a "spiritual dimension that was too great" as was the case with Marie-Louise von Franz.[11] The difficulty lies presumably, among other things, in the fact that in such a person the opposites are united, whereby "good" may bring about "evil" and "evil" bring about "good."[12] Marie-Louise von Franz noted that:

> The problem is that the opposites are too close to each other in me. When I do something evil, good may come out of it and then I no longer know whether I should stop it or continue. And when I do something good, evil may come out of it and then I no longer know whether I should save it. It is a paradox.[13]

I asked whether this made her sad. She answered, "No, because I try to see the criminal in me. My criminal [shadow] is to think that when I say something, this is of some use . . . . Hence my problem with speaking."[14]

Like every human being, Marie-Louise von Franz naturally also had her shadow, an all too human darkness.[15] If it is true that great personalities have great shadows, then—at least, according to my own personal experience—this is certainly true of von Franz. Thus it was on account of a dispute with her—during which von Franz reacted with a powerful outburst of affect along with an unexpected vehemence and forceful dynamism—that I had the darkest, emotionally most overwhelming, quasi-crucifying, soul-shattering experience of my life. It was numinous and painful, but at the very end, it was a redeeming experience of the *coincidentia oppositorum* where I was forced to experience a darkness in von Franz that was as overpowering as the light of her individual spirit.[16]

The encounter with von Franz's shattering rage was a violent "revelation" that was so crushing it almost drove me to the borders of madness. Yet I was grateful to the unconscious for this painful experience and the impact with which the opposites collided in my encounter with von Franz. I was also truly thankful to the unconscious for a subsequent archetypal dream that helped me come to terms with this profound transcendental experience of the paradoxical inner world opposites, an experience that reaches down into the depths of the psyche and gives the latter a wholeness in keeping with the projected ideal.

It is only after such an experience, so it seems, that a relationship between two human beings becomes personal, real, human, and complete.[17] Such an encounter allows one to be profoundly touched through the psychic connection. It enables one to relate consciously to the other individual, not as an idea or an image or a superhuman entity, but as a human being. And it helps one come close to the meaning of the projected—or venerated—value and to realize the ideal on one's own account as well as in one's own individual life. Jung writes: "It is conceivable that by virtue of this total effort a man may even catch a fleeting glimpse of his wholeness, accompanied by a feeling of grace that always characterizes such an experience."[18]

It is a well-known psychological fact that an intensive relationship to an other—whether it be a human being, the unconscious itself, or the Deity—lays the person open to an invasion far transcending anything personal and opens one's eye to the immensity of God.[19] The fact that I felt the effect of the *numinosum* in connection with my relationship to Marie-Louise von Franz does not astonish if we consider Jung's idea, discussed in "Psychology of the Transference," that of late the *numen* has immigrated (*eingewandert*) in the personal relationship and the soul "where the whole weight of mankind's problems has settled."[20] It is *here* that Jung sees the *magnum opus* of modern man "laying an infinitesimal grain in the scales of humanity's soul."[21]

According to my own personal experience of Marie-Louise von Franz, she was, like Jung, relatively conscious of her shadow, had integrated a considerable quantum of it, and, even more important, she *stood up* to her shadow.

No Festschrift or commemorative publication can ever do justice to the person honored. This is particularly true if the person is a woman such as Marie-Louise von Franz, a woman who for many people embodied true eros, that is, *feeling-relatedness to the deeper inner values and love for the genuine spirit of truth, the inner truth, the Self.* I would like to conclude with a quote from Jung expressing his view of eros and "love":

> Eros was considered a god whose divinity transcended our human limits, and who therefore could neither be comprehended nor represented in any way. . . . I falter before the task of finding the language which might adequately express the incalculable paradoxes of love. Eros is a kosmogonos, a creator and father-mother of all higher consciousness. I sometimes feel that Paul's words: "Though I speak with the tongues of men and of angels, and have not love" might well be the first condition of all cognition and the quintessence of divinity itself. Whatever the learned interpretation may be of the sentence "God is love," the words affirm the complexio oppositorum of the Godhead. In my medical experience as well as in my own life I have again and again been faced with the mystery of love, and have never been able to explain what it is. Like Job, I had to "lay my hand on my mouth. I have spoken once, and I will not answer."[22] Here is the greatest and smallest, the remotest and nearest, the highest and lowest, and we cannot discuss one side of it without also discussing the other. No language is adequate to this paradox. Whatever one can say, no words express the whole. To speak of partial aspects is always too much or too little, for only the whole is meaningful. Love "bears all things" and "endures all things."[23] These words say all there is to be said; nothing can be added to them. For we are in the deepest sense the victims and the instruments of cosmogonic "love." I put the word in quotation marks to indicate that I do not use it in its connotations of desiring, preferring, favoring, wishing, and similar feelings, but as something superior to the individual, a unified and undivided whole. Being a part, man cannot grasp the whole. He is at its mercy. He may assent to it, or rebel against it; but he is always caught up by it and enclosed within it. He is dependent upon it and is sustained by it. Love is his light and his darkness, whose end he cannot see. "Love ceases not"—whether he speaks with the "tongues of angels" or with scientific exactitude traces the life of the cell down to its uttermost source. Man can try to name love, showering upon it all the names at his command, and still he will involve himself in endless self-deceptions. If he possesses a grain of wisdom, he will lay down his arms

and name the unknown by the more unknown, *ignotum per ignotius*—that is, by the name of God. That is a confession of his subjection, his imperfection, and his dependence; but at the same time a testimony to his freedom to choose between truth and error.[24]

NOTES

1. In 1959, Jung was asked what recommendations he could make for the passage from the Age of Pisces to the Age of Aquarius. He answered: "A spirit of greater openness toward the unconscious . . . , an increased attention to dreams, a sharper sense of the totality of the physical and psychical, of their indissolubility; a livelier taste for self-knowledge." *Spring: A Magazine of Jungian Thought* (New York: The Analytical Psychology Club of New York, 1960), p. 9.
2. Marie-Louise von Franz was a member of the Psychological Club from 1944 to her death. She was an associate member from 1941 until 1944. She also acted as its librarian from 1942 until 1952. At that time, C. G. Jung was also a member of the library committee together with C. A. Meier and F. Allemann. Her very first professional appearance at the Club was when she lectured on the visions of Perpetua ("Einige Bemerkungen zu den Visionen der Heiligen Perpetua") on June 7, 1941. The lecture later became the theme of her first book, *The Passion of Perpetua,* published in 1949 by Spring Publications. There followed many other lectures at the Club, which later constituted the basis of many of her numerous books.
3. Marie-Anne von Franz studied history at the University of Zürich, where she received her PhD in 1939. From 1940 through 1948, she worked for the Red Cross in Geneva and from 1948 to 1972, she worked in the department of social sciences of UNESCO in Paris. In her function as senior program specialist, she assisted in the publication of a great number of books in the field of the social sciences. Since 1972, she has lived in Bubikon, a small village near Bollingen, Switzerland, where Marie-Louise von Franz spent a great part of the year in her country house. As Bubikon lies in the vicinity of both Bollingen and Küsnacht, Marie-Anne von Franz had easy access to both residences of her sister, with whom she had regular contact.
4. Unfortunately a few addresses were illegible.
5. Marie-Louise von Franz's tower in Bollingen was her "life's elixir," as she once said, and frogs and toads were her favorite animals. Like Jung, she considered animals as being naturally more sublime than human beings, who all too often disappointed, exploited, betrayed, or deceived her.
6. In another version of this story, a kiosk woman told Jung that she had read his books

with great joy. Jung purportedly responded: "But my books are difficult to read, they are full of old Greek and Latin." The woman replied: "Yes, but they touch the heart" (personal communication from Alfred Ribi). In Bollingen on November 23, 1959, Jung himself related to Eric and Elisabeth Hutchinson the following two stories: "There is an old woman in the village nearby who told me she had read one of my books once through and was going to read it again. She said to me, 'I don't understand it yet, but I know you are right.' A small old Jew with a little green box on his bicycle came to my door one day in Küsnacht and, opening the green box, demanded to see the man who wrote 'these books.' He would not be put off, and when I met him the Jew said to me, 'You are right, I know'" (stories rendered from Eric Hutchinson's private notes of his meeting with Jung; as William Kennedy had arranged the meeting, Mr. Hutchinson was kind enough to send him a copy of the notes). More extensive accounts of this and other similar stories are found in Jung's lecture, "Ueber Psychologie" (*Neue Schweizer Rundschau,* 1. Jahrgang, Mai 1933, Heft 1, p. 21ff). This lecture was given in the Zürcher Rathaus on December 18, 1932, on the occasion of the presentation of the Prize for Literature of the City of Zürich. The lecture is published in the *Collected Works* (vol. 10, par. 276ff). These three incidents, with which Jung tried to demonstrate that his work finds echo in the hearts of simple inconspicuous people, were not included in this text. See also *Spring* (1960, p. 14), where Jung tells the following story: "I always remember a letter I received one morning, a poor scrap of paper, really, from a woman who wanted to see me just once in her life. That letter made a very strong impression on me, I am not quite sure why. I invited her to come and she came. She was very poor—poor intellectually, too. I don't believe she had even finished primary school. She kept house for her brother; they ran a little newsstand. I asked her kindly if she really understood my books which she said she had read. And she replied in this extraordinary way: 'Your books are not books, Herr Professor, they are bread. . . .' And the little traveling saleswoman [peddling] women's things, who stopped me in the street and looked at me with immense eyes, says, 'Are you really the man who writes those books? Are you truly the one who writes about these things no one knows . . . ?' Yes, in the long run I am very optimistic. The people do follow it. . . . Who reads [my books]? Not the professors." See also Barbara Hannah, *Jung, His Life and Work: A Biographical Memoir* (Wilmette, Ill.: Chiron Publications, 1997), p. 323.

7. William McGuire and R. F. C. Hull, eds., *C. G. Jung Speaking* (Princeton, N.J.: Princeton University Press, 1977), pp. 443ff.
8. In *Memories, Dreams, Reflections,* Jung writes: "What we are to our inward vision, and what man appears to be *sub specie aeternitatis,* can only be expressed by way of myth." Jung's statement suggests that being has meaning, "divine" meaning. *Memories, Dreams, Reflections,* A. Jaffé, ed. (New York: Random House, 1963), pp. 3 and 316ff.
9. *Spring* (1960), p. 10.
10. These eulogies are published in *Jungiana: Beiträge zur Psychologie von C. G. Jung.*

Reihe A, Band 8, *Verlag Stiftung für Jung'sche Psychologie,* 1998, pp. 14ff, and reprinted here with permission.

11. The spiritual dimension being "too great" was indicated in a dream of hers shortly before her death.
12. In the summer of 1997, one of the caretakers assisting Dr. von Franz dreamed that von Franz was "lying in bed, half covered with a duvet on which the sun and moon were depicted."
13. Personal communication.
14. This was an allusion to a dream of mine with a criminal shadow figure. As a Christian burdened with the tendency to condemn the darker human side of my personality, it was a crucial help to me in dealing with the vital problem of the shadow when von Franz said to me: "It is very important to forgive one's shadow." This statement is in accordance with Jung's idea that the best "formula" to deal with the shadow is to hate it *and* love it at the same time. And due to the Parkinson's disease, her ability to speak gradually diminished; at the end she could hardly speak at all.
15. In all the years of our acquaintance, Marie-Louise von Franz related to me dozens of dreams of hers with shadow figures of all imaginable kinds. Shortly before her death, she dreamed of a negative shadow figure. Her comment on the dream was: "It is amazing how the unconscious never ceases to confront one with one's own shadow right up to the very end . . . until one dies a miserable death [*verrecken*] on the way."
16. See C. G. Jung, *Answer to Job* (1952) in *Collected Works,* vol. 11 (Princeton, N.J.: Princeton University Press, 1958).
17. Barbara Hannah once made the remark that one can only begin to really love someone if you also begin to hate that person as well (personal communication).
18. See C. G. Jung, *Psychology and Alchemy* (1944), *Collected Works,* vol. 12 (Princeton, N.J.: Princeton University Press, 1953), par. 7.
19. See Jung, *Answer to Job,* par. 731.
20. Jung defines *numinosum* as "a dynamic agency or effect not caused by an arbitrary act of will." C. G. Jung, "Psychology and Religion" (1940) in *Collected Works,* vol. 11 (Princeton, N.J.: Princeton University Press, 1958), par. 6. Also "The Psychology of the Transference" (1946) in *Collected Works,* vol. 16 (Princeton, N.J.: Princeton University Press, 1954), pars. 449, 539.
21. "The Psychology of the Transference," par. 449.
22. Job 40:4.
23. 1 Cor. 13:7.
24. C. G. Jung, *Memories, Dreams, Reflections,* pp. 353ff.

Chronology

1915	January 4: Marie-Luise Ida Margareta von Franz born in Münich to Baron Erwin Gottfried von Franz (1876–1944) and Margret Susanne, née Schoen (1883–1962). Her father was Austrian by birth and was serving as a member of the Joint Chiefs of Staff in the Austro-Hungarian Army. Her mother was German by birth. Both died and were buried in Zürich. At the time of birth, her mother and her two-year-old sister, Marie-Anne, were visiting the paternal grandmother at her summer residence, Bishoffswiesen, in Berchtsgaden, Bavaria, thus Marie-Louise von Franz was born in southern Germany. Her mother's family also had a summer residence (Pointlehen) in Berchtsgaden. Her father and mother had known each other since childhood. For many years Marie-Louise von Franz's family remained citizens of Vienna where they had their proper residence.
1919	The family moves to Rheineck in the canton of St. Gallen, Switzerland.
1920	Her father buys a house on February 1.
1921–1928	Primary school in Rheineck.

1923–1931 Ski holidays with her mother and sister from the end of February to the middle of March in Zuoz, Upper Engadin, Switzerland. From 1926 to 1929, she spent her winter sports holidays with her sister and/or friends in the Engadin, primarily in Zuoz and Sils Maria.

During her childhood and early youth, summer holidays were usually spent with the family and occurred primarily in the Swiss Alps, of which von Franz was very fond: San Bernadino (1927), Simplon Pass (1928, 1929), Lucerne (1928), Zermatt, Riffelalp (1928, 1929), Monte Rosa (1928), Bella Tola, Chandolin, Goernergrat (1929), Furka Pass (1929), Castle Vaduz and Kyburg (1929), Rapperswil, near Bollingen (1929), Sils Maria (1931).

1928 Matriculation at the Freies Gymnasium in Zürich (a high school specializing in languages and literature). Her sister, Marie-Anne, was also enrolled in the same high school. Both lived in a pension at Bärengasse 19 in Zürich, run by Mrs. Bachofner-Hess, wife of a pastor.

1931 The whole family moves to Dolderstrasse 107, Zürich, where her father had purchased a villa.

March 29, Palm Sunday: Confirmation at the Fluntern Church, Zürich. The confirmation's motto was: "He stores up sound wisdom for the upright" (Proverbs 2:7).

1933 During the summer between gymnasium and the beginning of her university studies, she meets C. G. Jung in Bollingen. She was eighteen years old.

On September 22, she graduates from the Freies Gymnasium, and in October, she begins her studies at the University of Zürich, where she majors in classical philology and minors in Latin and literature, and ancient history.

1933–1934 November 3 to February 23: she attends Jung's lectures on modern psychology at the E.T.H. Zürich (Eidgenössische Technische Hochschule, or Swiss Federal Institute of Technology).

1934 May 8 to July 20: she attends Jung's lectures on basic psychological concepts.

She begins analysis with C. G. Jung.

1935 May to July: she attends Jung's lectures on modern psychology and his psychological seminar.

She also launches her work on the symbolism of fairy tales (*Symbolik des Märchens*) which was to continue for nine years. (This three-volume monumental work was published under the name of her collaborator, Hedwig von Beit. Apart from a couple of stylistic corrections, the book was written solely by Marie-Louise von Franz.)

1936 February: the E.T.H. in Zürich grants her a scholarship of SFr 500.00 for symbolic historical research. Prof. C. G. Jung sponsored this application.

May 22 to July 28: she attends Jung's lectures on the association experiment and on psychology.

1936–1937 November 5 to March 3: she attends Jung's psychological seminar and his lectures on modern psychology.

November 10 to February 22: she attends Jung's psychological seminar.

She also participates for the first time in the Eranos Conference, Ascona, Switzerland. According to a letter to her mother dated August 29, 1937, she decided to attend the conference after Jung wrote to her that he would be very pleased to see her in Ascona. Toni Wolff took Marie-Louise along with her in her car.

1938–1939 November 22 to July 7: she attends Jung's lectures on the introduction to the psychology of the unconscious and his psychological seminar.

1939 April 4 to August 4: she resides in Ortenstein (a private castle in Switzerland) with friends of the family both as a holiday and to teach their children Latin.

June 3: she receives Swiss citizenship.

July 27: she becomes a citizen of Zürich.

1940 February 24: she receives her Ph.D. in classical philology *magna cum laude;* thesis title: "Die aesthetische Anschauungen der Iliasscholien" ("The Aesthetic Opinions in the Iliad Scholia"). Prof. Dr. Ernst Howald, her thesis advisor, writes: *summa diligentia et magna sagacitate conscripta.*

1941 She becomes an associate member of the Psychological Club of Zürich.

June 7: she gives her very first lecture at the Psychological Club of Zürich.[1]

ca. 1942 She has a decisive dream which indicates that it is her destiny to become an analyst. She discusses the dream with C. G. Jung, and she begins to see her first analysands.[2]

1944	She becomes a member of the Psychological Club of Zürich. (She was also a member of the SGAP and the IAAP.)
	Her father dies.
1945	Her mother sells their house at Dolderstrasse 107 and moves into an apartment at Zürichbergstrasse 47. Marie-Louise rents a small room, first at Jupiterstrasse 47 and later at Englischviertelstrasse 35 in Zürich.
1946	August: she spends her holidays with Barbara Hannah in Zuoz, and in the fall moves to a small apartment along with Barbara Hannah at Hornweg 2, Küsnacht. Barbara Hannah had been renting a room at the Hotel Sonne in Küsnacht.
1950	Trip to Paris.
1951	She lectures in Chaux de Fonds, Switzerland.
1953	Trip to United States of America, for three months, delivering lectures and sightseeing.
1955	Trip to Egypt.
1956	Trip to Greece.
	December 6: she becomes a training analyst at the C. G. Jung Institute, Zürich.
1958	She builds her tower in Bollingen.
1962	Her mother dies.

1963	July to August: she journeys to Scotland with Barbara Hannah.
1965	She moves with Barbara Hannah to Lindenbergstrasse 15 in Küsnacht.
1968	August: she participates in the second Baily Island Conference held in honor of Dr. Esther Harding's eightieth birthday and presents her paper "Number Games of the Universe," later published under the title, "Symbols of the *Unus Mundus*."
	She lectures in the United States.[3]
1970	Four-week long journey with Mrs. Ariane Rump to Bangkok, Angkor Vat, Phnom Penh, Tokyo, Nikko, Hakone, Toba, Nara, Kyoto, Hong Kong, Bali, and Singapore.
1971	She lectures in Bremen.
1972	She lectures in Elmau.
1973	May: trip to Rome.
1974	She lectures in Herrenalb/Baden Baden and in London.
1975	She delivers the lecture, "Psyche and Matter in Alchemy and Modern Science," at the opening of the Jung Centennial Pro Helvetia Exhibit in Zürich.
	She lectures in the United States and in Montreal.
1976	She lectures in Panarion.
1977	She lectures in Lindau, Graz, and Rome.

1978 She lectures in Panarion.

1979 She lectures in the United States.

1981 She lectures in Paris.

1984 March: she takes a two-week trip to Florence.

She lectures in the United States and, at the E.T.H., delivers the lecture "Archetypal Experiences Surrounding Death."

1985 August to September: she attends the Eranos Conference, Ascona, and delivers the lecture, "Nike and the Waters of the Styx." This was the last time that she attended the conference.

From this point on, she begins to lead a more introverted life in her house in Küsnacht and retreats ever more frequently to her tower in Bollingen, where she spends up to five months a year. She continues to see friends and analysands from all over the world and dedicates herself to her creative work, focusing especially on Arabic alchemy.

1986 She lectures in Garmisch, Partenkirchen: "Some Historical Aspects of C. G. Jung's Synchronicity Hypothesis." Participants in the conference included Carl Friedrich von Weizsäcker, the Dalai Lama, Joseph Needham, Raimon Pannikar, and Chungliang Al Huang.

November 25: she delivers her last public lecture: "C. G. Jungs Rehabilitation der Gefühlsfunktion in unserer Zivilisation" ("C. G. Jung's Rehabilitation of the Feeling

Function in our Contemporary Civilization") at Küsnacht.

1998 February 17: Marie-Louise von Franz dies in her home in Küsnacht around 2 A.M.

NOTES

1. Von Franz gave the majority of her lectures at the Psychological Club of Zürich and at the C. G. Jung Institute in Zürich.
2. In her passport—even as late as 1979—she declared her profession to be a "language teacher" with no mention of being a psychoanalyst.
3. Von Franz lectured in such cities as Chicago, Houston, New York, San Francisco, and Los Angeles.

The Fountain of the Love of Wisdom

PART ONE

Reflections on the Death of Marie-Louise von Franz

Death Announcements

Neue Zürcher Zeitung, February 18, 1998

Küsnacht ZH
Lindenbergstrasse 15

OBITUARY

Yesterday, after long and arduous suffering, my dearest sister, our cousin and relative passed away.

Marie-Louise von Franz
Ph.D.

4th January 1915–17th February 1998

Marie-Anne von Franz
Also in the name of all relatives

The memorial service will take place in the Reformed Church in Küsnacht on Thursday, February 26th at 2:15 P.M.

PSYCHOLOGISCHER CLUB
ZÜRICH

8032 Zürich
Gemeindestrasse 27

I have the painful duty of informing you of the passing away of our honorary member

Marie-Louise von Franz, Ph.D.

January 4, 1915–February 17, 1998

She died a quiet death after a prolonged and consuming illness which she mastered with venerable patience, utter dignity and full mental clarity.

With her departure, a chapter of the history of Jungian psychology comes to a close. Not only was she one of the last direct students of C. G. Jung, but due to her publications and her eminent pedagogical gift, she made it possible for a broad spectrum of the population worldwide to understand analytical psychology. Our Club, as well as many students of the Jung Institute, also profited from her marvelous flair for presenting complicated psychological experiences and events in a way that everyone could understand them without their deeper meaning succumbing to oversimplification. The wealth of her inner resources coupled with an extraordinary intelligence allowed her to be effective in many different areas although her interpretation of fairy tales remains her unsurpassable masterpiece. Her profound knowledge of symbolism made her interpretation of dreams so evident that her analysands as well as her audience were able to grasp their accuracy and genuineness. Her contribution to the meaning of numbers as a link between psyche and matter is to this day unrecognized in the momentousness of its consequences.

A person who incorporated the very essence of Jungian psychology in every vein of her body has departed from us and left us with a painful gap.

In the name of the Board of Trustees
Dr. Alfred Ribi, M.D.

C. G. JUNG INSTITUTE
ZÜRICH

To all
Analysts active in Switzerland
And all Students,
Patrons and Donors

Küsnacht
March 5, 1998

Dear Colleagues
Dear Students
Dear Patrons and Donors,

Today in Küsnacht, amidst a large congregation of mourners, we bid farewell to Marie-Louise von Franz. With deep regret we heard of her passing some days earlier. In view of her severe suffering during the last years, death may have brought deliverance; but it leaves an irreplaceable gap in the community of all those who feel connected with Jungian psychology.

Our Institute mourns this extraordinary woman who, with C. G. Jung, must have contributed most to the development of analytical psychology. In her unique way, Marie-Louise von Franz knew how to explain and deepen the works of C. G. Jung. For decades she was a decisive member of the Zürich C. G. Jung Institute—which the painful distance of recent years does not alter. To many of our analysts, she will remain in vivid memory as training and control analyst as well as lecturer. To many students and to all readers, she continues beyond her death to convey in her numerous books a deep knowledge of the human soul. To us all, she taught modesty when encountering the strength of the unconscious, always with alert spirit and in tireless pursuit of truth. She was richly talented and drew upon an immense fund of experiences.

We thank Marie-Louise von Franz for so very much. Her death signifies an irreplaceable loss for all Jungians. However, in our grief we are full of gratitude for all that she gave us during her long, richly fulfilled life. And with these feelings we also know that we are very connected with our colleagues of the "Zentrum."

With sympathetic greetings,
C. G. Jung Institute

For the Curatorium
Dr. Brigitte Spillmann, President

Neue Zürcher Zeitung, February 18, 1998

"With admirable modesty and an untiring love of the truth she dedicated her life to exploring and researching the human soul—and to carrying on the work of C. G. Jung. Her life remains for us today both as exemplary and as a duty."

Forschungs- und Ausbildungszentrum für Tiefenpsychologie nach Carl Gustav Jung und Marie-Louise von Franz

Marie-Louise von Franz-Stiftung für Grundlagenforschung in Analytischer Psychologie
Stiftung für Jung'sche Psychologie

Neue Zürcher Zeitung, February 17, 1998

Zürich
February 17, 1998

After prolonged illness, our founding member

Marie-Louise von Franz

has passed away. During many years she accompanied us with her animate and creative spirit.

Stiftung für Jung'sche Psychologie

Neue Zürcher Zeitung, February 18, 1998

Münsterhof 16
8001 Zürich
February 17, 1998

RESEARCH AND TRAINING CENTER
IN DEPTH PSYCHOLOGY
ACCORDING TO
C. G. JUNG AND MARIE-LOUISE VON FRANZ

Today, after a long illness, our Honorary President

Marie-Louise von Franz

passed away. With noble modesty and an untiring love of truth she lived her life in the services of investigating the human soul and carried on the work of C. G. Jung.

In gratitude
The members of the Center

The memorial service will take place in the Reformed Church in Küsnacht on Thursday, February 26th at 2:15 p.m.

Neue Zürcher Zeitung, February 17, 1998

Zürich
February 17, 1998

In the early hours of the morning

Marie-Louise von Franz

was released from her long,
courageously borne illness.

Till the very end her spirit—crystal clear—was vitally animate. Her life in the service of the Creative germinating from within the Unconscious was for us exemplary and remains for us a duty.

Marie-Louise von Franz Stiftung
für Grundlagenforschung in analytischer Psychologie

Tages Anzeiger, February 18, 1998

Zürich
February 1998

On February 17, after a long protracted illness, our honorary president

Marie-Louise von Franz

passed away. Her love, her spirit and her untiring search in the service of the unconscious will remain a guidepost for us forever.

In deep mourning and gratitude,
The members of the
Marie-Louise von Franz Institute
for Studies in Synchronicity

Obituaries

Obituary

DR. ALFRED RIBI

Early Tuesday morning on the 17th of February 1998, one of the last direct students of C. G. Jung passed away in her home in Küsnacht, Switzerland. Marie-Louise von Franz endured a particularly protracted and progressive illness with venerable patience and complete mental vitality despite the ever-advancing deterioration of her physical health. Although she loved independence above everything, she became increasingly dependent on household help, almost all of whom accepted her with graciousness in order to help her endure the path of suffering that she had to traverse. Several years before, as she felt her end approaching, she sent her analysands to those students who trained with her. Nobody could have then predicted that her body would hold so tenaciously onto life. During this time of such travail she actively participated in the events occurring around her, supported her students with advice as well as in deed, worked with her assistant on the publication of her final work, and even prepared an unedited seminar transcript

Published in the *Zürichsee Zeitung,* March 3, 1998.

on the cat in fairy tales for publication. Her unresting heart has now found much deserved repose; and a multifaceted life's opus its completion.

Marie-Louise von Franz was born in Munich on January 4, 1915. She descended, as she often noted with a grin, from minor Austrian nobility. Her father was a distinguished military officer who courageously proved himself on the Isonzo Front in the First World War.[1] Out of the fear of communist upheaval after the conclusion of the war, her family moved to the Rhine Valley in Switzerland where her father worked in the lumber industry.[2] She spent her youth in an agricultural environment from which her love of nature and of the simple life arose. The family first settled later in Zürich when both daughters chose to attend the secondary school track in preparation for the university. Marie-Louise von Franz then attended the Freies Gymnasium in Zürich. (Her sister Marie-Anne von Franz, two years older, attended the same.) As she was an excellent student, yet found school tediously boring, she decided to complete all of her homework assignments during school hours so that she would be able to freely spend more time out in nature. During her entire life she had a phenomenal memory that was—as Jung himself admitted—superior to his own. After the completion of her gymnasium studies she could not decide between either mathematics or antique languages. A dream in which "the gods of Greece paraded past begging alms" determined her choice: she studied ancient philology at the University of Zürich.

At the age of eighteen, while she was attending the Free Gymnasium, she met C. G. Jung. He had invited several of her friends for an excursion to his tower in Bollingen on the upper lake of Zürich where psychology was avidly discussed. Jung related the story of a mentally ill woman who lived on the moon. Marie-Louise commented that this was certainly to be taken symbolically; Jung looked her sternly in the eye and emphasized: "No, she [actually] *lived* on the moon." The student returned home with disparate feelings: either the professor was nuts, or he had said something terribly important that she could not yet understand. It was the latter, the reality of the soul, that then began to captivate her. She dedicated her entire life to the service of the soul and Jungian psychology. Years later in 1971, in gratitude for her long and close relationship as a collaborator of C. G. Jung, she was called to write a book on the meaning of Jung's myth in our time.

When still a student she asked Jung to take her into psychoanalysis. [As remuneration] he assigned her the highly responsible task of critically interpreting and publishing an enigmatic alchemical text, the *Aurora Consurgens,* attributed to Saint Thomas Aquinas. (This authorship is heftily disputed by Thomist scholars.) How could such an eminent theologian, who St. Thomas unquestionably was, busy himself with such an obscure alchemical text? Even her Latin professor—whom she had asked to assist her with the critical evaluation of the six extant manuscripts from that time—dismissed her with the comment that he would not involve himself with such trash. Her critical work, which was enriched—but not altered—by a newly discovered handwritten manuscript, was published along with a commentary as the third volume of Jung's *magnum opus, Mysterium Coniunctionis* on which she also collaborated.[3] She was able to conclusively prove—to those who were not prejudiced—that the text was in fact dictated by St. Thomas Aquinas in a state of agony. It was thus proven that in the Middle Ages alchemy was considered by respected scholars to be a serious science.

In that she was a rather impoverished student, she accepted an offer from Hedwig von Beit to write an encyclopedic work on the interpretation of fairy tales using von Beit's library and publishing it under von Beit's name. The three-volume work is still not published today under the name of the true author. Although at that time Marie-Louise did not have the necessary practical experience to bring the interpretations down into daily reality, this work remains today an inexhaustible source of information on symbolism. Years later in her lectures at the C. G. Jung Institute she was able to bring this material down to earth and illustrated to her audience time and again that folk and fairy tales are genuine unconscious products of the collective soul. She possessed a unique pedagogical skill—from which not only her Latin pupils profited—and was able to "cast a spell of fascination" on the students attending her lectures. Her gift lay in the fact that she could bring her public so close to extraordinarily subtle psychic contiguities that one had the impression that it was all very clear. When one attempted to reproduce the train of thought oneself, then one got stuck and noticed that she had first completed all of the work of becoming conscious herself. Her extraordinary level of consciousness was achieved by unremitting and continual research, and she was never satisfied alone with that which she had accomplished. She can be designated—and rightfully so—as the *discoverer of the psychological wisdom inherent in fairy tales.* In collaboration with Jung on his researches of alchemical philosophy—whose psychological content Jung himself discovered—her profound knowledge of symbolism was of great benefit, and it opened the very portals to her understanding of the unconscious.

These outer endeavors were accompanied by the conscientious observation of the manifestations of—and the guidance from—her own unconscious. There within lived the "gods and demons" who delivered the decisive impulse to her life and work, and from these she could not deviate even when they stacked up hardship upon hardship. She was a prolific dreamer who oftentimes had such rich, comprehensive, and complicated dreams that Jung himself had to wipe the sweat from his brow after succeeding with a dream interpretation.

Her childhood dreams predicted that the world of dreams, that is, the unconscious, would be her fate and she would not be able to lead an average sort of life. She never married, and her publications were her children. Following Jung's advice, she lived with Ms. Barbara Hannah, also a student of Jung's, where she found a cozy home life and the necessary protection from the world.

It was a stroke of good fortune for Jung to have found among his associates such a gifted and multifaceted student. For Marie-Louise, he was the first person who took her seriously. And she thanked him with her loyalty. For her creative work she often retreated to her tower in Bollingen. Yet in no way did she live in an "ivory tower." Quite the contrary: she was actively involved in the social and political events of her day, she was a member of the AUNS (committee for an independent and neutral Switzerland) and was a better proponent of democracy than many a Swiss, and she loved a good meal and a fine bottle of wine, heartily welcoming the company of her students and acquaintances. She entertained a lively correspondence with people from all over the world who read her books. And she was invited to speak in many countries where she was held in esteem as a lecturer.

Despite her renown, Marie-Louise von Franz remained modest. She simply ignored her aristocratic past and was humane, caring, helpful and open to everyone who had an honest concern. During the three and a half decades that I knew her, she was for me the only person who never did anything disingenuous and who never did anything to me behind my back. She occasionally had to tell me some unpleasant truths which I futilely tried to deny before I was able to find enough honesty within to accept their candor. Thanks to her own uprightness she was oftentimes able to say the most shameful truths without hurting a person. All of her scientific merit was outshone by the magnitude of her personality. Every person who came in contact with her with honest intentions was impressed by her exceptional character. Her foes consisted of those who could not measure up to the ethical demands of this woman. She opened her wealth of knowledge, experience, and humanity to all who earned it. At the same time she had a profound sense of humor that flowed from a true love of people and was characterized by a sense of the relative insignificance of the ego. Inflated peers were revolting, for she held to that sentence from alchemy which noted that, in contrast to the outer glimmering common gold, the true gold lies within.

Shortly before his death, Jung gave her a handwritten note on the symbolism of numbers with the comment that he was too old to follow through on all of his creative ideas. She took up this note as impetus for future work for it was contiguous with her second love, her love of mathematics which she had set in the background at the beginning of her university studies. During a period of over ten years she researched and prepared her pioneering text, *Number and Time,* wherein she elucidated the meaning of number as a link between psyche and matter. (This was a problem with which the old alchemists had also grappled.) On the one hand, the background of this theme today is well disclosed. On the other, it is still insufficiently understood. During the decades to come, the legacy of this highly significant book will entail the working out of all the details of her groundbreaking approach.

Everyone who knew Marie-Louise von Franz is deeply moved by the loss of this unique woman. Our world today, not particularly renowned for its enlightenment, has lost one of its sources of light. A lighthouse of humanity on the shores of the inhumane has been extinguished. This light now radiates all the more from those who were able, in one way or another, to come to her, tap this wellspring, and drink from its water. Each in their own way carries her light in their hearts. They have the responsibility and the task of carrying on that torch of "love and becoming conscious" that she lit for them in the darkness and coldness of the world. And now it is time that she, Marie-Louise von Franz, can receive from us something of this light in turn.

Erlenbach
February 26, 1998

NOTES

1. Slovenia, south of Austria.—*Ed.*
2. On the border of Switzerland, Germany, and Austria.—*Ed.*
3. In German, *Mysterium Coniunctionis* is published in two volumes. Thus *Aurora Consurgens* is the accompanying "third" volume of the work.—*Ed.*

Obituary

Analytische Psychologie

With the death of Marie-Louise von Franz, the last direct student and collaborator of C. G. Jung has passed away.

Her collaborative efforts with Jung began in 1934—analysis in exchange for the translation of Greek and Latin texts—a collaboration that continued as a colleague and coworker and which, after his death, expanded into carrying on his work. She elaborated many of Jung's seminal ideas and developed them into her own theory which can be observed in her depth-psychological interpretation of fairy tales and myths (which she herself established), the extension of Jung's thoughts on the subject of synchronicity, and her research regarding the relationship between psyche and matter. . . .

Fascinating were her lectures that she held at the C. G. Jung Institute in Zürich. Inspired by the results of her research that she presented, she awakened considerable enthusiasm. In her lectures one felt her alert intellect connected with her impressive intuition and the down-to-earth

V. Kast, I. Riedel, and R. Hinshaw, "Nachruf," *Analytische Psychologie* 29 (1998), pp. 342–343.

manner of her formulation. Una Thomas, always sitting in the first row, let nothing by and transcribed the lectures along with the discussion. Several of these transcripts were published by Spring Publications. In these books, one met Marie-Louise von Franz "live": her intellectual agility, her humor, and also her convictions that she did not let be questioned lightly. The fascination of her lectures was also due to the fact that she thought in terms of a vast psycho-socio-historical context.

This was also experienced in analysis with her: even relatively simple dreams were set in a cultural-historical context that lifted the person or the fate of the dreamer in an unforeseen manner. . . . But along with this elevation was her deep awe of the unconscious that she awoke in analysands.

Marie-Louise von Franz spoke openly about her life, yet was of the opinion that the essential nature of her life occurred in her dreams. She certainly saw, however, connections between the inner and outer worlds. As helpful as the animals in fairy tales were the animals in daily life. She was seldom seen without her English bulldog and occasionally found with a worm in her hand that she had rescued from certain death in traffic. And an analysand who could pick up a toad was ascertained of her sympathy.

Her lifelong passion—researching the objective psyche—is seen in her studies of alchemy, synchronicity, and in her critical dialogue with Christianity from which she attempted to interpret many phenomena of the collective unconscious, for instance, the transformation of the archetype of the feminine.

Decades before her death she occupied herself with the theme of dreams occurring within the dying process as statements of the unconscious in regards to this liminal event. Herein she was mostly interested in the correlation between psyche and matter at this particular point of transition. After she completed her work *On Dreams and Death,* she said that she no longer feared death.

Anne Maguire reported at the memorial service that Marie-Louise von Franz had told her a dream in which her illness had been healed and her body completely restored to health. She felt extraordinarily happy in the dream and deduced that she would soon die. As her caretakers report, she nonetheless passed along a difficult path up until her death on February 17, 1998.

As a philologist of ancient languages, Marie-Louise von Franz grasped first and foremost the importance of communicating the cultural-historical implications of Jungian theory—although the relationship to the practice of analytical psychology was always in the foreground. Through her lecturing in Europe and above all in the U.S.A., as well as through her books and their translation into many languages, she was in the position to bring to fruition on an international scale both her own researches and her understanding of Jung's work.

—VERENA KAST
—INGRID RIEDEL
—ROBERT HINSHAW

Obituary

Zürcher Oberländer

Marie-Louise von Franz has recently passed away. She was the last and most significant student of C. G. Jung with whom she worked for twenty-seven years until his death [in 1961]. Born in Munich on the 4th of January 1915, Marie-Louise von Franz was the daughter of a high-ranking Austrian military officer. As a three-year-old child, she moved with her family to Switzerland where she lived until the end of her days. She carried on the work of C. G. Jung in her own independent manner.

Marie-Louise von Franz became best known for her extensive series of books on the interpretation of fairy tales that arose out of her lectures. Remaining unsurpassed to this day are works such as *Individuation in Fairy Tales, Shadow and Evil in Fairy Tales, The Feminine in Fairy Tales, The Interpretation of Fairy Tales, Redemption Motifs in Fairy Tales,* and several others.

Many students who studied at the C. G. Jung Institute will long retain the unforgettable memory of the examinations she gave during her

Regina Abt-Baechi, "Letzte Schulerin von C. G. Jung," in *Zürcher Oberländer,* March 24, 1998.

many years there as a training analyst. She had a great pedagogical skill and a special talent of presenting complicated issues in such a simple and inimitable manner that one believed that one could have said it themselves. One quickly lost this illusion when one tried later on to write it down. Then one soon grasped how little one actually knew and how much work there was still to be done!

The far-reaching work of Marie-Louise von Franz imparted substantial impulse to themes such as synchronicity, alchemy, the relationship between psyche and matter, and finally, in her [second to] last work, *On Dreams and Death,* she addressed the question of life after death. She was frequently in touch with physicists, mathematicians, and proponents of other branches of the sciences whose recent research was utterly of interest to her and, in turn, she opened new perspectives in their fields of study for them.

In our modern society oriented in affluence and progress one believes that we can get things under control with outer measures if we can only finally do it right and make it universal enough. One then forgets that all that mankind has achieved has arisen out of the psyche including our contemporary potential of destruction. The highest form of heedfulness must be given to this colossal force in human nature—and not just in the practices of psychotherapists, for it concerns everyone!

Marie-Louise von Franz always focused her attention on the deeper causes lying beneath the current of outer events in politics, the economy, and culture. She remained vitally involved with the essential events in the world up until her death. In her profound concern about the fate of Switzerland she attentively followed political developments that she oftentimes felt to be unfolding in a direction threatening dissolution.

For her, Switzerland was always a land of intellectual and spiritual freedom, an image of the individual in a time of mass agglomerations who, in the best sense of individual consciousness, was able to stand up and out against the dangerous storm of mass tendencies arising out of the collective unconscious.

To all those who knew her, Marie-Louise von Franz will remain unforgettable. Through her direct, honest, and at times, blunt manner of expression one felt both a world of experience and knowledge and yet the finest sensitivity to the psychic background of the person she was with. Nothing was artificial, prefabricated, empty intellectualism, abstract, feigned-healer, or mothering. When one departed from her company, one felt clear, simple, and enriched at the same time with meaning having been conferred to one's life. Time and again I was amazed at her ability to explain complex issues so lucidly and to apply them so concretely to one's personal life. This was, in a sense, great art. C. G. Jung also considered her ability to be exceptional. Marie-Louise von Franz, we hope, will forever remain the patroness of the creative impulse out of the unconscious.

Obituary

Die KLEINE Märchenzeitung

The psychotherapist Marie-Louise von Franz, one of the last direct students of C. G. Jung, has passed away in Küsnacht, Switzerland. Her life was lived dedicated to researching the psyche and to the continuation of Jung's work. As a young university student of philology she was already translating texts for him. The relationship between psyche and matter was a great concern of hers throughout her life.

Marie-Louise von Franz became internationally known primarily in the field of depth-psychological research of fairy tales where she was a pioneer. All of the interpretations of fairy tales in Hedwig von Beit's profound work *Symbolik des Märchens* were analyzed and written by von Franz. To this day, these volumes are a treasure trove for the researchers of fairy tales. Her first books on this theme were published in English in the U.S.A. and appeared later in German translated by Kösel Verlag in Munich: *Creation Myths* (1972), *Shadow and Evil in Fairy Tales* (1974), *Individuation in Fairy Tales* (1985), *Redemption Motifs in Fairy Tales*

"Marie-Louise von Franz (4.1.1915–17.2.1998) zum Gedenken," *Die KLEINE Märchenzeitung der Schweizerischen Märchengesellschaft SMG.* 8, Ausgabe, 3. Jg. Mai 1998, p. 3.

(1986), and *The Interpretation of Fairy Tales* (1986). *Puer Aeternus* (1987) was an interpretation of Saint-Exupéry's *Little Prince.* In 1977, Bonz in Stuttgart published *The Feminine in Fairy Tales,* and in 1980 Insel Publishers published *The Golden Ass of Apuleius: The Liberation of the Feminine in Man.* Also *The Visions of Niklaus von Flüe* (1980), from Daimon publishers in Einsiedeln, Switzerland, will be of interest to students of fairy-tale interpretation.[1] Also well known is her article "The Unknown Visitor in Fairy Tales and Dreams" in *Archetypal Dimensions of the Psyche* and her essay "In the Black Woman's Castle: Interpretation of a Fairy Tale" in *Märchenforschung und Tiefenpsychologie* from the Wiss. Buchgesellschaft, Darmstadt (1965), with a foreword in the fifth edition by Verena Kast.[2]

All of these books are based on her true-to-life and humorous lectures at the C. G. Jung Institute and the Adult Education Programs of Zürich. Analysands came to her from all over the world and from all social classes. And she had an immense grasp of cultural history. This made it possible for her to interpret the symbolic content of fairy tales and to bring these interpretations in correspondence with the daily lives of contemporary men and women. . . . She experienced time and again the powerful effect that the archetypal images of fairy tales and dreams had on individual lives both in a positive as well as in a negative sense. Her experiences with patients and students showed her the same as what fairy tales teach us: the person who can reverently and courageously stand unbiased vis-à-vis the powers of the unconscious—symbolized in these fairy-tale figures—can hope for help from them. The person who rejects them or who only has egotistical goals in mind is rebuked.

NOTES

1. This work is presently being translated into English.—*Ed.*
2. For both essays, see M.-L. von Franz, *Archetypal Dimensions of the Psyche* (Boston: Shambhala, 1997).—*Ed.*

Obituary

Marie-Louise von Franz, Jungian Theorist, Dies

ROBERT McG. THOMAS JR.

NEW YORK: Marie-Louise von Franz, 83, hailed by many as the queen of Jungian psychology, died Feb. 17 at her home in Küsnacht, Switzerland. She was an expert on fairy tales who had been both Carl Gustav Jung's most brilliant and inspired disciple and the one who had done the most to illuminate the flame since his death in 1961.

Dr. von Franz began making her legend early. As a brilliant and independent-minded schoolgirl, for example, she proved so resistant to religious education that a priest was assigned as her personal tutor. The arrangement ended when the priest became so dazzled by his pupil that he lost his faith and abandoned his calling.

In time Dr. von Franz came to regret the episode. For it was Freud, after all, who regarded religion as poppycock while Jung embraced religion as every bit as authentic as fairy tales themselves.

Robert McG. Thomas, "Marie-Louise von Franz, Jungian Theorist, Dies," *The International Herald Tribune,* March 24, 1998, p. 2.

In Jungian theory, those primordial stories provide compelling evidence of [Jung's] central notion that all humanity shares a collective unconscious of genetically replicated archetypal forms reflecting and embodying the entire spectrum of human aspirations, feelings, fears, and frustrations.

For those who doubted, Dr. von Franz conducted a worldwide study of fairy tales and turned out a stream of rigorously researched and influential books on this subject.

As Jung had sensed, along the way she found too many common themes and symbols in too many isolated cultures for the similarities to be dismissed as mere coincidence.

After obtaining a doctorate in 1940, Dr. von Franz threw herself into Jung's work which became increasingly her own. She began as a student, patient, and research assistant, later became his colleague and collaborator, and eventually emerged as his successor at the C. G. Jung Institute in Zürich. During his lifetime, she made major contributions to his major studies, particularly his inquiries into the psychology of medieval alchemy.

After his death she extended his work, turning out a torrent of books including her fairy tale series and a 1980 study linking psychology and modern physics: *Number and Time.*

Known as a compassionate analyst who interpreted more than 65,000 dreams, she lectured widely around the world, all the while insisting that the goal of Jungian thought was not to become a Jungian but one's own unique Self.

Obituary

Marie-Louise von Franz

CHUCK SCHWARTZ

Marie-Louise von Franz was renowned on several counts. She was a first-rate and compassionate analyst. She was the closest colleague of C. G. Jung with whom she worked for over thirty years and contributed a great deal to his major works, particularly his monumental studies on psychology and alchemy. She was also the author of a number of books including a whole collection on the psychology of fairy tales and was a leading authority in this field.

What is exceptional about her books on fairy tales is their readability. She possessed a few theoretical formulations, and her direct and colloquial style of English (not her mother tongue) makes her writings easily accessible and as fascinating to read as the tales themselves. Through [her books and lectures], people from all walks of life have been made aware that these timeless tales are not the sole preserve of children and are struck by how relevant they are to their daily lives.

Chuck Schwartz, "Marie-Louise von Franz," *The Independent,* February 23, 1998, p. 15.

The first of these books, *The Problems of the Feminine in Fairy Tales,* was published in 1972; it was followed by *An Introduction to the Interpretation of Fairy Tales* (1973), *Shadow and Evil in Fairy Tales* (1974), and several others. They are still bestsellers in the psychology world and seem set to remain so.

There are many other books by her on a variety of subjects. Among the most distinguished are *Number and Time* (1980) on the connection between psychology and modern physics; a detailed scholarly work, in collaboration with Emma Jung (Jung's wife), on the symbolism of the Grail legend; *Aurora Consurgens,* a translation and exposition of an early alchemical text ascribed to St. Thomas Aquinas; and *Jung, His Myth in Our Time* (1972), a biography elucidating Jung's essential work.

Von Franz also wrote a landmark book called *The Problem of the Puer Aeternus,* a text on the "eternal youth," an increasingly common visitor to the consulting room, who lives his life as if his time has not yet come; a strictly provisional life which results in a refusal to commit to the moment, be it a job, a partner, or anything to do with the here and now. This is often accompanied by a fascination with flying or mountain climbing, the symbolism being to get as high as possible and as far away from the mundanities of ordinary life. She also published several other books on alchemy, dreams, classical mythology, and the psychology of projection.

Marie-Louise von Franz was born in Munich of Austrian parents, but spent most of her life in Switzerland.[1] Even in primary school she had a reputation for a formidable intellect. She was, for example, unwilling to accept the tenets of the religious education taught at her school. She so exasperated the priest who was teaching her class that he insisted upon giving her private lessons. The upshot, according to a repentant von Franz, was that he completely lost his faith and left the priesthood.

She went on to attend the University of Zürich and reached a stage where she had to choose between a doctorate in classical languages or study medicine. She had by now started analysis with Jung and told him about a dream that indicated that she should choose classical languages. It was a brilliant choice, particularly for Jung, who from then on got all the Greek and Latin texts he needed for his work translated for the price of free analytic sessions.[2]

When von Franz was forty-one, Jung permitted her to take on her first client. The client was a woman on the verge of a nervous breakdown. Von Franz was naturally eager to make a success of her first case, but the harder she tried to prop the woman up, the worse the woman became. In despair she turned to Jung who advised her to let the client have her nervous breakdown. Von Franz backed off and stopped straining to help, and the woman soon made a full recovery.

She said that this was the most important lesson she ever had on therapeutic technique, showing her the limitations of willpower and the ego, and the role of the unconscious at the center of the personality.

She likened this to Galileo's discovery that the Earth revolved around the sun, and not vice versa. Like the Earth, the ego is an important satellite revolving around a much larger and more powerful center. Galileo's discovery got him excommunicated by the ruling establishment, and Jung has suffered a similar fate at the hands of the scientific establishment.

For Jung, the structure of the psyche's center was made up of what he called "archetypes," the fundamental building blocks or anatomy of psychic life. Like every other part of the human anatomy, the archetypes were common to all people; this commonality he called the collective unconscious.

Some years ago, von Franz predicted that, like Galileo's discovery, future generations of researchers would discover these selfsame psychic structures without any reference to or acknowledgment of Jung. This she felt would be only right and proper. From the fact that they made this discovery independently would prove that Jung's work was not at all hypothetical but was based on the objective facts of psychic life.

In the last few years a whole new breed of evolutionary psychologists have indeed rediscovered these selfsame structures and rechristened them in such terms as "mental modules" often without any reference to Jung's work.

Working on this archetypal level, von Franz soon realized that, for her at least, the only effective and decent way to work with a client was to work on the material of her own life—both inner and outer—in other words, to set her own house in order.

Her model for therapy therefore, which she imparted to all of her pupils, was not at all modern or even postmodern. It was as simple as it was disconcerting: "Work very hard on your own psychic life, and hope for a synchronistic happening in the client's. In this way everything is kept open and alive and there are no set rules."

That is except perhaps one rule. Von Franz counseled that it would be wrong to become a Jungian. If you do that, you miss the whole point of his psychology, which was to become the one unique individual you are meant to be.

Everyone who knew Marie-Louise von Franz or her work can see to what remarkable degree she achieved her individuality.

NOTES

1. Marie-Louise von Franz's father was Austrian, her mother was born in Bavaria, Germany. See the chronology in this Festschrift.—*Ed.*
2. In the dream, the gods of Greece paraded by seeking alms. See the obituary by Dr. Alfred Ribi in this Festschrift.—*Ed.*

The Search for the Universal Self on the Death of Marie-Louise von Franz

LUDGER LÜTKEHAUS

Binary thought holds stubbornly to clear opposition also in the field of psychology which, like no other discipline in the natural sciences, questions the all too evident identities and with them the dualisms. Analytical psychology stands juxtaposed to the "complex" psychology, the "individual unconscious" juxtaposed to the collective unconscious, and, more than anything, Jung juxtaposed to Freud. However, in regards to the shadowless representation of the "anima" in the "animus" of the founders and their schools, at least one controversy is taken care of: that of the "Daughters of State," that concept of Klaus Thelweleits which made Freud's life easier when set among a horde of dissidents and renegades. The same phenomenon also decisively influenced the Jungian school.

Next to Aniela Jaffé, Jolande Jacobi, and Toni Wolff, Marie-Louise von Franz was one of the most important members of the "Daughters of

Neue Zürcher Zeitung, February 20, 1998.

State" and not just an "Anna-Antigone," but also highly devoted. The role of the borderliner was left over to Sabina Spielrein. Marie-Louise von Franz, born on the 4th of January 1915, in a "royal officer's" household, first met Carl Gustav Jung after the completion of her studies in ancient languages in 1934.[1] She was a non-medical lay analyst and thus all the more competent in regards to the cultural implications of Jung's depth psychology.

At this time Jung was fascinated with the theory of an "Aryan" unconscious which turned out not to be adequately complex. Arising from her interests in fairy tales and myths, von Franz, on the contrary, favored a universalism. She decoded a configuration of symbolic thinking in the fairy tales neglected by Freud (but not the entire Freudian school) in a series of books beginning with her *Individuation in Fairy Tales* and *Puer Aeternus*. Here it had mostly to do with a form of self-discovery and thus consequently did not arise out of the strict rationalism of the hard sciences but rather the need to be self-understood: the soul comprehending the soul.

Naturally this was also interpretation. The belief of all interpreters that they could let the thing itself—that is, the symbol—speak for itself remained here also an illusion. But von Franz found in the method of amplification both a universal "family of symbols" and a way—analogous to the reproducible experiments of the hard sciences—to unify the fairy tales and myths of all countries in all times, from Siberia to the Australian Aborigines, from the Valley of the Kings through to the lands between the Indus and the Ganges. The "Self" that she was searching for was once and for all the great "One."

After her book *Number and Time*, quantum physics and the genetic code also had to adapt to this passion of hers: in her own quantum leap in symbolism, von Franz sought to discover her parallels with the structure of the I Ching. Here even the more sober of spirits could no longer follow. The much promising *On Divination and Synchronicity* went indeed a bit too deep.[2] Yet her community and a fascinated readership she always found. As mentioned, she passed away at the age of eighty-three on February 17th in Küsnacht, the death place of C. G. Jung, where she taught at the Jung Institute.

NOTES

1. There are numerous errors in this report; see the chronology in this Festschrift for clarification.—*Ed.*
2. The author refers here to *Wissen aus der Tiefe*, which was the German title of *On Divination and Synchronicity.*—*Ed.*

On the Death of Marie-Louise von Franz

FELIX LEYER

I am disappointed that your newspaper has failed to appropriately report about Marie-Louise von Franz's life's work. The distorted and fragmented stub of [Ludger Lütkehaus's] report gives undoubtedly a clue to the psychology of the author. As your author correctly states, Marie-Louise von Franz was born in 1915 and met Jung in 1934.[1] She was eighteen years old at the time. Despite an ingenious mind and her ability to rapidly apprehend, she naturally had no university degree at this time. She met Jung before she began her university studies. Your author indicates among other things that von Franz's interest in fairy tales and myths favored "universalism." What "universalism"? Von Franz studied the unconscious in men and women her entire life and never ceased to emphasize that, in regards to things in the psyche of various individual human beings, there is hardly anything one can find that is universally valid. What was in her book *On Divination and Synchronicity* so pon-

Neue Zürcher Zeitung, no. 60, March 13, 1998, p. 79.

derously deep? Too deep in comparison to what? The book shows that the psyche sometimes knows of things which can be completely independent from our conscious knowledge. In Sunday school children learn of the existence of prophetic dreams, and this book deals with just this kind of knowledge. "De mortibus nihil, nisi bene" is a saying of the ancient Romans. It advises us to speak with respect and dignity about the dead, or keep our silence.

Adlingenswil, Switzerland

NOTE

1. See the chronology in this Festschrift.—*Ed.*

On the Death of Marie-Louise von Franz

ANDREAS SCHWEIZER

The article about Marie-Louise von Franz from Ludger Lütkehaus (*Neue Zürcher Zeitung* from February 20, 1998) bristles with a lack of knowledge of her work. . . . The phenomenon of the human psyche and soul is so complex and there is still so little scientific research done that even the researchers themselves are confronted with various and conflicting answers. Contrary to Lütkehaus's suggestion, it has nothing to do with identifying with the "wisdom from the depths." It has far more to do with making men and women take responsibility for the unconscious contents that confront their ego consciousness as these arise out of the very real depths of the soul. Such a scientific stance demands great modesty which Marie-Louise von Franz possessed to an admirable degree. . . .

Andreas Schweizer, "On the Death of Marie-Louise von Franz," *Neue Zürcher Zeitung*, no. 60, March 13, 1998, p. 79.

Internet Responses

After learning of the death of Marie-Louise von Franz, Daryl Sharp set up a Web site calling for personal responses.

It's understood that I really have no right to say anything at all about her, even now that she's gone. I never met her. I wasn't examined by her, analyzed by her, scolded by her. Yet I was taught, informed, even perhaps mentored from a great distance. Through her, as through no one else, did I get the clarity and force I sought for. Jung's ideas through her had a lucidity and power that made sense to me. Well, none of it really matters, except that I found an analyst in my area and started on the hard work. It's my doing. But it wouldn't have happened without her.

—REAGAN HEESE

I first had contact with von Franz through Joan Buresch who gave a talk in Santa Fe after showing [the film] *Matter of Heart.* It was my first introduction to Jung's world and led me into analysis and eventually to my developing the Institute for Archetypal Drama. I asked Joan that day whom she felt was the associate of Jung's who most clearly embodied his vision and without hesitation she said von Franz. Von Franz's particularly loving portrait of Jung in the film and her deep understanding of alchemy and the endearing story about Jung's tower will always stand in my mind as great and forceful homage to his spirit, as well as to her glowing capacity to think archetypally.

—BILL PEARLMAN

Yesterday, I searched my bookshelves for "von Franz"
and found a slim volume
Something about the Feminine and Fairy Tales—
a title that doesn't quite fit into
the 20th century career woman's lifestyle
but nevertheless has an ancient ring that stirs the soul
So, I started reading,
and long into the night and couldn't stop
"This lady is fantastic," I said to myself
"I can understand her,
She's putting it all together for me in a way I haven't found before
What great synthesis, a fantastic distillation of complex material"
Now this very day I find that this grand lady has died—
but you see, I have just really met her.
I just now have read about her death—how lucky you all were to actually know her
But this woman hasn't died—not for me—
I just really met her yesterday!
Tomorrow I will pick up her book and she will be alive for me—
and I will live differently because of that—
soul upon soul
Therein lies immortality

—JAN PEYTON, Toronto

I had the pleasure of writing my thesis in Zürich for Dr. von Franz. What I remember was the way she felt into me, into what I was trying to express, and into the importance the work had for the evolution of what might become my creativity. She liked the work because I was trying to be creative, even though now I see how incomplete the product was. It apparently didn't matter to her that the result was mediocre but that an honest-to-god attempt was being made to wrestle with the creative process. That is what she threw her weight behind.

I also knew her as a lecturer and examiner. No point in going on about her brilliance. But there was something even more impressive. The way her brilliance challenged my limited best in learning the analytic craft. Her intellect was keenly sharp, yet its force was based on love and not power. Thus her demand for competence never felt pushy, though it could have the might of a hurricane. She was saying: "Look at this civilization. Its story MUST be understood at depth to do the suffering human spirit justice."

I always felt I was being introduced—through rigor—to an excellence I had long been hungry for. Who wouldn't want to achieve that, and who wouldn't want to cooperate? It was the first time I ever felt authority really serve the essence of life. She was exacting for the sake of sufficient analytic response to the modern climate. This challenge is something I wanted to be a part of. I was struck by her balance of tolerance and precision. Others have well described her incredible mixture of distinction and simplicity. Probably above all I recall the intensity and humanity of her creative spirit which burned straight to the center inspiring in me a reevaluation of everything.

—J. GARY SPARKS, Jungian analyst

When I did my exams at the Zürich Institute in 1975, von Franz was one of my examiners in fairy tales. I did terribly. She let me pass saying: "He must have had a block. No one could be that bad." She was wrong; I was. At twenty-five I understood little of the depth of fairy tales. When we went to her house with our little study group and sat in her room, which by now has gotten mixed up with dream rooms in which I have met her since, her sharp voice told us not to pick at material like a piece of chicken, something here, something there. "Oh, intuitives!" she exclaimed. She was more methodical. I did not appreciate her much then, took her presence for granted. Now I find that I quote her more often than anyone else. What I learned from her was irony and devotion to the work. Dr. von Franz, wherever you are now, thank you.

—ROBERT BOSNAK, Jungian analyst

I am a lay person who never underwent depth analysis. However, in the circumnavigation of my own life experiences and in the development of a worldview which has meaning to me in midlife, reading both Dr. Jung and Dr. von Franz has been life altering. I am pleased to hear, as might be expected from one so fully individuated as she, that she was at peace with her coming death and accepted its place in the wholeness of the life process. She will be remembered as an inspiration in death as she was in life.

—RICHARD CURTIS

As an avid reader of Jung and a humble scholar, I thank Dr. von Franz, who, by virtue of her sex, was my grounding link to the works of Dr. Jung. Being a female myself, and accepting Jung's belief in incompleteness of the quaternity without the feminine aspect, I needed some role model for that feminine component. Whereas I understand that "feminine" does not refer to the female of the species of homo sapiens, yet in this predominantly patriarchal society, I personally needed a female to whom I can relate. Not having yet been able to incorporate a divine female, e.g., the Gnostic Sophia, in my striving for individuation, Dr. von Franz fulfilled that need. I will greatly miss her.

—LIZ FEESS

Marie-Louise von Franz was a rare woman who lived both on the moon and on this earth. Sixteen years ago, while in personal analysis with her student Fraser Boa, I had a dream which neither Fraser nor I could understand. Fraser was at the time working with Marie-Louise von Franz on the film series *The Way of the Dream* and he asked my permission to tell her my dream. I readily agreed.

This was my dream:

> *I was standing on the shore of a lake on a dark and clouded night with only a few rays of the moon shining through. In the middle of the lake a man in a small rowboat was fishing. I knew he was fishing for a gigantic two-headed sea serpent which lived at the bottom of the lake.*

Marie-Louise von Franz knew nothing of me, but said: "The dreamer is a man who is immersed in conscious psychologies. What does he think will happen if he ever hooks that serpent? It will pull him under!"

She was right, and from thousands of miles away she helped me to respect the power of the unconscious and learn how to live on the moon as she did. I will miss her presence on this earth, and her penetrating and all-encompassing vision will be sorely missed by us all. I wish her Godspeed on her journey into the mystery and trust that we will all carry on her work of caring for the life of the unconscious.

—DOUGLAS R. CANN, Jungian analyst

PART TWO

Eulogies

To many [people] death seems to be a brutal and meaningless end to a short and meaningless existence . . . . So it looks, if seen from the surface and from the darkness. But when we penetrate the depths of the soul, and when we try to understand its mysterious life, we shall discern that death is not a meaningless end, the mere vanishing into nothingness—it is an accomplishment, a ripe fruit on the tree of life. Nor is death an abrupt extinction, but a goal that has been unconsciously lived and worked for during half a life.

In the youthful expansion of our life we think of it as an ever increasing river, and this conviction accompanies us often far beyond the midday of our existence. But if we listen to the lower voices of our deeper nature, we become aware of the fact that already soon after the middle of our life, the soul begins its secret work, the getting ready for the departure. Out of the turmoil and terror of our life, the one precious flower of the spirit begins to unfold, and the four-petalled flower of the immortal light. [And] even if our mortal consciousness should not be aware of its secret operation, it nevertheless does its secret work of purification.

—C. G. JUNG

Eulogy

Given at the funeral service in Küsnacht on the 26th of February 1998

GOTTHILF ISLER

We are gathered here together to bid our farewell to Marie-Louise von Franz. Many of you here today knew her personally and were accompanied by her down longer or shorter paths in your lives. Others have come because they attended her lectures or were gripped by her books. Each one of us experienced her differently, each in his or her own personal manner.

One's "fate" was constellated during almost every encounter with her. I usually felt a bit of trepidation prior to each analytical hour, not because I was in any way afraid of her, but because I knew that, despite her benevolence and affection, I would be led to my own inner truth as it emerged from my dreams and active imaginations. The message of the unconscious always stood at the center of our encounters.

This unfaltering relatedness to the autonomous psyche (the indepen-

"Trauerrede in der reformierten Kirche Küsnacht," in *Jungiana, Beiträge zur Psychologie von C. G. Jung,* Reihe A, Bd. 8 (Küsnacht: 1998), pp. 14–22; translated by D. Eldred.

dent, self-acting "objective psyche"[1] contiguous to ego consciousness) determined her life like nothing else. Rather than speaking today about details and events of her outer life or about her comprehensive scientific works, I would simply like to share with you several dreams both from her earlier as well as final years, some that may help us reflect, and others that may help console us.

Many years ago Marie-Louise von Franz told my wife and me a childhood dream that she also mentioned in her essay, "The Unknown Visitor."[2] She had this dream shortly after her family fled from Berchtsgaden over Salzburg to the border town of Feldkirch and then into Switzerland. Fleeing the oncoming revolution in Austria, the family then settled in the village of Rheineck in the Rheintal. She was at that time almost four and a half years old.[3]

> *I was walking with my father and mother and sister through the streets of the village that we were staying in after having fled [Austria]. My father was holding my hand. Suddenly at a distance an older and a younger man appeared in the street and rapidly approached us. My father called out, appalled, "There they are!" I asked, "Who?" He answered, "The gods, they are coming to test us. Each person has an iron plaque inscribed with his name, his birthday and his day of death. One must preserve one's plaque unharmed. Whoever's plaque is broken falls into the hands of the gods."*
>
> *We ran back into the room of the hostel where we were staying. My father opened the chest in which the family silver was kept and withdrew these plaques. They were enameled in white with black letters. The inscription on my plaque looked like it had been shattered by a hammer. I was horrified. I showed it to my family but they began to back away from me. I then stepped out of my body and hovered up on the ceiling near a bright round light into which I entered. From there I looked down and saw myself below sadly holding my plaque. At this point, I came to the decision that I wanted to live and returned to my body. And I wanted to go and meet the gods. So I then approached the door. As I went to open it, the door handle began to move. They had come. I awoke screaming.*[4]

As Marie-Louise von Franz explained, she had had a traumatic war shock. Household help had reported to her of the atrocities occurring at the time in World War I. And these descriptions had eliminated any belief that she had had about a good and loving God since "a loving God could not allow such appalling events to occur." Thus she felt compelled to confront this unknown God, and this fact—occurring already in earliest childhood—influenced and determined her entire life. In a later active imagination she believed that these two figures had been the gods Wotan and Loki. Wotan played a major role throughout her entire life.

Wotan was, however, a nature god. At the seaside, when she was sixteen years old, she was overwhelmed by an experience of the divineness of nature. Thereafter, nature (in a comprehensive sense) was a divine force for her both as emotional/inner psychic nature and as the nature of the earth, plants, and animals. This was one of the reasons why she studied philology, because in antiquity nature still lived. In her book, *The Visions of Niklaus von Flüe,* she writes that Wotan has two characteristic features that are missing in Yahweh of the Old Testament, namely, the intense relationship to cosmic nature and, through the art of divination (that is, oracles), his bearings in the principle of synchronicity. These two characteristics are apparently

> nonetheless parts of a wholistic God-image which seems to encompass not only darkness and evil but also cosmic nature and its meaningful revelation in synchronistic events. Only within the context of these two features is it possible to have an individual encounter with the divine in the *hic et nunc* [here and now] in which the *genius loci* and *surrounding nature can be meaningfully integrated into the psychic sphere of the individual* where it then appears to him in its totality as the "one cosmos." This entails *an immense elevation of meaning lying within the life of the individual*—an increase in the meaning of the individual person . . . imparting greatest weight to his or her conscious comprehension and ethical behavior.[5]

In an active imagination much much later in life, Marie-Louise von Franz realized that this new divinity did not actually have to do with

Wotan but with the *puer aeternus,* the eternal youth, the eternally youthful creator god.

In a traumatic dream during the Christmas holidays just prior to her nineteenth birthday (which she mentions in her book, *C. G. Jung: His Myth in Our Time)* she finds herself in a chamber in the middle of the earth where she sees the "face of God with an expression of such despondency and sorrow that no human being could bear looking at it." At the end, this dream also deals with the birth of the new god experienced by her as the birth of Aphrodite rising out of the sea. She interpreted this birth of a feminine divinity as the manifestation of the Self since it was her own dream, the dream of a woman.[6]

Her life was, in a sense, ordained by the highest form of love. Yet beyond the individual meaning of this dream, the psychology of the unconscious entails the deepest form of feminine science. (That is, the symbolic understanding of images brought forth by the unconscious is of a synergic, feminine nature.) She once wrote that "symbolic thinking is a form of loving understanding, a light that does not dispel the god Eros."[7] The psychology of the unconscious is always involved with uniting the opposites, the union of consciousness with the unconscious, masculine and feminine, the above and the below, spirit and matter, heaven and earth. This is not a random or coerced unification but rather a new birth which necessitates the bearing and enduring of the suffering entailed in the emergence of a new symbol, a new point of view thus enabling both sides to uphold their vested rights while they are simultaneously comprehended as unified in oneness. Marie-Louise von Franz repeatedly said that as the world falls apart we can be genuinely creative, we can work to form and shape the messages of the unconscious, we can struggle to grasp and realize the *mysterium coniunctionis,* that is, the union of the opposites. Within the personal realm, this new birth enables a meaningful cooperation between consciousness and the unconscious in which neither side is lessened or harmed.

A great moment of fortune in the life of Marie-Louise von Franz was her meeting C. G. Jung when she was still an eighteen-year-old student at the gymnasium in Zürich. Soon thereafter her collaborative work with Jung ensued. Carried by a deep veneration and love for him—

coupled with inconceivable discipline and incredible rigorousness—she rendered her life's work prolific and profound. When we read her essays and books, we often have the impression that, thanks to her vast knowledge, she just wrote those things down. She confided to one of her caretakers that every sentence that she wrote was like lifting a heavy stone. She once said to me that a man can dedicate his entire life working for some cause (or toward some objective), but a woman could accomplish the superhuman for a person she loved. When Jung died, she thought that she could no longer write a single word. She had to learn from the ground up to write toward some objective. I believe, however, that till the end of her life she still wrote out of her love for Jung.

Her incurable illness and her dependence on caretakers which endured so many years repeatedly raised for some of us the question of the meaning of life. Probably she actually had overworked herself. But the question of God still stands in the background. Why did God let this woman suffer so long, a woman who was so religiously dedicated to His own divine process of struggling toward consciousness and salvation, and who sacrificed to Him so many of the comforts of life?

On numerous occasions and in various ways she showed an admirable ability to take on her own fate. She once told me that in her younger years Jung had cast an African oracle with her. The prophesy set forth that, in the end, the Highest Judge would come. (This was a sign of great good fortune, and she actually experienced many incredible things; yet many had to remain secret which is why she could not talk to me about them.) But subsequently an "After Judge" would come, and this predicted great misfortune. This calamity was her illness. She was nevertheless glad that she had cast this oracle because she knew that this misfortune belonged to her fate. She had no illusions. She knew that God was not only loving but that one had to live in fear of Him as well. One time when I spoke to her about her illness I mentioned that men and women who felt passion and pity were in a way more loving than God, and she answered, "Yes, nature is incredibly intelligent, but fearfully cruel as well."

She carried her fate not only stoically. Four years ago, as she had a bout of flu and could not eat anymore, she thought that her solution had come; she would simply stop eating and the problem would then take care of itself. Subsequently she dreamed:

> *She was at Bahnhof Enge.*[8] *She set her leg on the track, thinking that the train would now run over her. But as the locomotive drove out of the tunnel she began to scream loudly for help. Somehow she was rescued. But then a dark cloud enshrouded everything so that she could no longer see. In this darkness she felt the coat of a large dog and grasped onto it. The dog then spoke in a human voice saying: "Don't do that. Everything is organized."*

As she then told this dream, she laughed mischievously: it is all organized, the ticket ordered, the hotel reserved. She now knew that she had to carry her suffering and would still have to wait.

Prior to and after this dream, she had captivatingly beautiful dreams that pointed to her completion. These were dreams that made her profoundly happy. I would like to share with you a few of these images. For example, she dreamed that

> *she was near a farmhouse where there were many people dressed in black. A young farm laborer was digging a hole for a coffin. Out of the casket rose an old man who was suffering from the same illness as she. He wanted—unconditionally—to live. The farm laborer argued with him, saying that he belonged in the casket; he threw him back into the coffin and closed the lid. I stood passively on the side, thinking, "This has nothing to do with me." In the farmyard stood a tree, probably a horse chestnut. But it was a magnificent tree with passion flowers the size of dinner plates. And she herself had once planted this tree. In each flower there was a little tomato. She plucked one, ate it, and knew that it was the* cibus immortalis, *the food of immortality.*[9]

She commented to me then that the old man was the will to live, a willpower that does not want to give in and which just extends her suffering. The laborer thinks that it is time to die. (Years later, as it became increasingly difficult to take in nourishment, she said that she still wanted to eat, the will to live generally being the strongest drive.) And she then added that tomatoes in Austria are called "paradises," and that tomatoes are often considered to be aphrodisiacal fruits from the Tree of Knowledge.

In the summer of 1994, a woman visited her who wanted to convince Marie-Louise to collaborate with her. This woman, who was a medium, was convinced that the Christian and Buddhist spirit were uniting in the beyond in order to save the world. Marie-Louise von Franz promised nothing, saying that she would first like to consult her dreams. The following night she dreamed that

> *she was working in the laundry at the monastery in Einsiedeln. She was told that Jung would come down from heaven to the wedding of the Black Madonna. She belonged to the one hundred elect who would be allowed to participate in the marriage festivities.*

She said at that time that the unconscious was indeed preparing a form of help for the world and a union, not in the heavenly spiritual realm, but rather a union of above and below, a union of spirit and matter. The Virgin Mary was considered very early to be "the earth" and the Black Madonna a nature goddess. And yet the union occurs within the Christian framework, which Marie-Louise von Franz had never been able to accept. Nevertheless, the dream filled her with such happiness.

Two years ago, she dreamed that she saw a tree in marvelous bloom. It stood in water with little earth around it.[10] In all earnestness she said to me that she wanted us to know that the wind could easily topple it.

In August of last year, Marie-Louise told me that she had dreamed that she

> *had written an eight-volume work on Arabian alchemy. The eight volumes were there in front of her and she was very pleased.*[11]

She understood the dream as saying that her life work was now completed.

Last November she dreamed:

> *It is evening and she still had to rake together the hay so that the dew of the night would not moisten it. And in the dream, she knew that night would rapidly come.*[12]

She then told me that she now had to set her estate in order. On this past Christmas, she said that she was no longer fighting and this was something which was new for her, for up till now she had always fought. She was still mentally alert and crystal clear, and she was interested in every individual who visited her as well as in what was happening in the world. And she remained so till the very end. It was, however, often difficult to understand her because at times she could hardly speak at all.

She wanted to die, and of death she had no fear. Many years ago she said that, with her book *On Dreams and Death,* she had convinced herself that, after death, life still continues. One of the women who helped take care of Marie-Louise for many years—at times with considerable self-sacrifice and to whom we cannot be grateful enough—had a dream while she was there spending the night just a couple of weeks before Marie-Louise's death. The woman dreamed that she

> *descended the stairs down to the ground floor where Marie-Louise was sleeping. There in the entrance stood C. G. Jung, aged, well-dressed, the very manifestation of wisdom. He smiled at the dreamer, went into Marie-Louise's room and sat on her bed. They then had a long amiable conversation.*

Marie-Louise was so happy when she heard the dream because she knew now that Jung would come to take her to the beyond. She would then be together with him and possibly with the people to whom she really belonged.[13]

She had already "known" for a long time that Jung lived there. She had once given him a gift of a precious Chinese frog carved from jade. He had found the gift so valuable that he specified that this "jewel" would be returned to her upon his death. A few weeks after his death, she dreamed that *she was looking into a brook and saw what she took to be a bit of human excrement, something "made by man." As she got get closer, she saw that it was this little frog. It suddenly lifted its front leg and waved at her.*

This dream was a sign for her that Jung lived on, and it was with this frog in her hand that she passed away. (The frog, by the way, is a symbol of resurrection.)

Marie-Louise von Franz died at 2:15 A.M. on February 17, 1998. A few years prior to her death, she dreamed that

in an old city a new building had been built with a perimeter of seventeen regular sides, a construction that was earlier believed to be impossible.[14]

In Arabian alchemy, the seventeen-sided geometric form symbolized the union of psyche and matter which was the very center of the research that she performed. In addition, the number 17 is the number of completed individuation, the accomplishment of totality.

Nevertheless, we must not forget: death is always an experience of something terrifying and full of awe. But these dreams from the close proximity of death show the merciful face of God. It is for us, as well as for the world, an immeasurable piece of providence and good fortune that a woman like Marie-Louise von Franz lived, and that we were able to meet her. Her spirit lives on among us . . . as well as in her numerous works.

NOTES

1. A term Jung gave to this nonsubjective aspect of the unconscious.
2. Marie-Louise von Franz, *Archetypal Dimensions of the Psyche* (Boston: Shambala, 1997), p. 71.
3. For the details reported here I wish to thank Marie-Anne von Franz, Marie-Louise von Franz's sister.
4. Told to me on March 28, 1988; this dream is discussed in *Archetypal Dimensions of the Psyche*, p. 71f.

5. M.-L. von Franz, *Die Visionen des Niklaus von Flüe* (Zürich, 1959), p. 129f.
6. M.-L. von Franz, *C. G. Jung: His Myth in Our Time* (Toronto: Inner City Books, 1998), pp. 205ff.
7. M.-L. von Franz, *Erlösungsmotive im Märchen* (München, 1986), p. 142.
8. One of several train stations in Zürich; trains arrive and depart through tunnels.
9. Told to me on May 12, 1993.
10. Told to me on March 22, 1996.
11. Told to me on August 29, 1997.
12. Told to me on November 6, 1997.
13. See C. G. Jung, *Memories, Dreams, Reflections* (New York: Vintage Books, 1989), p. 291.
14. Told to me on November 3, 1994.

Eulogy

In tribute to Marie-Louise von Franz at her memorial service
on February 26, 1998

NORA MINDELL

Dear ladies and gentlemen: As members of a foundation dedicated to supporting Dr. Jung's and Dr. von Franz's studies in synchronicity, we would like to pay tribute to Marie-Louise von Franz today by sharing with you excerpts from a personal conversation that we had with her three summers ago at her lovely round *Stube* table in Bollingen.[1]

As most of you know, Dr. von Franz was not only well versed in Chinese mythology, eastern divinatory techniques, diverse mathematical systems, and the arcane wisdom of the I Ching, but her knowledge sprang from a well of profound experiences and insights accrued during her lifelong study of the objective psyche.

Toward the end of her life, this great lady even cheerfully proclaimed that Jung's ideas were *so* "mind-boggling" that she was *just* beginning to grasp them herself!

One summer's afternoon at Bollingen over tea, Dr. von Franz spoke with us about the Lo-shu and Ho-t'u mandalas considered to be cosmic plans of the universe that underlie the basic structure of the I Ching.[2] The Ho-t'u, "Older Heavenly Order," she pointed out, is quaternarian, a picture of absolute totality outside time and space—totality as it ever was and ever will be! By contrast, the Lo-shu, "Younger Heavenly Order," wanders along like the numbers 1, 2, 3, and 4. The meaning that it embodies is the same as the Ho-t'u, but the Lo-Shu is clothed in the manifestations of material and psychic processes.

Whenever you ask a question of the I Ching, these two matrices of energy dynamically interact, setting in motion an answer on two levels: one relating more to issues emerging in the foreground of reality and the other to eternal patterns, values, and states of mind. For example, after Dr. von Franz first met Jung, she wondered if she should try to see him again. She consulted the I Ching and got hexagram no. 17, Following. The text reports: "An old man defers to a young girl and shows her consideration. By this he moves her to follow him." This image prophesied the unswerving direction that her life would take at the same time that it responded to the momentary question utmost in her mind.

This double mandala pattern is a *coniunctio* of heaven and earth, time and timelessness, spirit and matter, the transcendental mystery which plays a central role in C. G. Jung's and Marie-Louise von Franz's works. Dr. von Franz devoted her life to writing books which shed light on this arcane opus, but it is a mark of her greatness that she struggled to experience what she wrote and taught, always consulting the clear, unspoiled spring of the unconscious for guidance.

Speaking of the interaction between the Lo-shu and the Ho-t'u in relation to the divine marriage on that afternoon, her voice took on a special quality of eros as she commented: "Jung once said that what is happening now is forever. So when we sit here now it is transient, and at the same time it is the Self—we will sit here together forever."

None of us spoke for quite a while afterward. I am sure that all of you have had experiences of the Self in which eternity and the here-and-now spontaneously come together in a numinous way. As Dr. von Franz talked, we entered another time dimension that was inexplicable; by means of her capacity for relating to the collective unconscious, the opposites came together miraculously.

In closing, we wish to send you a message, dear Marlus. "Please do not forget that so many of us sitting here are immensely grateful and touched by the good fortune we had of becoming acquainted with you. We have experienced your dedication, your wisdom, your love, your loyalty, and your enduring search for a deeper understanding of the living psyche."

We have been together.

We are together today.

We shall remain together for all time. . . .

Nonetheless, we shall miss your earthly presence intensely.

NOTES

1. This eulogy was delivered at the memorial service by Dr. Roy Freeman.
2. M.-L. von Franz, *Number and Time: Reflections Leading toward a Unification of Depth Psychology and Physics* (Evanston, Ill.: Northwestern University Press, 1974), pp. 22ff.

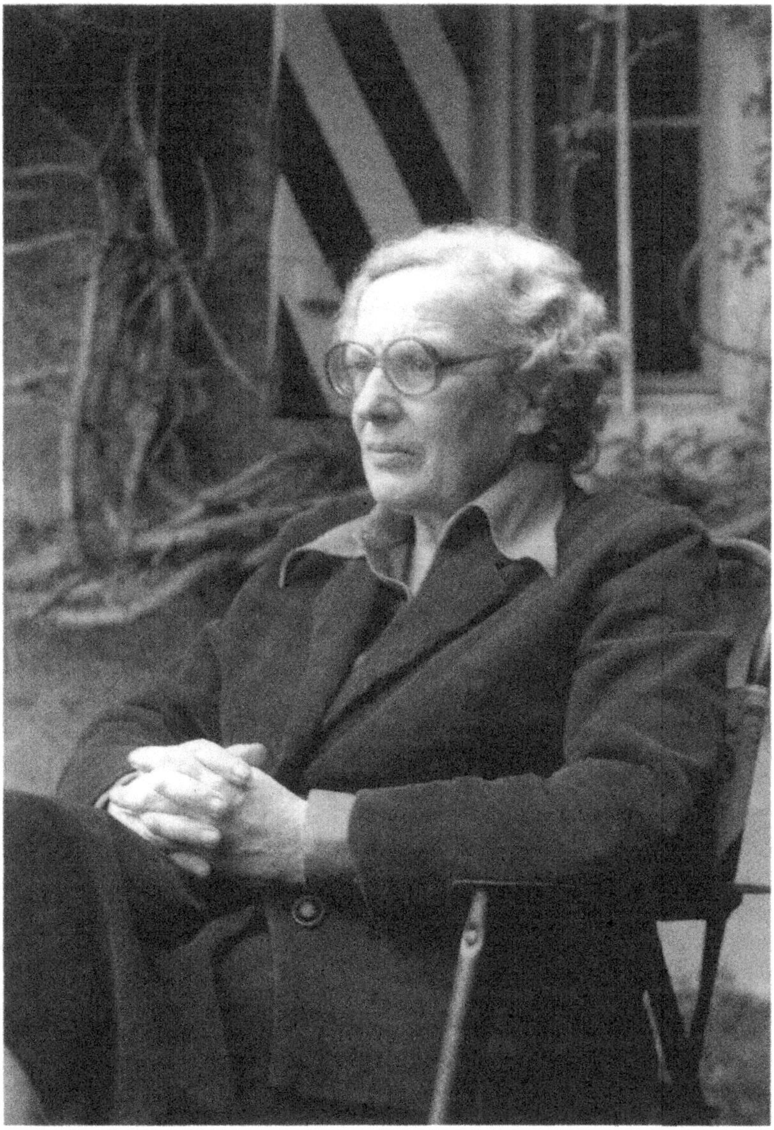

Plate 1. Marie-Louise von Franz in Bollingen. Courtesy of Françoise Selhofer, 1982.

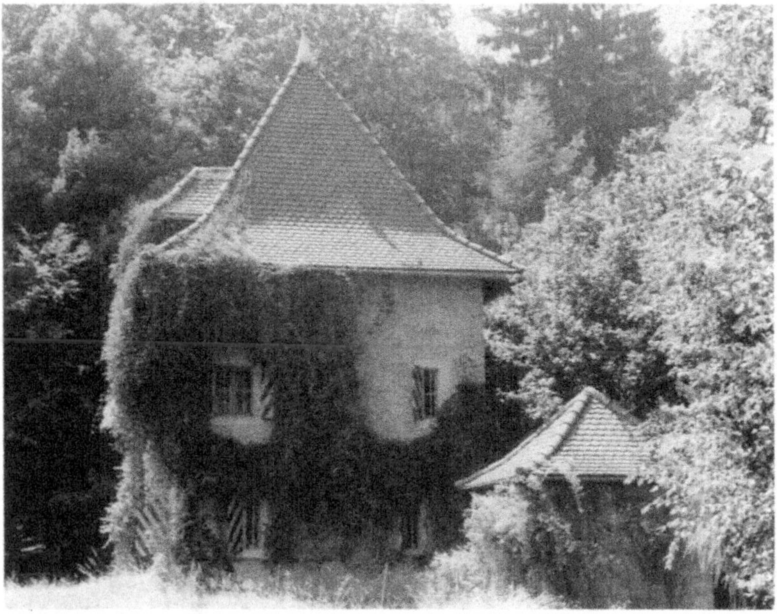

Plate 2. The "tower" of Marie-Louise von Franz in Bollingen. Courtesy of Robin Lea Hutton.

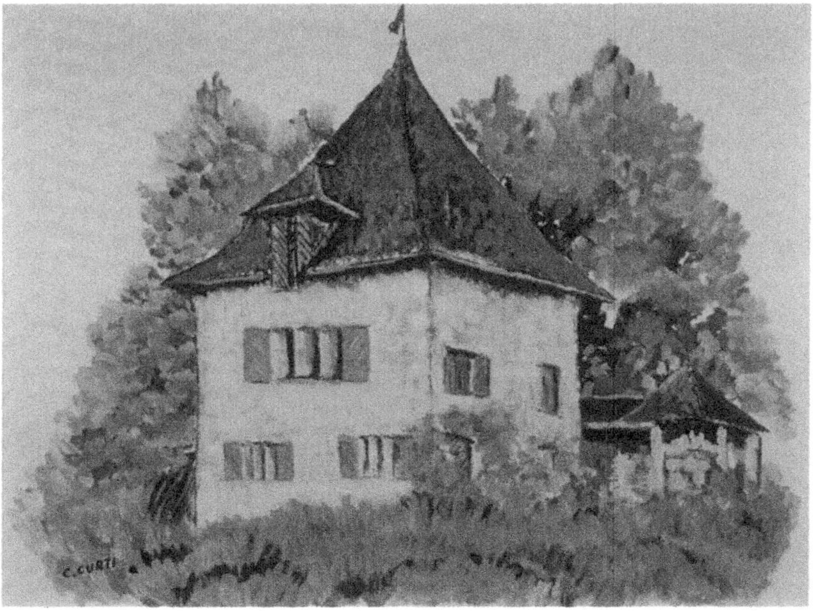

Plate 3. The "tower." Oil, 60 cm x 45 cm. Courtesy of the artist, Costanza Boss-Curti.

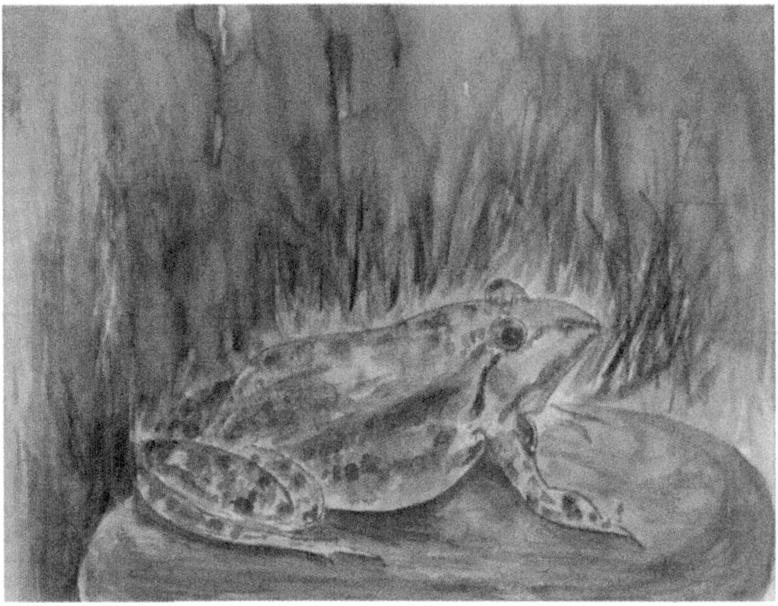

Plate 4. Frog. Watercolor, 32 cm x 25 cm. Courtesy of the artist, Costanza Boss-Curti.

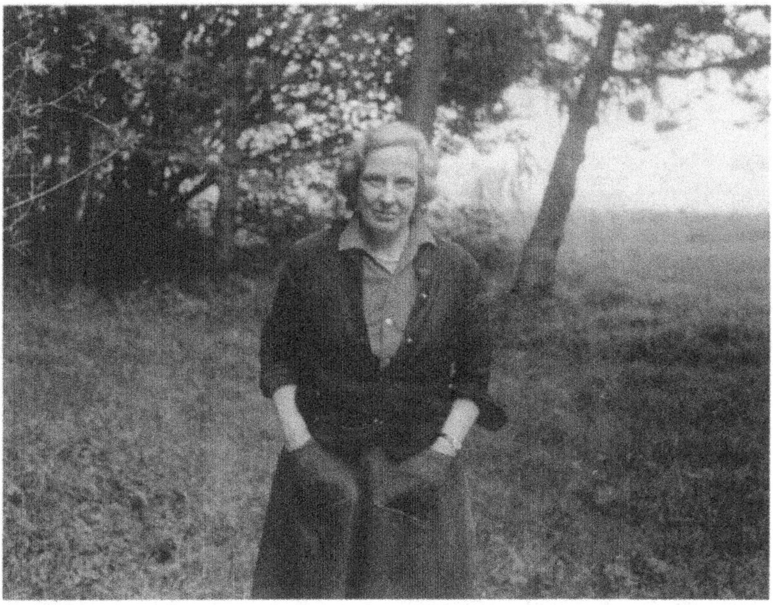

Plate 5. Marie-Louise von Franz in Bollingen. Photographed by William H. Kennedy.

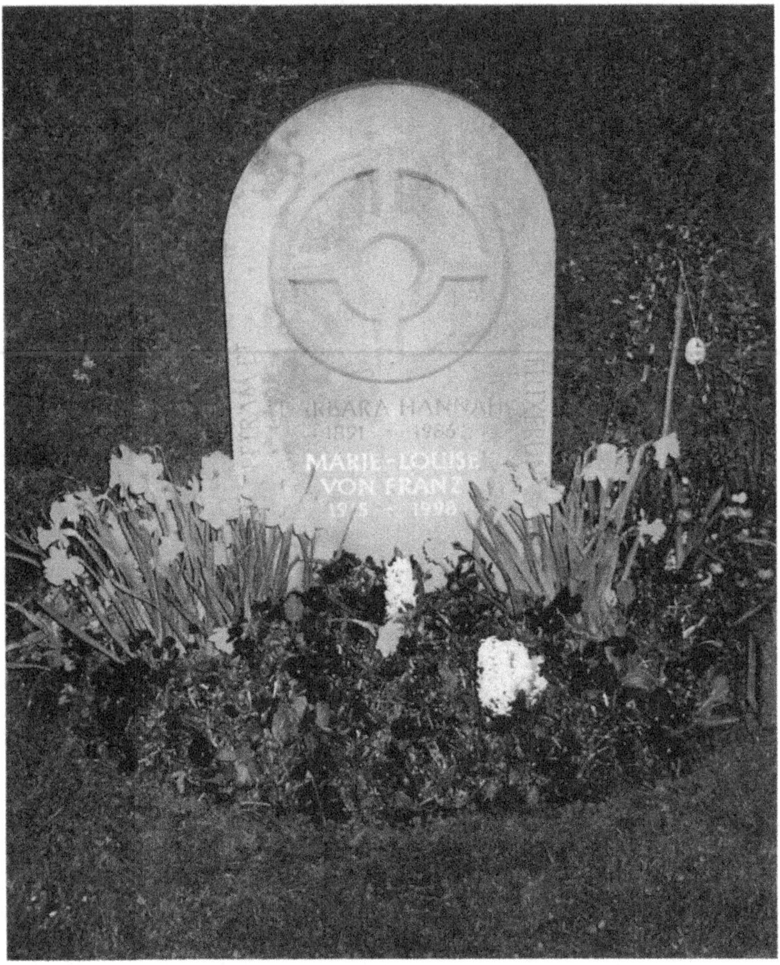

Plate 6. The grave of Barbara Hannah and Marie-Louise von Franz in Küsnacht. Courtesy of Marie-Anne von Franz.

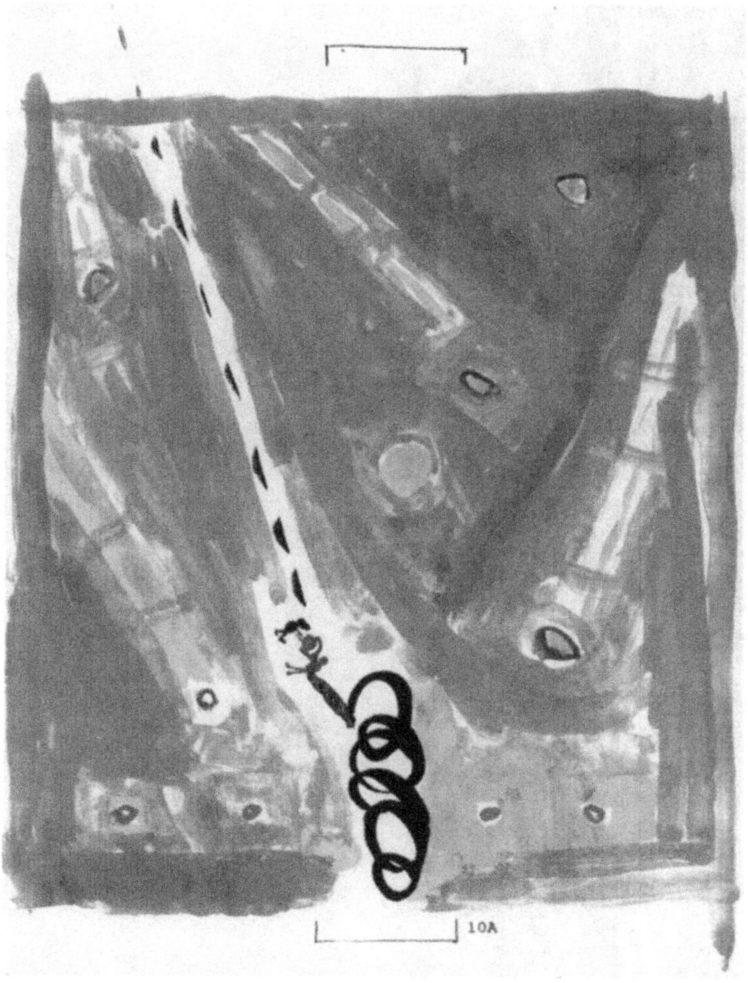

Plate 7. Diagram of a play in field hockey, from Roger Lyons, "Dream Analysis with Marie-Louise von Franz" (see p. 349).

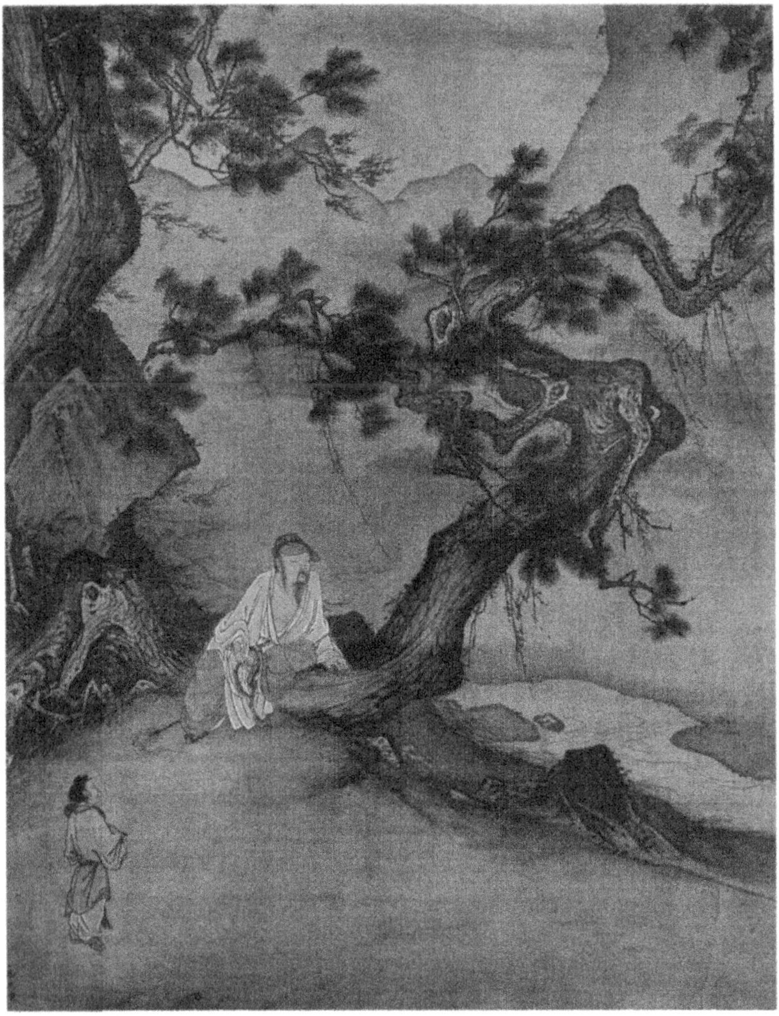

Plate 8 (from Lara Mindell, "On the Tao of Uselessness," p. 386). "Listening in the Wind to the Pines," by Ma Lin. Seal dated 1246, hanging scroll (cropped at the top and the bottom), width 43.5 inches, ink and colors on silk. National Palace Museum Collection, Taipei, Taiwan. Taken from J. Cahill, *Treasures of Asia: Chinese Painting* (Ohio: The World Publishing Company, 1960), p. 64. Reproduction courtesy of the National Palace Museum, Taipei, Taiwan, Republic of China. Reprinted by permission.

Eulogy

Valedictory address for Marie-Louise von Franz at the burial service held in the Reformed Church, Küsnacht, Switzerland, on February 26, 1998

ANNE MAGUIRE

I am deeply honored to receive the singular invitation to deliver this valedictory address for our dear departed friend, Marie-Louise von Franz, a truly great lady whose passing is marked by those of us gathered here on this sad day, a day when the reality of our loss is realized as we bid her earthly self adieu.

I doubt not that each one of us present this day has had his or her life transformed in some way either by personal contact with her, or through knowledge of her literary creative work, which in turn has introduced her to a vast world audience.

She was born at a momentous time, in the first terrible winter of the Great War, in the German city of Münich, itself a city under the aegis of the little hooded *kabir*, the *Münchener kindt*—the child. A cloaked figure akin to the phallic *kabir* of the ancient world—Telesphoros, a companion and guide of Asclepius, the god of medical healing. At the same time he was a youthful double of Asclepius and was known as "the one who brings to completeness," the god of inner transformations.

Three years after her birth, toward the end of the war, she was brought by her Austrian parents to Switzerland; eventually she became a citizen of her adopted country and lived her life here. At the age of eighteen years, one afternoon in 1933, the year that Adolf Hitler seized power in Germany, she was invited by a friend to meet Carl Gustav Jung. The meeting was portentous, for on that day she was introduced to the reality of another realm of reality—the hidden inner world. As the unconscious presented itself to her through the medium of Dr. Jung she was utterly astounded. During that afternoon Jung had described a young woman he had treated who "lived on the moon." When Marie-Louise heard this, she decided to approach the professor and ask him if he meant that it was "as if" the girl lived on the moon. Dr. Jung answered her and told her that it was not "as if" but the girl did live on the moon. She told me that at that moment she thought either "he is crazy or I am." That meeting circumscribed the fateful moment of transformation in her life. The following year, in 1934, she began to work with C. G. Jung and did so until his death in 1961.

The statement made by Jung and which had so perplexed her led to a lifelong search for the inner truth as concealed in the unconscious world of objective psyche. It was then that she learned of the importance of the dream as a message from that interior world. She had a splendid rational intellect with an incisive mind, which enabled her to become a deep, and later an inspired and inspiring, thinker. Her ability to grasp and to discern had a rapierlike character, yet she was always able to explain a point or enlarge an aspect of a problem, with an exquisite but immensely patient clarity. This aspect of her personality belonged to the archetype of the teacher for she was, in my view, unassailable in that particular field. She retained, it seems, this lucid clarity of mind until she died.

As a multilinguist and medieval Latin scholar, she collaborated with Jung in the study of alchemy, she contributed related studies to two of his major works, *Aion* and *Mysterium Coniunctionis*. In her early years as a psychotherapist, she dreamed that she was walking upon ground where "no one had trodden before." Some time later she was to begin her monumental creative work upon the fairy tales and later with the archetypal world of numbers. These previously unexplored fields were to occupy her energies for many years.

Perhaps for a moment may I speak of the fairy-tale studies. Today they are so much a part of Jungian training and psychotherapy that one forgets the immense primary work undertaken by Marie-Louise in those early years.

As a young woman she enjoyed the natural world, particularly the mountains where she liked to walk in summer and ski in winter. She liked nothing better than to be immersed in nature with the greenness of its trees, the flowers under foot, and the splendid mountains themselves. She had an exceptional knowledge of animal lore and a profound sympathy with that world. She held the present view that the natural world is in fact doomed by man's gross unconsciousness and ignorance of the spirit of wild nature, a spirit which if left alone could and indeed would bring about a reparation of the damage to which the earth and its seas have already been subjected, but only if left alone by man.

With such vital interests in the importance of the dream in an individual life and the domination of the spirit in the natural world, it is clear that the domain of the fairy tales, those age-old traditional tales, should call to her. She answered the call and was seized by the material. She read thousands of fairy stories from all over the world. This empowered her to perceive those hidden secrets held in them, which engendered their fascination. Thus she came to understand perhaps better than anyone else in the world the archetypal structure of the natural world in these tales and in unconscious psyche. She saw, as it were, the skeletal structure of psyche, inasmuch perhaps as one sees the singular distinctive skeletal shape and pristine beauty of a deciduous tree in wintertime when unhindered by its leaves. This immense work and the knowledge thus gained from her creative genius I am sure led her to become a master analyst and an incomparable interpreter of the dream.

There was, however, another facet to this multifaceted personality which she possessed, an aspect not usually immediately apparent because of her innate modesty and her primary introverted attitude. She had a dislike for the vulgarly ostentatious and unseemly power drivenness, and thus her eros to which I refer held a certain quality of reticence. In her lectures, one was always aware that behind her powerful intellect her eros was, albeit shyly, constantly palpably present. I always thought her eros to be totally genuine, all pervading and enveloping—the true *charitas.* She was a kind woman, and real love has much to do with kindness.

In her attitude to others, it seemed to me that she desired that all should benefit from her own knowledge and her experience which she gave freely and generously, just as she gave her hospitality. She endeavored to aid them to reach the hidden inner truth as she perceived it to be. This was the spirit by which she lived, always seeking to bring a soul to the light of illumination. I believe it is because of this true kindness that we have come gladly to remember her today with our love, albeit we are deeply saddened by our loss.

In the last years, she bore stoically, nobly, and with immense courage a devastating physical illness. She was indomitable until the end of her earthly life. Yet in spite of her suffering she retained her richly perceptive insights, her capacity to emit the trenchant asides, her kindness to others, and last but by no means least, her sense of humor. She astonished me, how in pain, disabled in body and sometimes with the speech difficulties which accompany this illness, she was able to joke, and to laugh with abandon, and express herself in her own inimitable way.

During one dark evening not very long ago, whilst recumbent on her bed, after we had discussed the *unus mundus,* she told me that she had dreamed a wonderful dream the night previously. In it, her illness was cured and had left her completely healed in body. She told me she was immensely happy in the dream, and she added that she would be leaving soon. The dream brought her great joy.

She strove throughout the years of her tribulation to participate consciously in her individual pathway to wholeness, as it unfolded in her dreams and outer life.

I see her as a woman who sought ever the inner spirit of creative truth and fought for justice in the acceptance of that truth.

This is the spirit which gathers us together today—we her many friends, who loved her, companions who accompanied her throughout her years of prime life, and those of her years of travail, caring, and looking after her. In particular, I would like to mention those nursing companions, faithful, devoted, and tireless in their love to ease her passage from this life and who served her so well, and also those who contributed to her comfort in diverse ways.

With respect I mention Barbara Davies, friend, assistant, and collaborator, who became her writing hand, Julia Brunner, Alison Kappes, Nomiki Kennedy, Vicki Reiff, Mary Scheinost, Regine Schweizer-Vüllers, Zita Tauber, and Anne-Marie Wöbel.

It was her wish to stay in her own home. I felt she would have liked to die in Bollingen, which she loved, but that was not God's will and so she died in her townhouse with all the good spirits of her past, and her students, analysands, and friends came to her, not forgetting her late dear friends, Barbara Hannah and Franz Riklin, and their regular gatherings together in that house. Her named devoted companions supported her and permitted her to have her wish in this respect.

I am very sorry that my dear friend of over thirty years, Marie-Louise von Franz, has died. She leaves the world a poorer place, and although in the years to come undoubtedly some will endeavor to emulate her work and perhaps even forget the originator, they will surely fail because none will possess the unique combined attributes contained in the creative genius of this great lady.

Because of her love and reverence for the soul, may I with respect quote a few lines from the beautiful poem, "Ode to the Soul," by the great Islamic physician-philosopher Ibn Sina who died a thousand years ago.

Ode to the Soul

Out of her lofty home she hath come down, upon thee
this white dove in all the pride of her reluctant beauty:
veiled is she, from every eye, eager to know her, though
in loveliness unshrouded radiant, unwillingly she came,
and yet perchance still more unwilling to be gone from thee—
so she is torn by griefs.

. . . .
Why then was she cast down from her high peak? to
this degrading depth?
God brought her low. But for a purpose-wise,
that is concealed even from the keenest mind
and liveliest wit.
And if the tangled mesh impeded her
the narrow cage denied her wings to soar freely
in heaven's high ranges, after all she was a
lightning flash that brightly glowed—
momently o'er the tents and then was hid as
though its gleam was never glimpsed below.
(translated by A. J. Arberry)

PART THREE

Birthday Addresses

Address Delivered at the May Festival of the Psychological Club of Zürich

Zunfthaus zur Meise, Zürich
May 10, 1975

J. TAUBER, M.D.

Marie-Louise von Franz [is a] pillar of Jungian psychology, proving time and again that she is its ingenious and indefatigable interpreter, an "Old—and 'Jung' philologist." In a dream she showed me an underground realm of roots. At first, I found it cold and unpleasant there, but then she pointed mutely to a picture of a rose on a wall and suddenly it dawned on me: all roses fade and pass away, but this archetypal picture of the rose never wilts, never withers.

(Marie-Louise von Franz celebrated her sixtieth birthday in January of this year.)

Address Delivered on the Occasion of the Seventieth Birthday of Marie-Louise von Franz

Hotel Bad, Schmerikon, Switzerland
May 4, 1985

VERNON BROOKS

Most of the activities this evening have been conducted in a foreign language. Now perhaps I might introduce another possibility. My own German is a bit spotty. I still feel a bit like Mark Twain, who asked, "What can you do with a language in which a young girl has no sex and a turnip does."[1]

Marlus, I had the most marvelous dream last night. I enjoyed it enormously. When I awoke I thought that perhaps I had been converted to a Freudian because there was nothing compensatory about that dream; it was pure wish fulfillment.

I dreamed that I had been given the duty, the opportunity, and I may say even the pleasure of prosecuting—for their sins—those friends of mine who became seventy years old in this calendar year. And you can imagine my excitement when I saw that the first name on the list was that of Dr. M.-L. von Franz, the first friend of mine to become seventy in 1985.

Now this event took place in a rather grand courtroom which was open at the top into the beyond. There were time and number symbols on the walls around the courtroom.

I was given a list of the sins of which you were accused, sins which you had committed at some time during your life. And if I went into all of them this evening, we would still be here when we come back to celebrate your seventy-fifth birthday. So I have to be very selective and choose only those which are the most interesting.

ACCUSATION ONE: You are accused of having written too many books.

Now, how many books are too many books? At one time I asked you how many books you had published so far, and you said, "Oh, eight or nine or ten perhaps." But when we started counting them up, they ran close to twenty.

Well, there was that book about the *puer,* which every American has read three or four times because Americans are very fond of *puers.*

And then there was the *Aurora Consurgens,* which nobody has read. We all own a copy, but how many of us have read it? Well, the Judge asked, "Is it really a sin to write a book that no one has read?" And then the Judge answered, "No."

Then there was that book that you wrote only half of.[2] And since Emma Jung was not on trial at the time, the question arose: "Is it a sin to write half a book?" And the Judge said: "Either it's a whole sin or it's no sin, there's no such thing as half a sin." So we had to eliminate that one.

Then there were all those seminar publications. And the defense brought in a witness from the publishing world who said that "technically those are publications, they are not books." So, on a technicality, you were declared innocent of having written too many books.

Now, let's see.

ACCUSATION TWO: You are accused of being impatient with people who are stupid.

And when I heard that word *stupid,* something began to clatter in the back of my head. And I thought: "On what occasion have *I* ever been so stupid as to provoke Marlus's impatience?"

Well there was an occasion when Bill Kennedy and I had invited Marlus and Barbara to have dinner with us in this hotel, Hotel Bad here in Schmerikon. Well, we were stupid enough to go to Germany that day for lunch. Then we lost our way coming back and couldn't seem to find Switzerland. When we finally located it again, we arrived here for dinner two hours late. And Barbara and Marlus were sitting in the room just above us at a table by the window patiently waiting for us.

So you are *not* guilty of impatience with stupid people, or at least so the Judge declared on hearing that shameful story.

ACCUSATION THREE: You are accused of squandering your affection on frogs.

This accusation was withdrawn very shortly when it was made clear that there had been a misunderstanding, that the accusation did not mean that you were especially fond of Frenchmen, but especially fond of a different kind of living creature.[3]

ACCUSATION FOUR: Now you are accused of having abandoned analytical psychology in favor of becoming a movie star.

The principal evidence produced in this instance was a ten-hour film in which you appear. Now, I am a great film fan myself, and I have sat through some very long films. But I have never sat through ten hours of film at one sitting.

The accused was called to the witness stand and the following question-and-answer testimony took place, which is taken *verbatim* from the records of the court:

Q: You are accused of having abandoned analytical psychology in order to become a film star. Is this true?

A: No.

Q: However, is it not true that you consented to appear in a film that lasts for ten hours?

A: Yes.

Q: Do you imagine that there is anyone who will sit still for ten hours to watch a film?

A: There were hundreds of Americans who watched that film for ten hours and they paid three hundred dollars apiece to see it.

Q: So you have gone into film business for financial reasons?

A: Don't be absurd.

Q: Then you will please tell us why you consented to appear in a film of such monstrous length?

A: Well that film was made by North Americans, and I figured that if I gave them ten hours of dream analysis they could show the thing over and over again instead of coming over here and asking me for analytic hours in person.[4]

She was found not guilty of this charge, too, and I began to feel very uncomfortable because she seemed to be innocent of all the sins she was accused of.

But I noticed one down close to the bottom of the list which gave me some hope. It said:

ACCUSATION FIVE: You are accused of analyzing too many dreams too quickly.

Well, I am perhaps the only person in this room tonight who has never had personal analysis with Marlus von Franz. But I have a friend, Manolis Kennedy, who does and who dreams by the yard. His dreams run three and four yards at a time, and he takes ten or twelve of these to Dr. von Franz and expects her to analyze all that yardage in one hour. And you know what? She does!

So I thought: "Well, at least we have found something that she is really guilty of."

But at that moment I heard a commanding and rather tremendous voice from somewhere up there in the beyond, which said: "Why are you persecuting one of the people I have loved the most?"

And I thought: "I've heard that voice somewhere before. It's not an American voice, it has a foreign accent."

I responded: "I was only doing my duty."

And the voice replied: "Ah yeah, that's what the Nazis said."

And I answered: "Well, who are you who asks this question?"

And the voice said: "Since you Americans are so fond of calling people by their first names, just call me Charley."

So I jumped out of the dream and back into what passes more or less for reality, and I thought: "Well, anyone who has a guardian angel like that doesn't need anyone's defense."

Marlus, there will be many people tonight who will say to you: "I love you." I am not going to say to you: "I love you." I am going to say to you, in your own language, "Ich liebe Dich."

NOTES

1. Referring to the gender of the German article before nouns: a young girl is preceded by the neutral article *das,* a turnip by the feminine article *die.*—*Ed.*
2. E. Jung and M.-L. von Franz, *The Grail Legend* (New York: G. P. Putnam's Sons/ C. G. Jung Foundation, 1970).
3. Although politically incorrect, this text, as throughout this Festschrift, has been altered only when it suffers from lack of clarity or grammatical error.—*Ed.*
4. In a letter to William H. Kennedy (March 28, 1973), she referred to the Americans as "soul tourists": "Summer is anyhow the time of the 'soul tourists' where I am always overburdened." Before she built her tower in Bollingen, she used to work analytically throughout the whole summer in her house in Küsnacht. This is evident from her appointment book for the year 1957, one year before she built her country home. In this sense, her tower was truly a *refugium.* See also "Films with Marie-Louise von Franz" in Part Eight.

On the Seventieth Birthday of Marie-Louise von Franz

Bad Schmerikon
May 4, 1985

GOTTHILF ISLER

EXCERPTS

Dear Marie-Louise, dear participants,
When I honor you here, I do so solely as an individual, out of my own experience.

Meeting you has fundamentally changed the lives of many people here. I know of many friends whose lives were totally turned about by the encounter with you. One could probably liken what we experience with you to what you experienced with Jung. I personally never knew him—although several of us here tonight did—but I do imagine that your experience of Jung meant much the same to you as our experience of you does to us.

You have led each of us to their own individual truth, to their own Self. And it seems to me that you are able of doing that only because you live this yourself and because what you say to us is totally, honestly you. This is possibly—at least in the foreground—my greatest and most intrinsic experience of you: the unconditional relatedness to the inner authority and to the objective psyche.

Maybe there is something still more important and this has to do with the manner in which you are related to the Self. Although difficult to put into words, it has to do somehow with this modesty and humaneness and honesty. One never has the feeling of being taken by the hand and led in some childlike manner, that is to say, a bit protected by some guru initiating the novice into the wisdom of Jungian psychology. . . .

When one sits with you in a room, then it always has to do directly with the Self, the *numen,* with the indomitable will of God as it is present in dreams or active imagination. And it never has to do with something of the ego. Even when sitting together with you, one kneels and you kneel, and the one who is with you kneels as well in front of the Great and Incomprehensible. This forthrightness of human existence vis-à-vis the numinous . . . this is the great experience I have of you.

From the Foreword to the Festschrift for the Seventy-fifth Birthday of Marie-Louise von Franz, 1990

[unpublished]

The life of [Marie-Louise von Franz] is . . . unique and for us, as well as humanity, of a meaning that goes beyond all measure.

—THE BOARD OF TRUSTEES, Stiftung für Jung'sche Psychologie

For the Celebration of Marie-Louise von Franz's Eightieth Birthday

Excerpts from a text from the Group of Analytical Psychology, Valencia

RAFAEL MONZÓ

Marie-Louise von Franz embodies the faithful devotion to the creative unconscious both through her work in the resolution of her own personal enigmas as well as in her genuine effort toward the realization of the unconscious itself. . . . She is a woman with profound human qualities, a scientific genius, and an enormous creative and working capacity, and she shows a unique loyalty to the unconscious and to analytical psychology whose spirit she has kept alive throughout her entire life. . . . Her work is the fruit of her love of truth. No doubt such a work is a watershed in the history of knowledge and science that opens the way and makes us advance even more into the enigmas of existence and the search for the personal collective meaning which underlies human experience. . . . We are grateful to von Franz for the enormous creative, scientific, and human task which she has tirelessly undergone. Through scientific knowledge of the depths of the psyche and thanks to her various discoveries she has assisted us toward a greater understanding of the mysteries of the psyche. With her paradigmatic personal commitment to analytical psychology, with her faithfulness to the spirit of our times, and with her openness to a more complete integrative and evolving humanism she put herself in the service of the human development of a science which includes love. . . . In the name of our small group which von Franz supported with her unsurpassed capacity for relatedness and personal affection, we express our most profound gratitude.

PART FOUR

Personal Impressions

Marie-Louise von Franz was the *spiritual daughter* of C. G. Jung.

—PETER JUNG, Jungian analyst

Marlus is *the* pupil of Jung whose name will be attached to Jungian psychology.

—BARBARA HANNAH

Without you [Marie-Louise] I would have never pulled through that ghastly darkness in order to accomplish what I had to accomplish in my life. It was your books and your insights and your personal help which put me over the top. Whatever failures you feel you have suffered in your life, you have succeeded with me. You spoke to me and it made a tremendous difference. It made the difference between life and death.

—AN ANALYSAND

Marie-Louise von Franz is the closest spiritual heir to Jung. She has brought about the flowering of his thought, and it is she who has most creatively understood his point of view and used it in her therapy and her books. In a personal and utterly individual way, von Franz has brought out the quintessence of Jung's work.

—MOLLY TUBY, Jungian analyst

In *Psychological Perspectives: A Journal of Global Consciousness Integrating Psyche, Soul and Nature,* no. 24, Spring-Summer 1991 (C. G. Jung Institute of Los Angeles), p. 54.

With the death of Marie-Louise von Franz, Jungian psychology has lost its greatest creative thinker.

—ROBIN ROBERTSON

"A Guide to the Writings of Marie-Louise von Franz," in *Psychological Perspectives: A Journal of Global Consciousness Integrating Psyche, Soul and Nature,* no. 38, Winter 1998–1999 (C. G. Jung Institute of Los Angeles), p. 70.

She was a woman with a brilliant spirit.

—FELIX LEYER

Neue Zürcher Zeitung, March 13, 1998, p. 78.

She was such a unique personality for all of us.

—ETHEL VOGELSANG, Jungian analyst

. . . . the brilliance of her mind, her deep and passionate attention to the unconscious, her clarity in putting forth her ideas, and her devotion to the writings of Jung. . . .

—JAMES KIRSCH

The Jungians: A Comparative and Historical Perspective (London: Routledge, 2000), p. 11.

At the center of my analytical work is the influence of Dr. von Franz. During my years in Zürich, I attended all her lectures, ingested her books . . . and occasionally worked with her privately.

—MARION WOODMAN

"A Legacy of Dr. Marie-Louise von Franz," in *Jung on the Hudson Seminar Series* (New York: Rhinebeck and Historic Kingston, 1999).

. . . . A brilliant scholar and analytical psychologist.

—DENNIS STILLINGS

"The Archetype of Apokatastasis," in *Artifex*, vol. 8, no. 2/3 (Summer/Fall 1980).

Dr. Marie-Louise von Franz [is] one of the giants in the field of analytical psychology. In all likelihood, no other Jungian analyst or author has contributed as much to explaining and expanding upon Jung's ideas as Dr. von Franz. Long acknowledged as Jung's leading student, her original approach to understanding the psyche has had a wide-ranging impact. Indeed, she has influenced such diverse disciplines as psychotherapy, physics, philosophy, theology, anthropology, and, of course, the areas she had been most widely acclaimed for: the interpretation and understanding of dreams, fairy tales, and myths.

Dr. von Franz's ideas influenced more people than any other Jungian of her generation. She took Jung's concept of the objective psyche and revealed its dynamic involvement in producing myths, fairy tales, and dreams. She was a brilliant exponent of the art of amplification which establishes the cultural and archetypal context of one's personal mythology.

"Jung on the Hudson," Seminar Series of the New York Center for Jungian Studies. In honor of Marie-Louise von Franz, this two-week seminar series was organized in 1999 and attended by a distinguished and international faculty which shared "ideas that had grown from their association with von Franz and/or her work as well as their personal reminiscences of shared moments with this special woman." The topic of the first week was "The Objective Psyche: The Wisdom of the Unconscious." The topic of the second week was "Archetypes and Mystic Patterns in the Family."

Marie-Louise von Franz first met C. G. Jung [in 1934] when she was [seventeen] years old. She went into analysis with him soon thereafter. . . . A classics teacher in school, von Franz paid for her analysis by translating Greek and Latin alchemical texts for Jung. In her late thirties, she became an analyst herself and began her lifelong work of exploring and expanding Jung's ideas. Recognized as one of the few who was Jung's peer in intellectual thought, von Franz was asked by Jung in his later years to carry out a task he cherished but could no longer execute: an exhaustive investigation of the archetypal significance of number. The result [was] *Number and Time,* a scholarly and brilliant book that integrates material from the divergent fields of mathematics, the natural sciences, ethnology, archaeology, psychology, and mythology.

Dr. von Franz has authored and co-authored numerous other volumes, each of which illuminates a particular facet of the psyche in both its personal and archetypal expressions."

—CHARLENE SIEG

Foreword to "Love, War and Transformation: An Interview with Marie-Louise von Franz," in *Psychological Perspectives: A Journal of Global Consciousness Integrating Psyche, Soul and Nature,* no. 24 (Spring-Summer 1991).

I cherish an intensive encounter with von Franz as memory, and the lifelong challenge from her book, *Number and Time,* still lies ahead of me.

—URSULA SEZGIN

The lectures of Dr. von Franz were brilliant and inspiring. I will never forget the first time I heard Dr. von Franz lecture (on the *puer aeternus*). It was a numinous experience. I thought God was speaking. She seemed to know everything. Never in my previous academic training had I heard such far-reaching and profound reflections. When I told this to my analyst the next day, he only smiled.

—MURRAY STEIN

Marie-Louise von Franz is a witch. When I read her book, *Puer Aeternus,* I feel she writes about *me*!

—AN ANALYSAND

She has been an important person in my life. She was my second mother. By writing *Number and Time,* she saved my life. The book helped me to survive the clash between physics and psychology in my interior life.

—HERBERT VAN ERKELENS

There are writings which are perfect but they don't touch me. When I read von Franz, it is as if something invisible lies between the lines and behind the words which touches me. This "invisible something" is what I understand as eros.

—VRENI SUTER

PART FIVE

Book Reviews and Publishers' Comments

Alchemy: An Introduction to the Symbolism and the Psychology

Alchemical texts are notoriously cryptic, virtually a secret language. In trying to understand them, one risks falling into what the practitioners themselves called "the madness of the lead." Jung's writings on alchemy are very perceptive, but many find them almost as difficult to follow as the texts he so diligently deciphers.

Enter Marie-Louise von Franz, Jung's longtime friend and co-worker, with her remarkable gift for translating esoteric symbolic material into everyday psychological reality. In 1959 she designed a series of nine lectures as an introduction to Jung's more detailed studies, and presented them to students at the Jung Institute in Zürich. . . .

Inner City Books has attractively packaged von Franz's brilliant, lucid lectures. They make fascinating reading. . . . In a lively and stimulating manner, von Franz traces the development of alchemical symbolism from one of the oldest known sources. . . .

On the way, von Franz sprinkles her discourse with her distinctive flair for what Jung called symbolic thinking and she herself describes as "listening to what the symbol itself has to say." It is a non-linear, right brain kind of thinking, an approach that immediately and satisfyingly reveals the psychological meaning of alchemical procedures that are otherwise virtually incomprehensible.

The images and motifs that so occupied the alchemists constantly crop up in the dreams and drawings of modern individuals. Those involved with their own psychological development are, in effect, alchemists, and this book is a practical guide to what is going on in the laboratory of the unconscious.

"Jung at Heart: Studies in Jungian Psychology by Jungian Analysts," *Spring*, no. 28, (Toronto: Inner City Books, 1998), p. 2.

Alchemy: An Introduction to the Symbolism and the Psychology

FROM THE BACK COVER:

It was the genius of C. G. Jung to discover in the "holy technique" of alchemy a parallel to the psychological individuation process. This book, by Jung's long-time friend and co-worker, completely demystifies the subject.

Designed as an introduction to Jung's more detailed studies, and profusely illustrated, here is a lucid and practical account of what the alchemists were really looking for—emotional balance and wholeness.

Once again, Marie-Louise von Franz demonstrates her remarkable gift for translating esoteric symbolic material into everyday experience. For the images and motifs that so occupied the alchemists were of an archetypal nature, and as such, they constantly turn up in modern dreams and drawings.

This is an important book, invaluable for an understanding of dreams and indispensable for anyone interested in relationships and communication between the sexes.

"The secret art of alchemy lay in the transformation of the personality. . . . Anyone involved with his or her own psychological development is an alchemist, and this book is first and foremost a practical guide to what is going on in the laboratory of the unconscious. I highly recommend it. . . ."

—DR. C. CONWAY SMITH, psychiatrist

Animus and Anima in Fairy Tales

Animus and Anima in Fairy Tales is, delightfully, the one hundredth title of Inner City Books. It is a diverse collection of tales, brilliantly commented upon by the late Marie-Louise von Franz (Inner City's Honorary Patron) and richly educational for those interested in learning more about Jungian psychology. It is also yet another sparkling gift from this magnificent twentieth-century literary scholar and Jungian analyst who continues to benefit others even after her death.

Reviewed by Eleanor Cowan in *The Montreal Jung Society Newsletter*, October 2002.

Archetypal Patterns in Fairy Tales

This delightful book is based on a series of lectures given in 1974 at the C. G. Jung Institute in Zürich. In her preface, von Franz states that she wanted to present stories from a variety of cultures rather than choosing a specific theme to focus on, as she had done in her previous books on fairy tales. She wanted to do this in order to demonstrate how Jung's method of interpreting archetypal fantasy material could be applied to all fairy tales, since they too relate to archetypal material.

This book is vintage von Franz. If you enjoy her writing, run, don't walk, to your nearest Jungian bookstore and buy it. Sit in your favorite armchair, perhaps by a cozy fire, savor and enjoy.

Perhaps what is so pleasurable about this book compared to some of von Franz's other writings is that it is based quite closely on lecture material; consequently the style is less dense and definitely easier to follow than her more academic studies. . . . As a result, her vivacious personality really shines through.

Here is the revered teacher chiding her students for mistakenly assuming that a fairy-tale character can automatically be interpreted as an ego—when that character is clearly an archetypal image—and then chiding herself for doing the same: "Now you see what a dirty trick I've played! I've slipped into treating the young man as if he were a conscious human being who is sharing what he has with the spirit. But that's not true, because the young man is an archetypal image, and the old man who represents the spirit is an archetypal image too. That's where students, in interpreting fairy tales, always 'slip off.' And now I've done it myself—consciously, because I noticed it, but I thought: 'I'll just carry on to show you how one slips off.'"

Von Franz more than makes up [in so many ways for stereotyping a few cultures], especially by her genius in amplifying the various elements of the stories. For instance who else can so clearly explain the difference between trolls (brutish nature figures), wizards (dark fathers, black magic figures), and ogres (generally evil beings that have a devouring quality like the unconscious complex); and differentiate between priests (preservers of rituals), shamans (soul specialists dealing with possession, and ensuring that souls find their proper place after death), and medicine men (who do the same as shamans, but don't have to put themselves into an ecstatic trance, since they have a natural access to the Beyond)?

And who else but Marie-Louise von Franz can take a simple little story about a piece of straw, a piece of coal, and a bean, all escaping from a woman's cooking pot, and through it teach us the essential wisdom of how to individuate?

Mary Harsany, "Vintage von Franz Demystifies Fairy Tales," in *Jung at Heart,* no. 31, Fall (Toronto: Inner City Books, 1999), p. 3.

Archetypal Patterns in Fairy Tales

FROM THE AUTHOR'S PREFACE:

"This book is a collection of fairy-tale interpretations I presented in a series of lectures at the C. G. Jung Institute in Zürich. I did not want to focus on a specific theme but rather to wander through many countries and types of fairy tales. I chose some that challenged me because they were unusual. I wanted to show both their diversity and their underlying similarities so that one could appreciate what is nationally or racially specific and what is common to all civilizations and all human beings. I wanted to show how Jung's method of interpreting archetypal fantasy material could be applied to these diverse tales."

Archetypal Patterns in Fairy Tales is the first new volume of Dr. von Franz's legendary Zürich lectures to be published since 1980. There are in-depth studies of six fairy tales—from Denmark, Spain, China, France and Africa, and one from the Grimm's collection—with references to parallel themes in many others. Featuring the symbolic, nonlinear approach she is famous for, it offers unique insights into cross-cultural motifs, as well as being an invaluable resource for understanding dream images.

"Dr. von Franz has the rare ability to ground her psychological theories and insights in practical examples from everyday life. This makes her work equally accessible to both the general reader and the professional."

—FRASER BOA, director of *The Way of the Dream*

Aurora Consurgens

Originally published in 1966 as a companion volume to C. G. Jung's *Mysterium Coniunctionis,* this scholarly gem is scattered throughout with insights relevant to the psychological process of individuation. *Aurora Consurgens* is a rare medieval alchemical treatise reputed to be the last work of St. Thomas Aquinas which was rediscovered by C. G. Jung in the course of his researches. It bears out Jung's long-standing view that the traditional practice of alchemy is best understood symbolically as an attempt to express conscious psychic contents through their projection onto matter. The analysis of *Aurora Consurgens* by Marie-Louise von Franz suggests that its author experienced a breakthrough of the unconscious while in an ecstatic state shortly before his death. History records that Thomas Aquinas died in a trance soon after expounding the Song of Songs, and *Aurora* ends with a paraphrase of the same biblical verses and a vision of the mystic marriage. Von Franz's penetrating commentary shows how Jung's analytical psychology may be used as a key to unlock the meaning of this cryptic but psychologically significant text.

C. G. Jung: His Myth in Our Time

EXCERPTS:

Each individual's life follows a pattern which, from the point of view of analytical psychology, represents the "myth" or archetypal outline of the inner and outer events of one's own biography. *His Myth in Our Time* refers to such a pattern in the life of C. G. Jung.

For most of us, however, the patterns of the myths we experience are limited to our immediate environments. Yet there are a few in each century who live lives of such wide-ranging, long-lasting effects that they serve as creative influences, not only within their own social and professional circles, but throughout a broad spectrum of fields of human endeavor.

Such a man was C. G. Jung. The effects of his life and work have profoundly influenced such varied disciplines as anthropology, atomic physics, ethnology, theology, and parapsychology, as well as his own fields of psychology and psychotherapy. Marie-Louise von Franz's study of Jung has as its theme the myth of Jung's life in the context of the twentieth century.

Jung was the first modern scientist to take seriously the reality of the unconscious *and* to remain in dialogue with it throughout his life. Since dreams are one of the primary means by which contact is made with the unconscious, he paid scrupulous attention to his dreams and to what they had to communicate concerning his personal development and the development of the collective life of his day.

Dr. von Franz, who worked closely with Jung for over twenty-five years, traces the development of basic Jungian concepts such as the collective unconscious, the archetypes, the psychological types, active imagination, the creative instinct and the process of individuation from their origins in specific dreams which Jung had throughout his life to their eventual empirical documentation in the voluminous books and papers he published over a period of sixty-five years. In this respect, *C. G. Jung: His Myth in Our Time* is a unique document, a portrait which relates inner and outer events to the development of the individual, both on the personal level of C. G. Jung the man, and on the more universal level, C. G. Jung, the twentieth-century prophet.

For Jung was one of those individuals whose sensitivity to the collective unconscious gave him dramatic insights into the problems of his time. His psychology is an attempt to order and give perspective to those problems and to indicate the measures which we must be prepared to take if we are to avoid the psychic dangers of our century.

This is not an academic biography of Jung, nor is it a primer of Jungian thought. Rather, it is a daring innovation in the literature of psychology: a history of the growth and development of one man's creative powers during a lifetime of dialogue with the unconscious—a dialogue from which emerges the "myth" of a great man in our time.

Dreams

These collected essays by the distinguished analyst and author Marie-Louise von Franz offer fascinating insights into the study of dreams, not only psychologically, but also from historical, religious, and philosophical points of view. In the first two chapters, the author offers general explanations of the nature of dreams and their use in analysis. In the first, she addresses the question of the development of self-knowledge. The second chapter describes the way in which C. G. Jung concerned himself with dreams and points out fateful ways in which they were entwined with the course of his life.

In the second part of this book, dreams of historical personages are recorded and interpreted: Socrates; Themistocles and Hannibal; Monica, the mother of Saint Augustine; the mothers of Saint Bernard of Clairvaux and Saint Dominic; and René Descartes. . . .

FROM THE BACK COVER:

Marie-Louise von Franz analyses these and other dreams of historical figures, illuminating the principles of Jungian dream interpretation and providing insights into the unique lives and destinies of these famous dreamers.

On Divination and Synchronicity

Marie-Louise von Franz, acknowledged authority on the psychological interpretation of fairy tales, dreams, myths, and alchemy, turns her attention in this book to the meaning of the irrational.

While conducting a comparative historical analysis of number theory in the East and West, von Franz uncovers the major patterns and archetypes which motivate and dominate Eastern and Western modes of scientific thought. She shows that Western scientists may for some time have been under the influence of an archetype—that of the divine gambler—which, she says, "is what makes people believe things that are not true."

Her comparison of various "magical" approaches with the generally accepted scientific method is particularly illuminating. Western science would throw out the single case (as when one unexpected deviation causes a researcher to fudge the data in order to prove a point about repeatability). Divination, on the other hand, is comfortable with the unique reality of any event. A particular throw of the I Ching, for example, has its effect according to one's psychic state at that very moment. No two divinatory events are alike, yet each one is equally valid.

Von Franz explores a wide range of topics in these fascinating lectures, concluding with an examination of the mandalic unity of inner and outer reality. She shows convincingly that number theories spring from the same unconscious sources that create religions and are influenced by similar presumptions and experience. Probability itself, the region in which we realize "fate," is seen as a vast playing field for human consciousness.

On Divination and Synchronicity is altogether intellectually exciting and emotionally satisfying. . . . Its scholarship mediated by its clarity of style.

FROM THE BACK COVER:

> This is a short book, but one with a big range, its scholarship mediated by its clarity of style. A fine introduction to the subject, as we would expect from this author.

—MARY WILLIAMS, *The Journal of Analytical Psychology*

> Highly recommended to anyone interested in Jung's thought and its responsible elaboration by one of his close collaborators.

—JAMES A. HALL, psychiatrist and Jungian analyst,
author of *Clinical Uses of Dreams*

> Dr. von Franz, more than any other author in the field, has the rare ability to ground her psychological theories and insights in practical examples from everyday life. This makes her work equally accessible to both the layman and the professional therapist.

—FRASER BOA, Jungian analyst

"On Meaningful Chance: A Review of Marie-Louise von Franz's *On Divination and Synchronicity: The Psychology of Meaningful Chance*," in *Jung at Heart,* no. 34, Winter/Spring (Toronto: Inner City Books, 2001), p. 5.

On Dreams and Death

Our dreams of death prepare us for a profound transformation and for a continuation of the life process which is unimaginable to everyday consciousness.

In this classic work of Jungian theory, reprinted with a new foreword by Emmanuel Kennedy-Xypolitas, Marie-Louise von Franz breaks completely new ground in the investigation of death and the unconscious.

Examining numerous case studies of actual death dreams, von Franz relates these to persistent themes in cultures from ancient Egypt to contemporary Europe, casting all our assumptions about death, life, and a possible afterlife in a surprising new light.

> "What is there in the end but dying? Our dying will not be a simple process; what do the dreams of the dying say about this process? Do we know what will happen? After death, the earthly soul descends and wanders away toward the West, and the diamond soul ascends and wanders to the East? Marie-Louise von Franz gives hints about the traveler we will each become. A precious book."
>
> —ROBERT BLY, author of *Sibling Society*

"*On Dreams and Death* is a fantastic book, full of the wisdom and insight which only a Jungian like Marie-Louise von Franz can write. It gives one a deeper respect for our inner knowledge, for the deep significance of dreams, and last but not least, for ancient and present customs whose origin we have long forgotten."

—ELISABETH KÜBLER-ROSS,
author of *Living with Death and Dying*

"*On Dreams and Death* is a rare and precious jewel, one of the very greatest books that our century has produced. I have re-read it many times, and each time I have thought: 'My God, I have never really read this book before.' Von Franz takes an entirely new approach to the questions of death, a possible life after death, and how these relate to the meaning of an individual life."

—THEO ABT

Projection and Recollection in Jungian Psychology

Projection and Recollection in Jungian Psychology: Reflections of the Soul, by Marie-Louise von Franz, is a brilliant delineation of the objective psyche and how it has been experienced through the ages—from primitive religion to nuclear physics and synchronicity. It is Jungian psychology at its finest.

—EDWARD F. EDINGER, M.D., author of *Ego and Archetype*

Dr. von Franz's new book sets an inspired standard for new works in the spirit of C. G. Jung. In these days, when the insights of modern physics and depth psychology begin to converge, this book and others to be presented in the "Reality of the Psyche" series will illuminate the way towards individuation in the context of an undivided universe.

—JUNE K. SINGER, PH.D.,
author of *Boundaries of the Soul* and
Androgyny: Toward a New Theory of Sexuality

Marie-Louise von Franz's important book is a comprehensive study of projection with far-reaching implications. Marie-Louise von Franz has extended Jung's research and concepts of projection in her own original and penetrating way. Some of the chapter headings may hint at the depth of this study: Projection and Scientific Hypothesis, The Hypothesis of the Collective Unconscious, The Evil Demons, The Great Mediating Daimons, The Inner Companion, Consciousness and Inner Wholeness.

—JAMES KIRSCH, M.D.,
author of *The Religious Aspect of the Unconscious*
and *Shakespeare's Royal Self*

Shadow and Evil in Fairy Tales

FROM THE BACK COVER:

In this book, Marie-Louise von Franz uncovers some of the important lessons concealed in tales from around the world, drawing on the wealth of her knowledge of folklore, her experience as a psychoanalyst and a collaborator with Jung, and her great personal wisdom.

The Cat: A Tale of Feminine Redemption

This small volume is an amazing gem containing an exciting, penetrating, and crystalline view of the very difficult psychic work that is required in developing the inner feminine. . . . Based on a lecture series given at the Jung Institute in Zürich, the writing flows in an easy, straightforward manner, as if von Franz were chatting with us about this quite challenging theme. . . . Von Franz presents this material in the most engaging manner. Her writing is light, clear and lyrical, continually drawing from the myth to illuminate the mystery of the redemption of the feminine. On one level, this little volume is easily read, yet on another level it is teeming with von Franz's extraordinarily deep insights into the archetypal workings of the unconscious. It is quite a nourishing meal—an amazing gift von Franz left behind for us, a book to read and re-read.

FROM INNER CITY BOOKS COMPLETE CATALOGUE, SPRING 1999:

[The fairy tale] is patiently dissected by von Franz with her characteristic erudition and earthy humor. . . . This is von Franz at her very best, theoretically lucid, sharply insightful and always grounded in lived experience.

Reviewed by Ann Walker in *Psychological Perspectives: A Journal of Global Consciousness Integrating Psyche, Soul and Nature,* no. 40 (2000), and reprinted in *Jung at Heart,* no. 38, Winter-Spring (Toronto: Inner City Books, 2003).

The Feminine in Fairy Tales

FROM THE BACK COVER:

In this engaging commentary, the distinguished analyst and author Marie-Louise von Franz shows how the Feminine reveals itself in fairy tales of German, Russian, Scandinavian, and Eskimo origin, including familiar stories such as "Sleeping Beauty," "Snow White and Rose Red," and "Rumpelstiltskin." Some tales, she points out, offer insights into the psychology of women, while others reflect problems and characteristics of the anima, the inner femininity of men. Dr. von Franz discusses the archetypes and symbolic themes that appear in fairy tales as well as dreams and fantasies, draws practical advice from the tales, and demonstrates its application in case studies from her analytical practice.

The Golden Ass of Apuleius

FROM THE BACK COVER:

"Today there is much discussion of the liberation of women," writes Marie-Louise von Franz, "but it is sometimes overlooked that this can only succeed if there is a change in men as well. Just as women have to overcome the patriarchal tyrant in their own souls, men have to liberate and differentiate their inner femininity. Only then will a better relationship of the sexes be possible." It is this timely theme that Dr. von Franz explores in her psychological study of a classic work of the second century, *The Golden Ass* by Apuleius of Madaura. The novel recounts the adventures of a young Roman who is transformed into an ass and eventually finds spiritual renewal through initiation in the Isis mysteries. With its many tales within a tale (including the celebrated story of Psyche and Eros), the text as interpreted by Dr. von Franz is a rich source of insights, anecdotes, and scholarly amplification.

The Grail Legend

The Grail, and the events involved in the search for it, is one of the most powerful symbolisms operating in contemporary man. It represents the quest for the supreme value which makes life meaningful, and it is modern man's special need to find meaning in a world where most conventional values have all but disintegrated.

The Grail legend is as psychologically rich and involved as its history. A product of the Middle Ages in both Britain and continental Europe, the legend of a vessel, or stone, which both nourishes and heals, reaches back into unrecorded Celtic and Eastern origins. Later it became associated with the stories of King Arthur, his court and his knights, and with the legends of Joseph of Arimathea and the eucharistic vessel.

Emma Jung, wife of C. G. Jung, worked for thirty years on this study of the deep-seated unconscious psychic processes which had kept the legend alive through the centuries. After her death in 1955, the project was completed by Marie-Louise von Franz, one of Dr. Jung's most creative followers.

Using the Chrétien version as a point of departure, the authors trace the principal events of the legend in all of their individual psychological implications. Perceval's relations to his shadow personality (the Red Knight), to his anima (the maiden Blancheflor and the Queen of the

Castle of Damsels among others), and to the archetype of the Old Wise Man (the hermit Gornemanz) are representative of the personal aspects. On the collective level, it is the symbol of the Grail itself which is richest and most rewarding.

The last chapters introduce the problem of the Trinity and the missing Fourth, and the relation of this problem to the question of evil, its meaning and its possible resolution. Merlin, the necromancer from Arthur's court, is particularly relevant to this aspect of the legend, and some of the most original and thought-provoking material in the volume centers around Merlin and his relations to the Grail, to the Trinity, and to the disappearance of the Grail from the psychic life of medieval man.

That the legend persists through the centuries in the unconscious of the west suggests that it still embodies a living myth. What Mrs. Jung and Dr. von Franz have to say about the meaning of this myth for us today constitutes the heart and relevance of this study of the psychological significance of the Grail legend.

The Interpretation of Fairy Tales

FROM THE BACK COVER:

Of the various types of mythological literature, fairy tales are the simplest and purest expressions of the collective unconscious and thus offer the clearest understanding of the basic patterns of the human psyche. Every people or nation has its own way of experiencing this psychic reality, and so a study of the world's fairy tales yields a wealth of insights into the archetypal experiences of humankind.

Perhaps the foremost authority on the psychological interpretation of fairy tales is Marie-Louise von Franz. In this book—originally published as *An Introduction to the Interpretation of Fairy Tales*—she describes the steps involved in analyzing tales and illustrates them with a variety of European tales from "Beauty and the Beast" to "The Robber Bridegroom."

Dr. von Franz begins with a history of the study of fairy tales and the various theories of interpretation. By way of illustration she presents a detailed examination of a simple Grimm's tale, "The Three Feathers," followed by a comprehensive discussion of motifs related to Jung's concept of the shadow, the anima, and the animus.

The Problem of the Puer Aeternus

EXCERPT FROM THE TEXT:

Puer Aeternus is the name of a god of antiquity. The words themselves come from Ovid's *Metamorphoses* and are there applied to the child-god in the Eleusinian mysteries. Ovid speaks of the child-god Iacchus, addressing him as *puer aeternus* and praising him in his role in these mysteries. In later times, the child-god was identified with Dionysus and the god Eros. He is the divine youth who is born in the night in this typical mother-cult mystery in Eleusis and who is a kind of redeemer.

The title *puer aeternus* therefore means eternal youth, but we also use it sometimes to indicate a certain type of man who has an outstanding mother complex and who therefore behaves in certain typical ways which may be characterized as follows.

In general, the man who is identified with the archetype of the *puer aeternus* remains too long in adolescent psychology; that is, all those characteristics that are normal in a youth of seventeen or eighteen are continued into later life, coupled in most cases with too great a dependence on the mother.

Generally great difficulty is experienced in adaptation to the social situation and, in some cases, there is a kind of false individualism, namely that, being something special, one has no need to adapt, for that would be impossible for such a hidden genius, and so on. In addition there is an arrogant attitude toward other people due to both an inferiority complex and false feelings of superiority.

Such people also usually have great difficulty in finding the right kind of job, for whatever they find is never quite right or quite what they wanted. There is always "a hair in the soup." The woman too is never quite the right one; she is nice as a girlfriend, but. . . . There is always a "but" which prevents marriage or any kind of definite commitment.

This all leads to a form of neurosis which has been described as the "provisional life," that is, the strange attitude and feeling that one is not yet in real life. For the time being one is doing this or that, but whether it is a woman or a job, it is not yet what is really wanted, and there is always the fantasy that sometime in the future the real thing will come about. If this attitude is prolonged, it means a constant inner refusal to commit oneself to the moment. With this there is often, to a smaller or greater extent, a savior complex, with the secret thought that one day one will be able to save the world; the last word in philosophy, or religion, or politics, or art, or something else, will be found.

The one thing dreaded throughout by the typical *puer aeternus* is to be bound to anything whatever. There is a terrific fear of being pinned down, of entering space and time completely, and of being the unique human being that one is. There is always the fear of being caught in a situation from which it may be impossible to slip out again. Every just-so situation is hell. At the same time, there is something highly symbolic—namely, a fascination for dangerous sports, particularly flying and mountaineering—so as to get as high as possible, the symbolism being to get away from the earth, from ordinary life.

In general, the positive quality of such men is a certain kind of spirituality which comes from a relatively close contact with the unconscious. Many have the charm of youth and the stirring quality of a drink of champagne. *Puer aeterni* are generally very agreeable to talk to; they usually have interesting things to talk about and have an invigorating effect upon one; they do not like conventional situations; they ask deep questions and go straight for the truth; usually they are searching for genuine religion, a search that is typical for people in their late teens.

FROM THE BACK COVER:

It is impossible to overstate the influence on both men and women of this classic study, originally a series of lectures at the Zürich Jung Institute. It is Jungian psychology in its more down-to-earth voice, telling it like it is so accurately and with such a depth of understanding that it is still much in demand even though it has been out of print for many years. This new edition features a bibliography and an extensive index.

Reviewed in *Jung at Heart,* no. 32, Spring (Toronto: Inner City Books, 2000).

The Psychological Meaning of Redemption Motifs in Fairy Tales

The great lesson fairy tales teach us is that things are not what they seem.

In dealing with fairy-tale themes, as in exploring the meaning of archetypal motifs in general, the broader the working knowledge of the field the better. Much of the significance of the material, as well as much of the necessary corrective on interpretations, can only emerge out of comparative study, and Dr. von Franz's knowledge of fairy-tale variants is unmatched.

Here she takes the redemption motif—the emergence of the fully human in ourselves and others—as the theme to be illustrated and amplified by a wealth of fairy-tale material: some tales almost fully retold, others used in fragments for comparison and interpretation. The result is a complex but flowing account of the problems of psychological redemption in therapy, illuminated by those extraordinary transformations that are at the very heart of fairy tales.

This is preeminently a practical book on dealing with complexes, for it helps us to understand that the guise in which the unconscious confronts us reflects the whole attitude of consciousness, including the *Weltanschauung* we unconsciously accept.

FROM THE BACK COVER:

Why are we often at odds with ourselves? What lies behind our conflicts and relationship problems? Have they any purpose? This book, originally a series of lectures at the C. G. Jung Institute in Zürich, explores these issues and many others. It is unique in its demonstration of the significance of fairy tales for an understanding of the process of psychological growth, especially in terms of integrating animal nature with human nature.

Readers familiar with Dr. von Franz's earthy appreciation of psychic reality will find here another gem. Her symbolic, nonlinear approach to the meaning of typical fairy-tale motifs (that also appear in dreams—bathing, beating, dismemberment, animals, clothes, etc.) and her clear description of complexes, projection, active imagination, and archetypes combine to make this a modern classic.

Reviewed by David L. Hart in *Jung at Heart,* no. 10, Fall (Toronto: Inner City Books, 1991).

PART SIX

Some Biographic Data

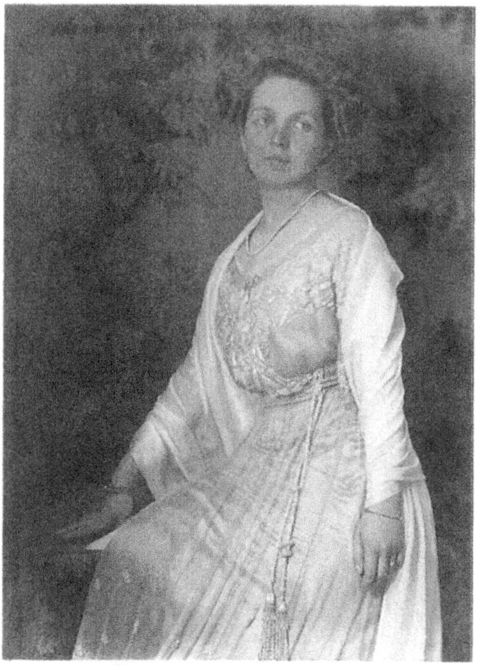

Figure 1. Margret Susanne (née Schoen) von Franz, mother of Marie-Louise von Franz. Courtesy of Marie-Anne von Franz.

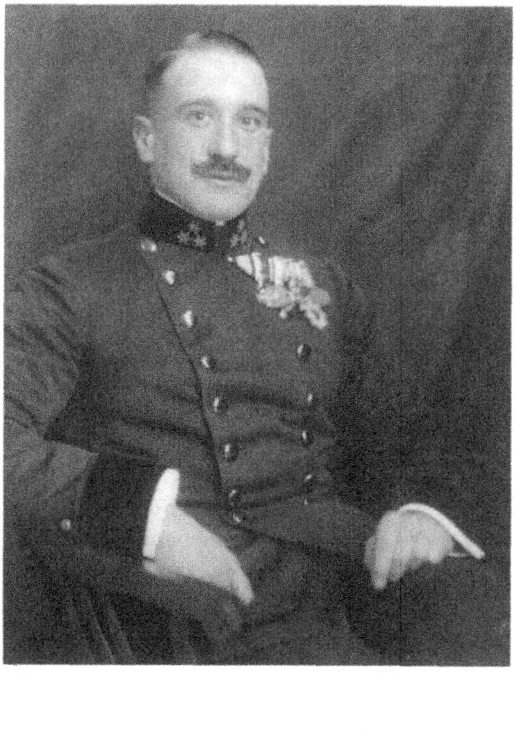

Figure 2. Baron Erwin Gottfried von Franz, father of Marie-Louise von Franz. Courtesy of Marie-Anne von Franz.

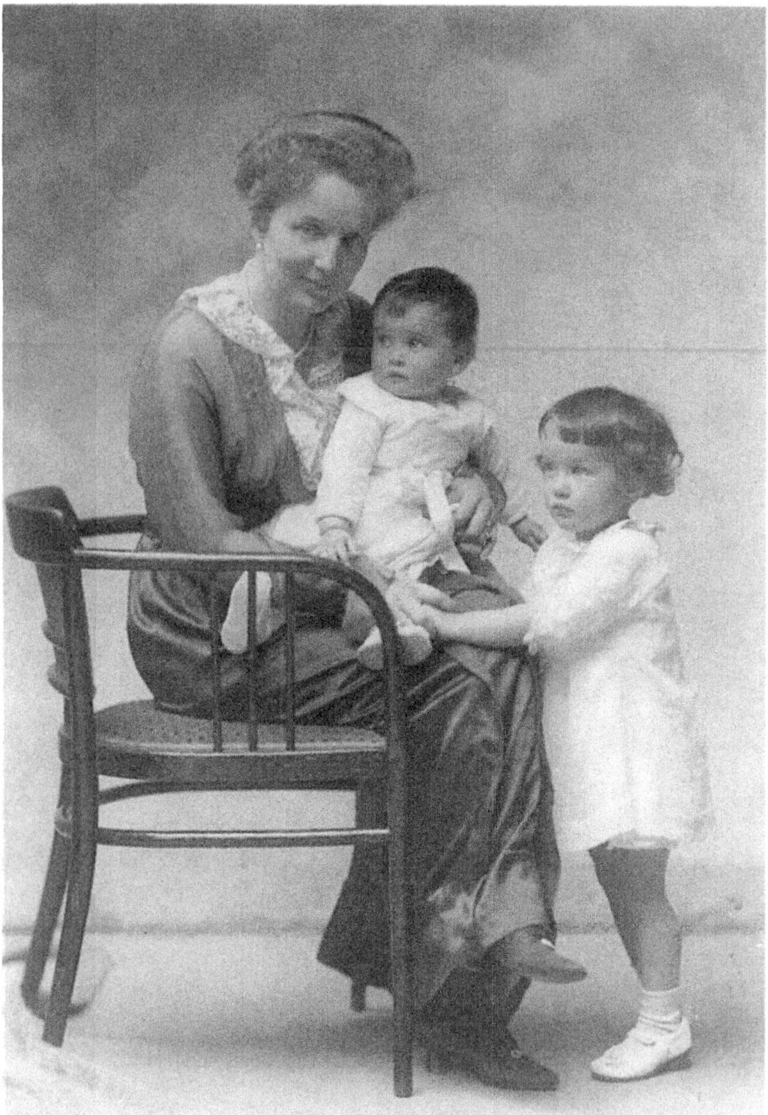

Figure 3. Marie-Louise von Franz with her mother and Marie-Anne (standing). Courtesy of Marie-Anne von Franz.

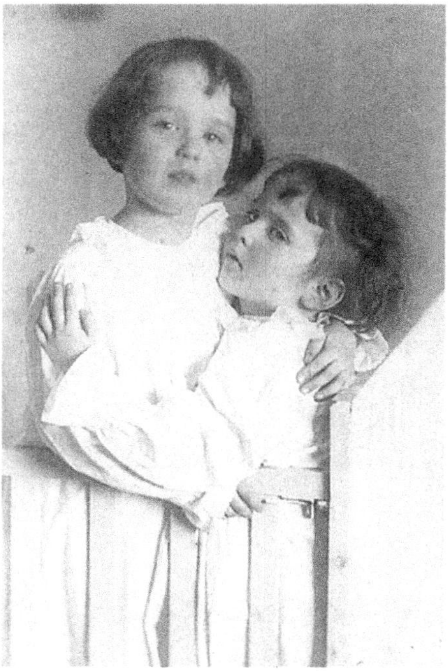

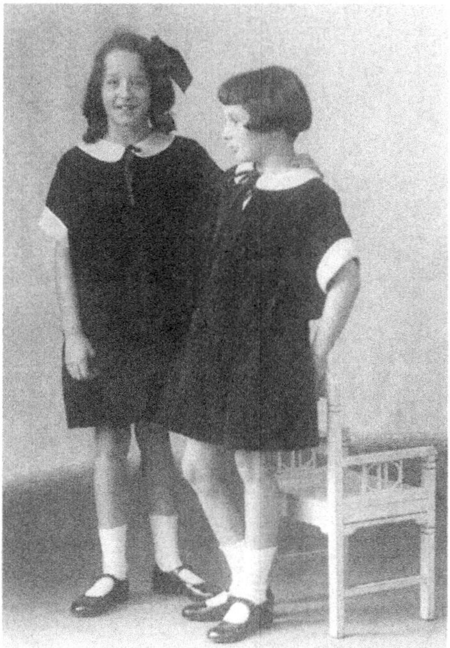

Figures 4 and 5. Marie-Louise von Franz with her sister (left). Courtesy of Marie-Anne von Franz.

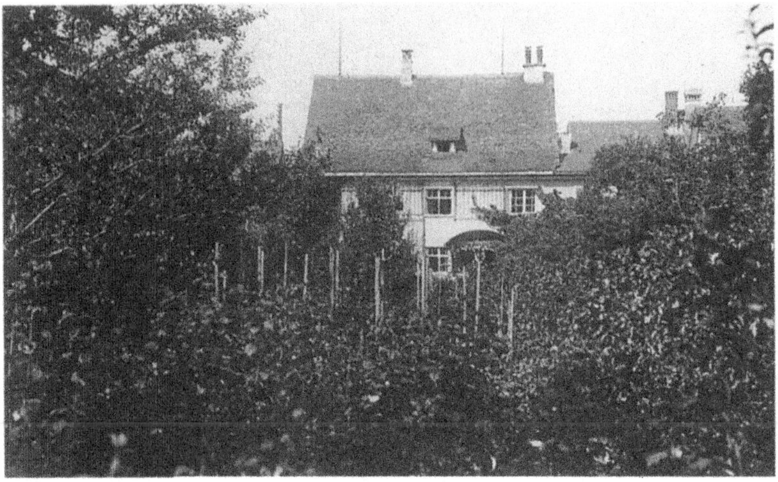

Figure 6. The house and garden at Rheineck. Courtesy of Marie-Anne von Franz.

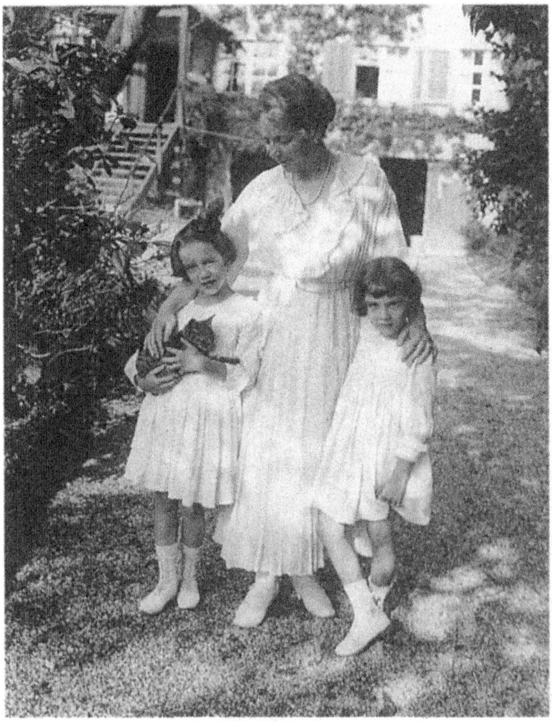

Figure 7. Marie-Anne (left) and Marie-Louise with their mother in Rheineck. Courtesy of Marie-Anne von Franz.

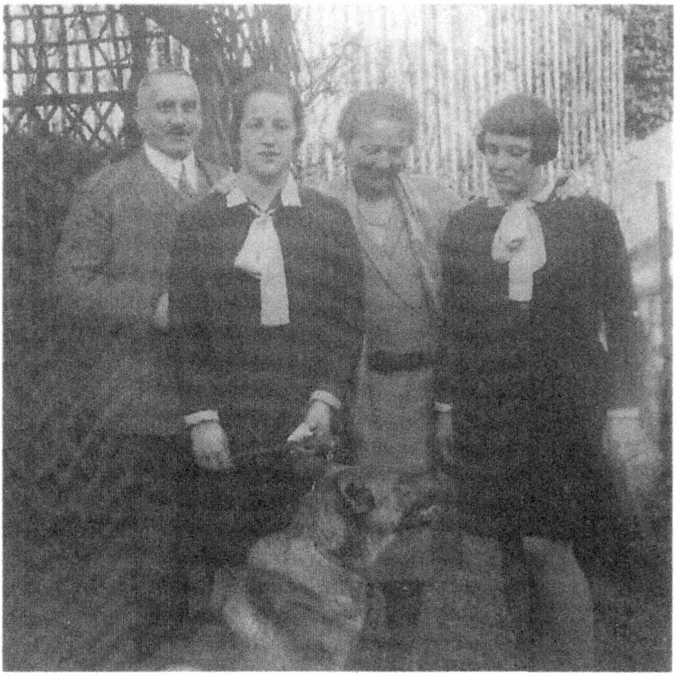

Figure 8. The von Franz family in Rheineck, ca. 1928. Courtesy of Marie-Anne von Franz.

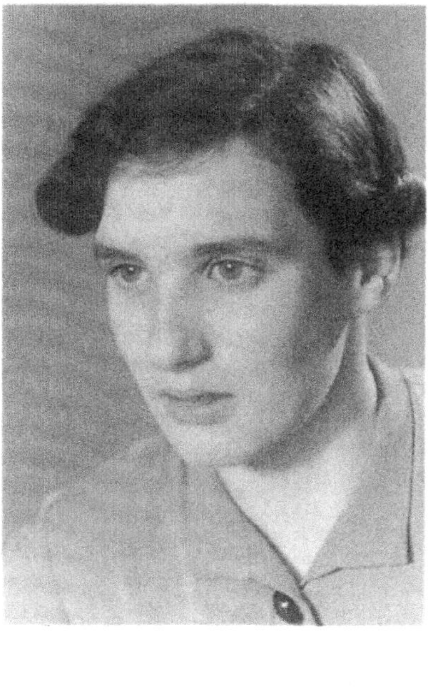

Figure 9. Marie-Louise von Franz. Courtesy of Marie-Anne von Franz.

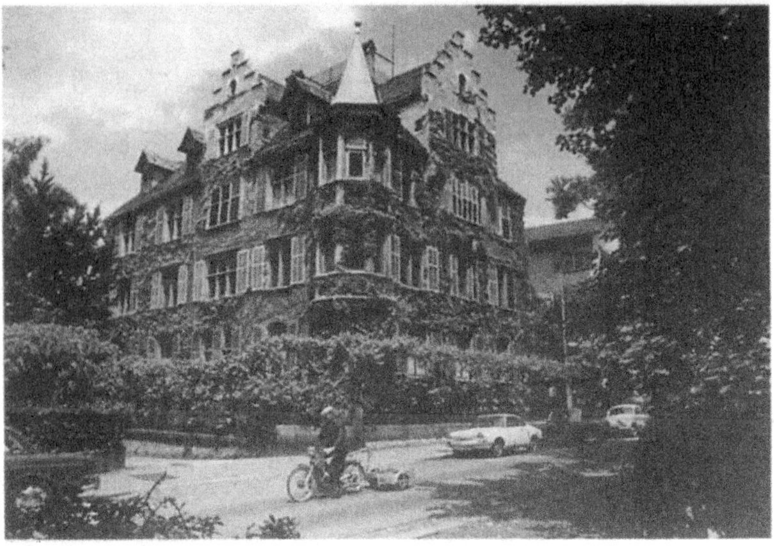

Figure 10. The Psychological Club of Zürich. Photo © Robert Hinshaw, 1971. Reproduced by permission of the photographer.

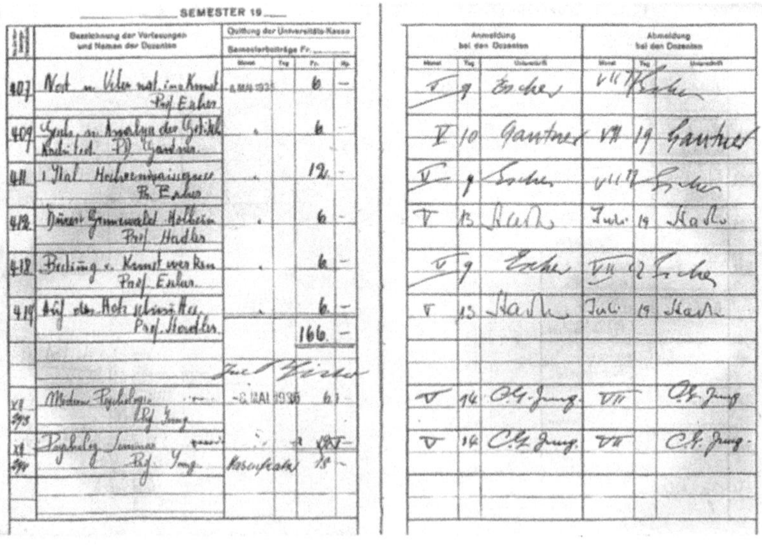

Figure 11. Marie-Louise von Franz's transcript, including courses she took in May 1935 at the E.T.H. (Eidgenossische Technische Hochschule, Zürich, or Swiss Federal Institute of Technology).

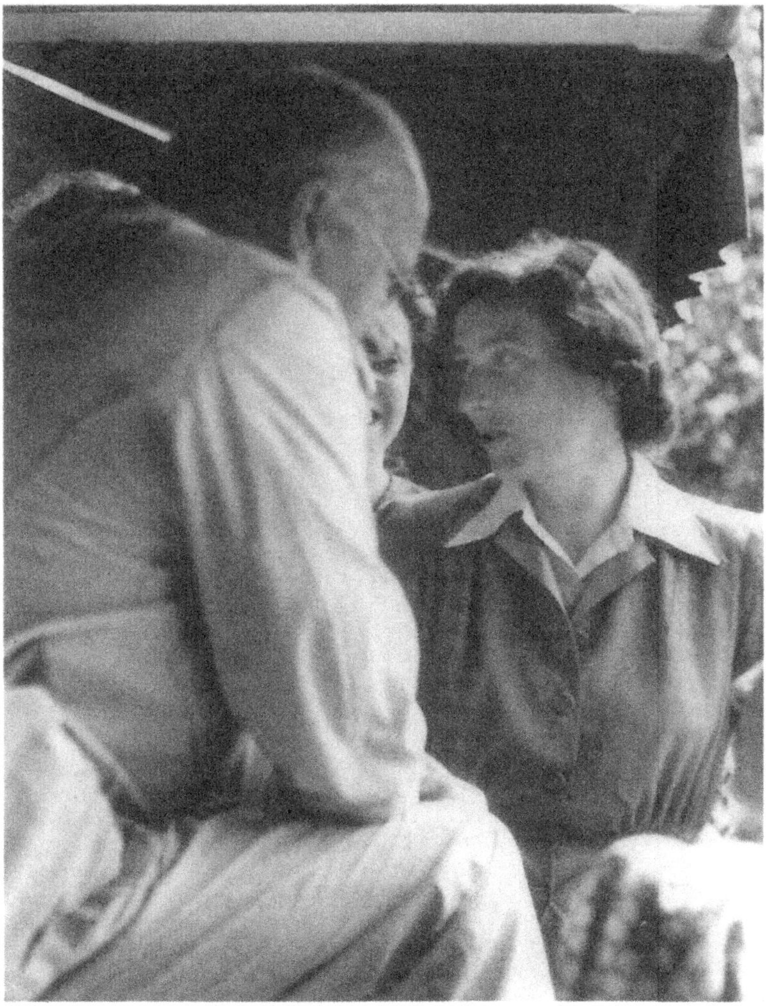

Figure 12. Carl Gustav Jung and Marie-Louise von Franz at the Eranos Conference. Courtesy of Marie-Anne von Franz.

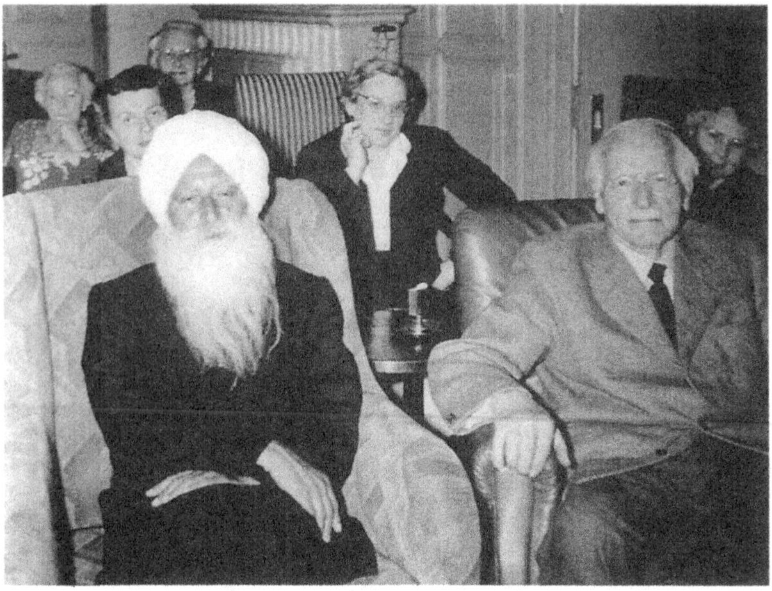

Figure 13. Carl Gustav Jung (right) and Marie-Louise von Franz (center), with others, attending a lecture at the Psychological Club of Zürich. Courtesy of Marie-Anne von Franz.

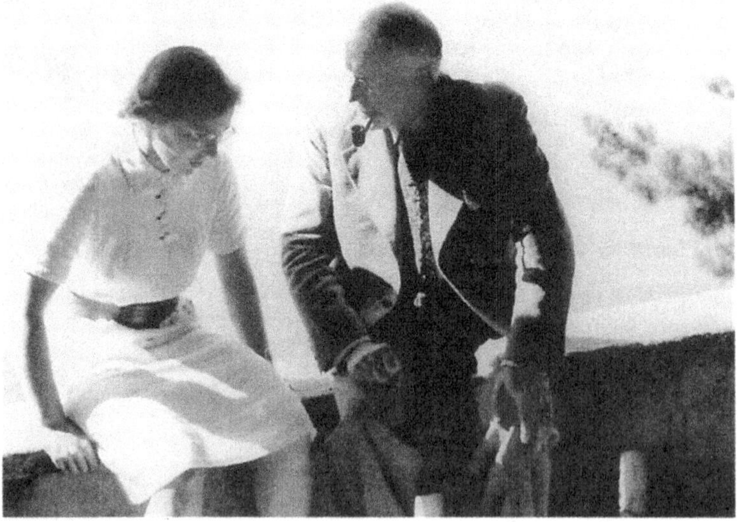

Figure 14. Marie-Louise von Franz and Carl Gustav Jung at the Eranos Conference. Courtesy of Marie-Anne von Franz.

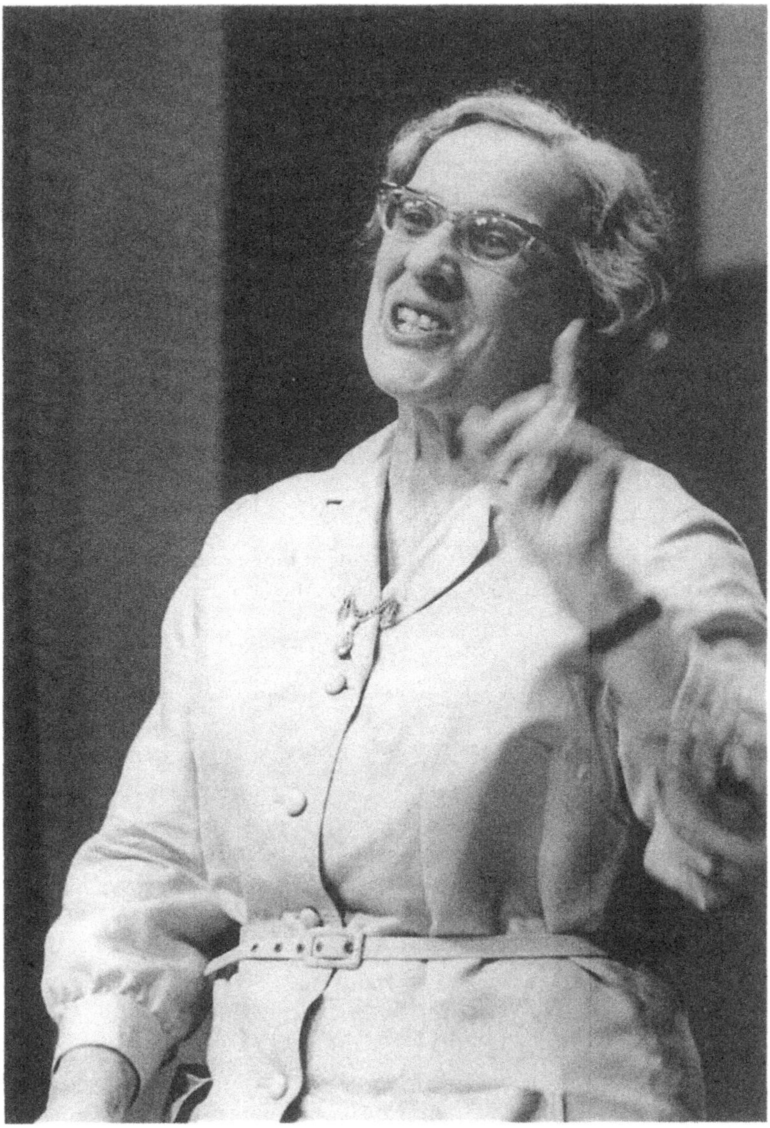

Figure 15. Marie-Louise von Franz delivering her lecture "Number Games of the Universe" in 1968, at the second Baily Island Conference, Maine, USA, held in honor of Dr. Esther Harding's eightieth birthday. Photographed by Edwin Snyder. Courtesy of Marie-Anne von Franz.

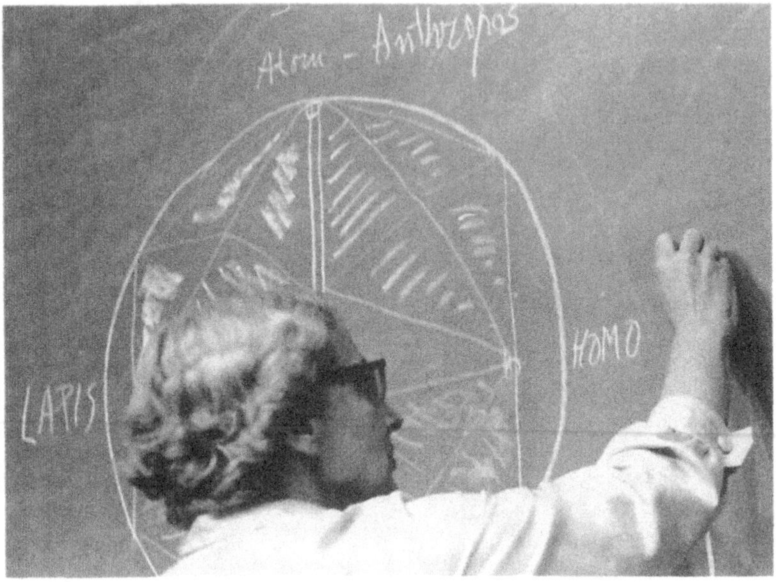

Figure 16. Marie-Louise von Franz, lecturing at the second Bailey Island Conference, Maine, USA. Courtesy of Marie-Anne von Franz.

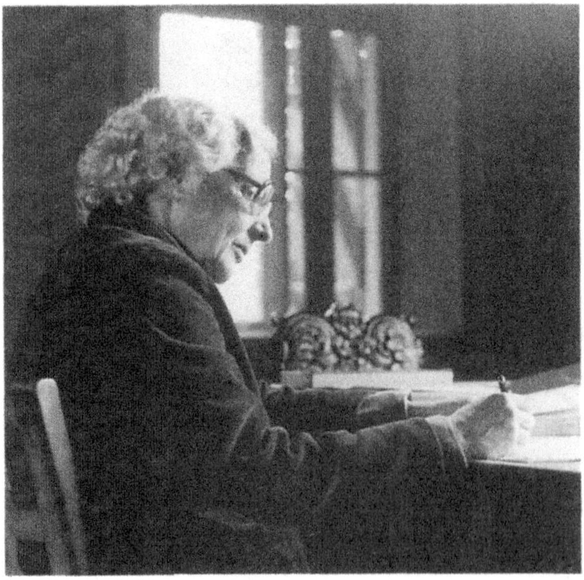

Figure 17. Marie-Louise von Franz at her desk in Bollingen. Courtesy of Françoise Selhofer, 1982.

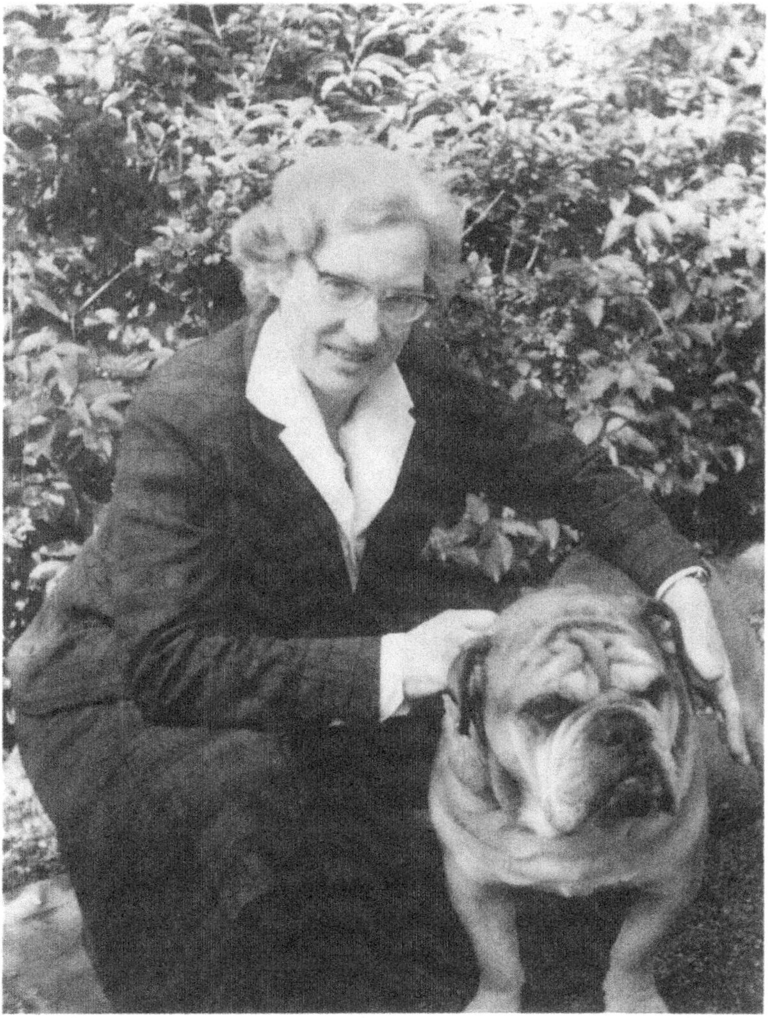

Figure 18. Marie-Louise von Franz with Nibby in Küsnacht. Courtesy of Marie-Anne von Franz.

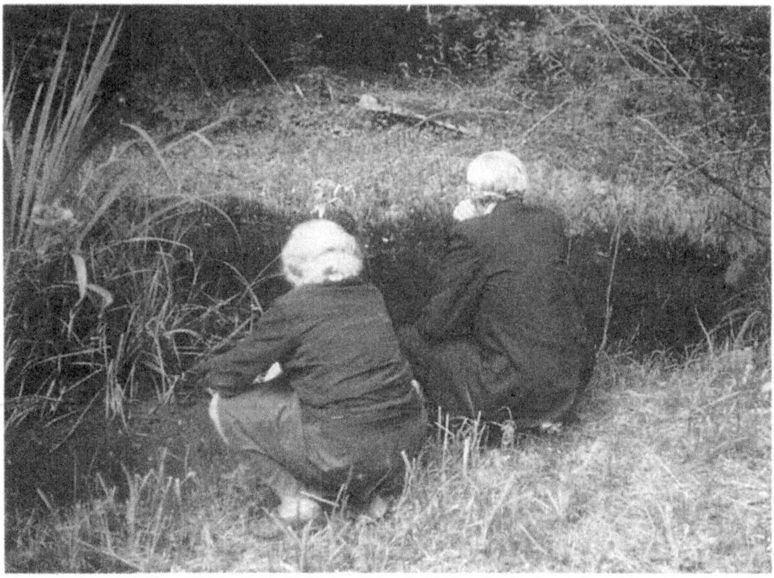

Figure 19. Marie-Louise von Franz with Vernon Brooks, watching the toads in her pond at Bollingen. Photographed by William H. Kennedy. Photo © Emmanuel Kennedy.

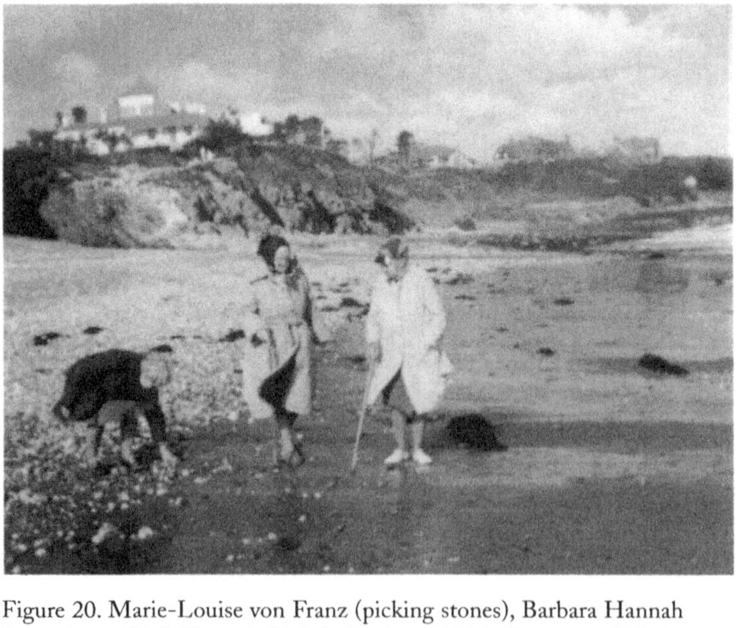

Figure 20. Marie-Louise von Franz (picking stones), Barbara Hannah (center), and E. J. Hannah (right), Scotland, 1963. Courtesy of Marie-Anne von Franz.

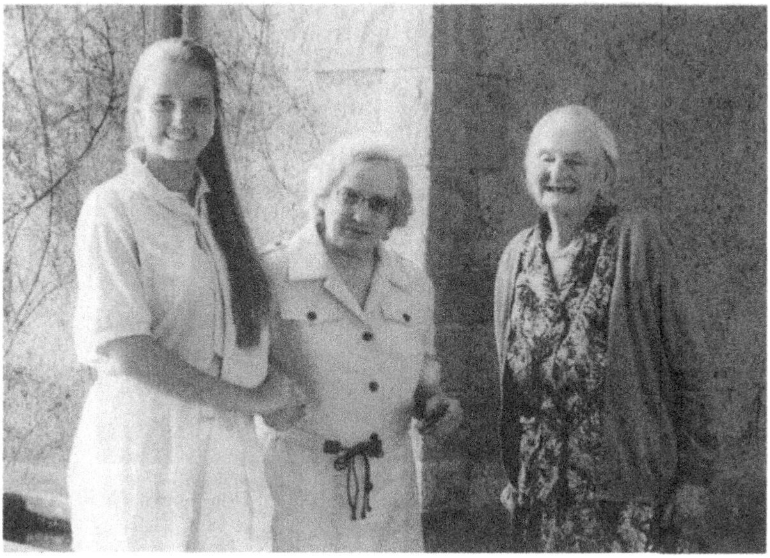

Figure 21. Robin Lea Hutton (left), Marie-Louise von Franz, and Barbara Hannah (right), at Bollingen, 1984. Photograph © Robin Lea Hutton. Reproduced by permission of the photographer.

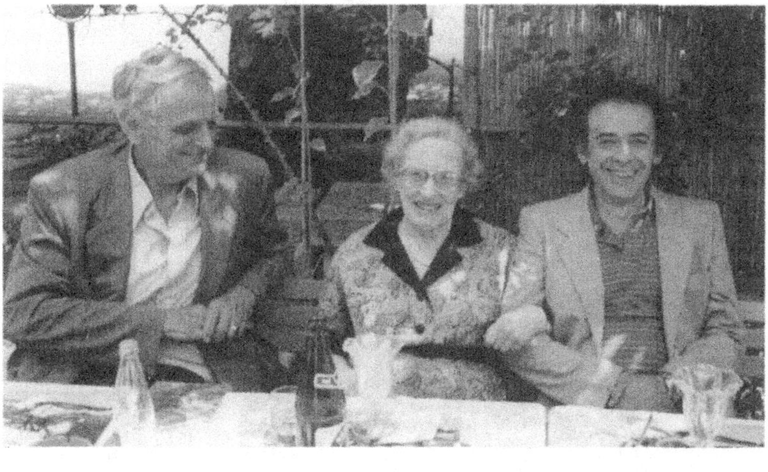

Figure 22. Dieter Baumann (left), Marie-Louise von Franz, and José Zavala (right), having lunch at the Ochsen-Hotel, Küsnacht, 1986. Photographed by Ramon Conell, courtesy of José Zavala.

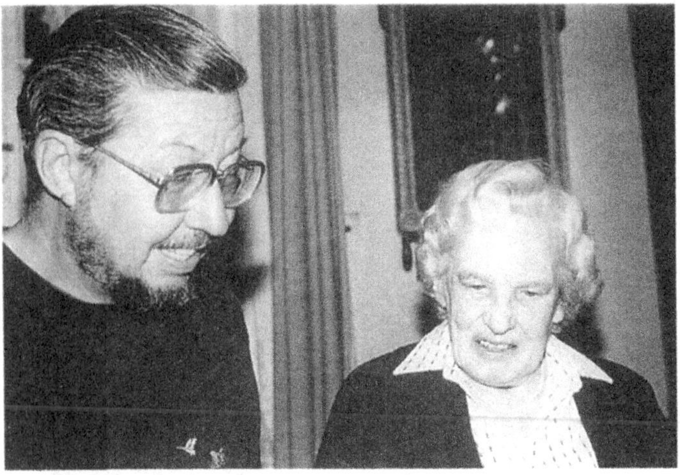

Figure 23. Alfred Ribi and Marie-Louise von Franz. Courtesy of Alfred Ribi.

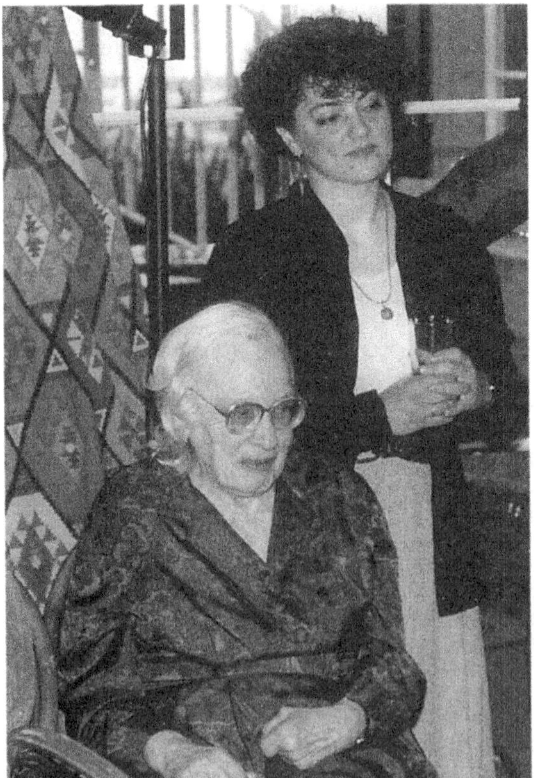

Figure 24. Marie-Louise von Franz and Lara Mindell. Courtesy of Lara Mindell.

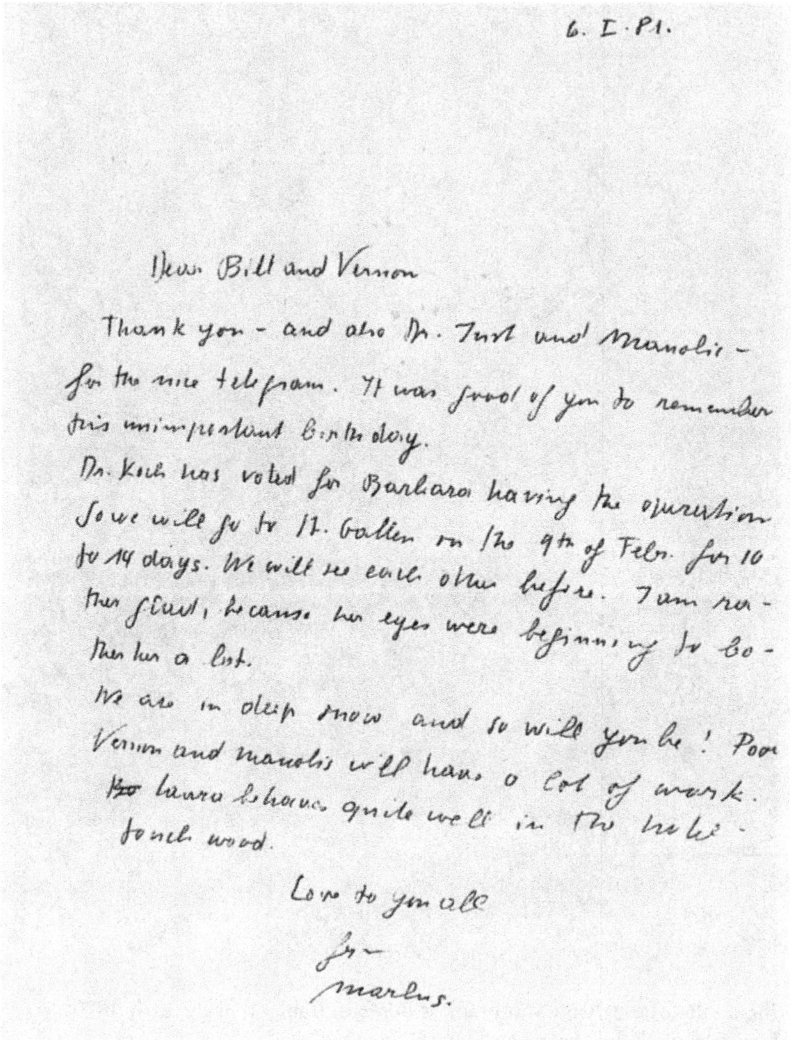

6. I. 81.

Dear Bill and Vernon

Thank you – and also Dr. Just and Manolis – for the nice telegram. It was good of you to remember this unimportant Birthday.

Dr. Koch has voted for Barbara having the operation So we will go to St. Gallen on the 9th of Febr. for 10 to 14 days. We will see each other before. I am rather glad, because her eyes were beginning to bother her a lot.

We are in deep snow and so will you be! Poor Vernon and Manolis will have a lot of work. ~~Bo~~ Laura behaves quite well in the hole – touch wood.

Love to you all

Yours

Markus.

Figure 25. Letter to William Kennedy and Vernon Brooks, January 6, 1981. Courtesy of Emmanuel Kennedy.

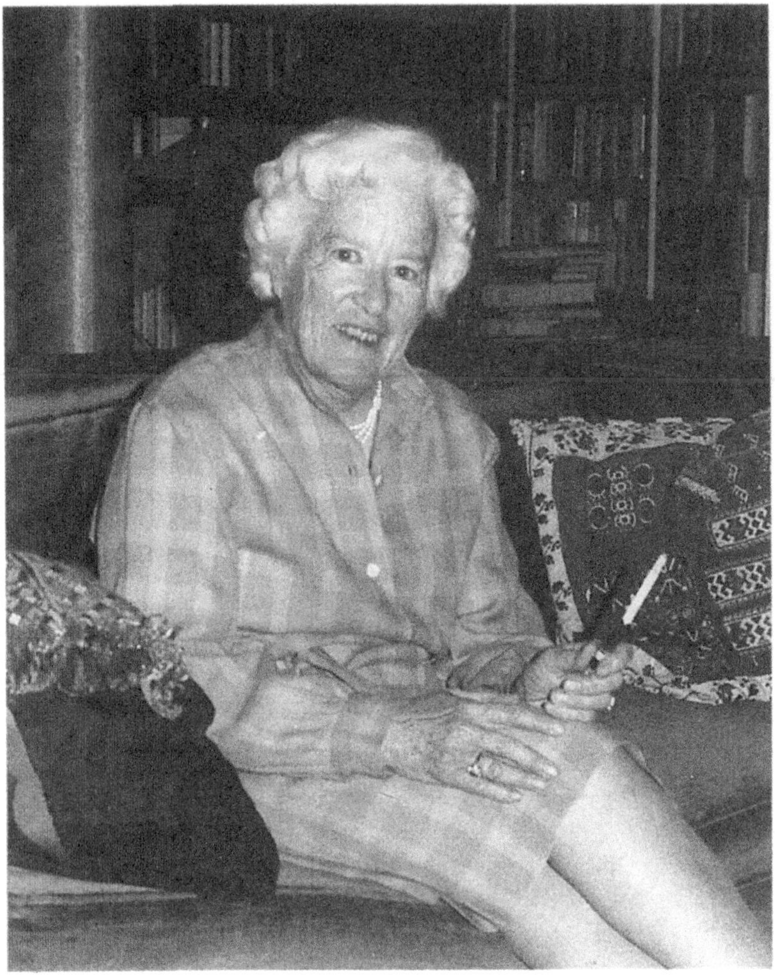

Figure 26. Marie-Anne von Franz at home in Bubikon in the early 1970s. Courtesy of Marie-Anne von Franz.

Some Biographic Data on Marie-Louise von Franz

MARIE-ANNE VON FRANZ

Marie-Louise von Franz was born in Münich on January 4, 1915, during the First World War. Our father served in military campaigns in western Russia and in the Dolomites while our mother stayed for the duration of the war with her own mother in Upper Bavaria. Shortly after my mother had given birth, I was taken by my grandmother's maid, Babette, to her room to see my new little sister. But all that I could see was a large white bed, my mother in a white nightshirt, and in her arms a white bundle with a bit of dark hair at the top. I wanted to climb up on the bed to see my sister, but the maid took me energetically out of the room.

I recall an incident four years later in which I actually really "saw" my little sister for the first time. I remember being on the balcony of the house on a wonderfully sunny day, the sunlight glistening in the frame of the open door, and there in the deep shade stood Marie-Louise. She looked at me with dark, large, lively, and incredibly enterprising eyes; I was absolutely enchanted. In my joy, I ran to the piano and started making as much noise as possible. But suddenly my mother stood behind me saying, "Come, I will show you how you should do it." She sat down at the piano, I leaned against her side, and Marie-Louise came running, yelling, "me too, me too." My mother turned and said, "No, you are still too small." And then, in the same second, Marie-Louise violently slapped her face. There was a moment of complete, petrified silence. Then my mother left the room, and Marie-Louise stood by my side, bewildered, holding back the tears in her eyes.

In the winter of 1918–1919 our parents were with us in our paternal grandmother's house at Bishofswiesen near Berchtsgaden. We were waiting for visas for a holiday in Switzerland. My father, who had undergone a severe operation at the end of the war in 1918 and then caught the flu, an epidemic sweeping through Europe, was still quite invalid. He was going every week to the municipal offices of Berchtsgaden to ask whether the visas had come. And in the spring of 1919 they finally arrived. Our parents left with us immediately, taking a train from Salzburg to Buchs, a village on the border of Switzerland. There we had to get out of a wagon full of howling and singing Austrian soldiers and walk over to an empty train in the station in Buchs. Our parents left us alone on the rails carrying our suitcases from one train to the other. My sister and I were trying to follow them but were unable to keep up because of the heavy cobblestones between the rails. A half century later my sister told me that she had a bad shock from this episode. For me, aged six, it was difficult but acceptable.

In the summer of 1919 [at the age of four], my sister had to undergo a second heavy operation in Bern. (At the age of two, she had had acute appendicitis which, in order to save her, could only be settled provisionally by the surgeon.) At the same time, my father was gradually recovering from his own operation and came slowly to the conviction that it would be best for the whole family to stay longer in Switzerland and to try to obtain a job. In the autumn of that year, some friends in Vienna put him in touch with an Austrian wood dealer who was importing enormous quantities of lumber into Switzerland to be sawed and milled for the construction of buildings of every kind in the entire eastern part of the country. Some time later, he was employed as a director, working in the office of the same Holzindustrie AG, a large sawmill in the border village of St. Margrethen, northeast of St. Gallen. Our parents bought an old house in Rheineck, the little neighboring town.

And here we settled in. The house had a lovely garden, not too big and not too small, and my sister and I could play every day in a garden for the first time in our lives. In the autumn of 1921, Marie-Louise began elementary school in Rheineck, and in the spring of 1928, our parents decided to send us both to the Freies Gymnasium in Zürich.

We finished the gymnasium and then immediately started our studies at the university. That is, Marie-Louise finished high school in 1933 and completed her doctorate in classical philology and classical languages (Greek and Latin) seven years later. (Our father, however, had lost the greatest part of his money in the early 1930s, so when we started our university studies, he told us that we had to earn the entire matriculation fees and expenses ourselves.)

It was in the summer of 1933—between the gymnasium and the university—that a classmate of Marie-Louise (a nephew of Toni Wolff) invited her along with seven boys to pay a visit to Professor C. G. Jung in his tower in Bollingen. Late that evening, I went to my sister's room to say good night and naturally also to hear about the visit. She sat at her table and told me of the entire visit from beginning to end. When I got up to say good night and leave the room, she added, "This was the decisive encounter of my life." I realized only many years later how true this was.

Marie-Louise asked Professor Jung for a training analysis and agreed with him that she would repay his time by investigating two major alchemical manuscripts. Although Marie-Louise had spontaneously envisioned her profession and future life, she was just beginning her university studies. To her major in classical philology and languages, she added Arabic because the alchemical manuscripts lent to her by Professor Jung included numerous documents which had originated in the Islamic treatises from Persia as well as the southern Mediterranean and Spain. Possibly the two most important manuscripts were *Aurora Consurgens* and the *Museum Hermeticum.* And during her university studies, she attended all of Jung's lectures held at the E.T.H., the Federal Technical University of Switzerland in Zürich.

In fact, during her lifetime, Marie-Louise had three major fields of research and was in contact at different periods with many people from various walks of life and cultural backgrounds. One field of interest was the investigation of fairy tales, which became the basis for much of her later interpretation of dreams. The second was the innumerable problems connected with the world of alchemy. And the third was her interest in synchronicity, psyche and matter, and numbers.

When Marie-Louise was twenty years old, a lady contacted her who was looking for a part-time assistant in writing a book about fairy tales.[1] Marie-Louise devoted many years and innumerable hours to this research, which became well known and highly respected in practically all parts of the world. On the other hand, the alchemical studies also required that she continuously reorganize the concepts, interpretation, and translation of the material, which then slowly became increasingly relevant to psychological issues.

Marie-Louise left home when she was twenty-five and lived in a single room, first on Jupiterstrasse and later on Englishviertelstrasse in Zürich. The 1930s were economically difficult years, and the war then added to these problems. After the sudden death of our father in the autumn of 1940, our mother eventually had to sell the house.

Marie-Louise then moved to a small apartment herself in 1944 and, generally speaking, lived frugally for many years, supporting herself as a tutor of Latin and Greek for gymnasium and university students, working on fairy-tale texts.

Almost immediately after the Second World War, Miss Barbara Hannah returned to Küsnacht to again meet Professor Jung, whom she had come to know quite well before the war. (She, in fact, first met him in 1929.) She then resided at the Hotel Sonne in Küsnacht and very much wished to stay and work again in Switzerland. Professor Jung had seen that my sister found it difficult to pursue all of her professional and scholastic commitments while managing a household as a single woman. Knowing both women rather well, he suggested to them one day that they join and try at least to set up a common psychotherapeutic practice.

So, in 1946, they rented a three-room apartment in Hornweg next to the Hotel Sonne in order to give this possibility a try. Despite an age difference of approximately twenty-five years, and being very different personalities, the two worked well together. My sister realized very soon that it was essential for them to find more space. But the finances were such that it was not until 1965 that Marie-Louise saw the ad in the newspaper regarding the sale of a house on the slopes of Küsnacht.

It took her no time at all to fall in love with the house and sign the contract. It was first in her home on Lindenbergstrasse 15 that my sister's life as a psychologist and a woman of research came together as one and began to flourish.

Like so many people after the war, Marie-Louise became increasingly interested in traveling abroad, and from that time onward she regularly visited our neighboring countries. In addition, she discovered many different parts of England and Scotland on holidays with Barbara Hannah. She also went twice to the United States for professional visits and for holiday stays. During one of these tours, she wrote me from a short holiday in the northwestern part of the States, saying, "Here nature is still wild."

Marie-Louise had a passionate interest in nature and gardening. So it was not long after she moved to Lindenbergstrasse that she realized her hunger for nature was not stilled in the rather tiny garden there. She thus acquired a piece of land on the borders of a large forest above Bollingen, which she came to know through her visits to Professor Jung there. With his agreement and advice, she decided to build a tower on the crown of the hill. This house became her refuge in nature and gave her the possibility to escape modern civilization with all its unrest. It also gave her the physical strength to write the innumerable books that she had planned very early on in her life, books that she realized one after the other throughout the decades.

It is an odd story of how Marie-Louise noticed and identified her Parkinson's syndrome sixteen years before her death. One day, she was working in her Küsnacht garden, a hobby that she loved, when she suddenly fell head first down the slope of the garden, sliding about six meters before being stopped by the fence high above the street. She then spent weeks, even months, reflecting on what had happened to her because the fall had no rational cause. It was only a very short time later that she diagnosed herself as having Parkinson's. Then one day she told this to her doctor while she was at the baths in Bad Ragaz. Marie-Louise died from the side effects of her illness on February 17, 1998.

NOTE

1. This was the work on the symbolism and the interpretation of fairy tales by Hedwig von Beit.—*Ed.*

PART SEVEN

Contributions

The Tao of Primal Chaos—*Hùn Dùn*

A Remembrance of Marie-Louise von Franz

CHUNGLIANG AL HUANG

I met Dr. von Franz for the first time when we were both presenters at the International Transpersonal Conference in Davos, Switzerland, in August 1983. We became instant friends. And our mutual admiration grew into deep friendship on multiple levels by further sharing as colleagues at various conferences and symposiums in Europe. But for me, throughout the years, the most memorable meetings were those very special occasions, being with her as kindred souls, when I came through Zürich. Invariably, I would be invited to visit her at her house on Lindenbergstrasse in Küsnacht, where we would have the most stimulating conversations on all subjects, sipping ginseng tea together (in earlier years, always with Ms. Barbara Hannah and their beloved dog nestling close by!). One special time, I was invited by Marie-Louise to share a lecture for the Friends of Jung at the Hotel Sonne in Küsnacht. Dr. von Franz suggested the subject of *Hùn Dùn* (the Primal Chaos) and invited me to share the Taoist perspective on it, particularly from the illuminating writings of Chuang Tzu. Here is the text of this specific gem, from his Inner Chapter #7, "The Sage King":

> The ruler of the South Sea was called Light; the ruler of the North Sea, Darkness; and the ruler of the Middle Kingdom, Primal Chaos. From time to time, Light and Darkness met one another in the kingdom of Primal Chaos, who made them welcome. Light and Darkness wanted to repay his kindness and said: "All men have seven openings with which they see, hear, eat and breathe, but Primal Chaos has none. Let us try to give him some." So every day, they bored one hole, and on the seventh day Primal Chaos died!

Both Dr. von Franz and I appreciated this deeply insightful Taoist parable, written over two and a half millennia ago, warning us of this prophetic disaster looming in the world and threatening all human endeavors, as a result chiefly of our arrogant interference with nature, especially with human nature. As the old saying goes: "The road to hell is often paved with good intentions." So much of our troubles in the world are caused by unwarranted interference through neurotic anxiety and ignorance. It would seem wise for all leaders, teachers, and therapists to help ourselves, together with our people, students, and clients to learn to understand and exercise the art of noninterference (*wu wei*) in the Tao, and to share the discipline and practice of *tai ji*—balance in everyday living.

As I recall, that specific evening, with the wit and wisdom of Dr. von Franz guiding us through the animated discussion and insightful dialogues, we were able to share the excitement of having experienced a few glimpses of a genuine *satori*—the sudden enlightenment in Zen and Tao. I shall always treasure the pleasure of that evening and the subsequent occasions of inspired learning from her.

Another time, Dr. von Franz, who was especially fond of one of my books, *Quantum Soup: Fortune Cookies in Crisis*, suggested the wonderfully metaphoric German title *Tao Wetter*, which we cherished and which was much appreciated by our readers for the first Swiss edition. She and I shared a fondness for the humor in human incongruities and a trust in the latent coherence in the midst of chaos and uncertainty, in the ambiguities and contradictions in all our lives. We shared a belief in the universal wisdom in the primal chaos (*Hùn Dùn*): the potential growth with dormant inertia state in which order is latent in human nature. It is with this undisturbed and unadulterated essence, the "wilderness" in nature's original condition, human beings become most creative and vital. And it is in the understanding and embodiment of the concepts of *tzu ren* (self-so-ness spontaneity) and *feng liu* (the flow of wind and water) in our daily awareness that the Tao can be fully realized in human activities.

I shall always think of Dr. von Franz with great admiration during her final years, dealing valiantly with her failing health. She maintained her dignity and integrity through the end with such clarity of mind and spirit. We managed to share quality time whenever possible, even if only for a few moments of mutual silence when I was able to reach her by phone while she was often much too weak to converse audibly.

Her final communication with me was in a brief note replying to my letter, shortly before her passing:

> Dear Chungliang Al Huang,
>
> Thank you for your kind note. I am OK but
> packing for the big journey.
>
> Love, Marie-Louise von Franz

In my Chinese mind's eye, I can visualize her "big journey"—riding on a white stork, soaring in the wind, safely landed at the celestial kingdom, joining all the international immortals, including her mentor-friend, Carl G. Jung, and mine, Joseph Campbell, with Lao Tzu and Chuang Tzu toasting them with rice wine and ginseng tea, having a most passionate discussion on *Hùn Dùn*—the primal chaos.

Frau Holle in the Depths of Our Souls

CHRISTINE ALTMANN-GLASER

My first encounter with Marie-Louise von Franz was at a lecture series on fairy tales at the C. G. Jung Institute in the beginning of the 1960s. I was so enthusiastic about her lectures that I mustered up the courage to ask if I could do an analysis with her. Because I was particularly interested in fairy tales, they played an important role in my analysis. Soon I was asked to attempt to interpret one myself.

Marie-Louise von Franz was a stringent teacher and tolerated no interpretations that did not consider the archetypes to be living forces in life. Archetypes such as the animus, the anima, the shadow, and the Self were as observable as the goings-on of daily life; they were not theoretical constructions but experiential phenomena. In that she highly valued creative work, I would like to honor her with an interpretation of a fairy tale.

As it is my wish to bring the spirit of Marie-Louise von Franz and C. G. Jung more to everyday people, I organize regular symposiums for the Swiss Fairy Tale Society, at which a representative of Jungian psychology is present whenever possible. The theme of the first of these symposiums, which provides the basis of this essay, was "Frau Holle and Her Sisters and Brothers." As this lecture was given to psychological laypersons and scientific skeptics, Jungian terminology was avoided. I had also learned from Marie-Louise von Franz that when one interprets fairy tales, one should draw on different versions of the story. I assume that the reader is acquainted with the fairy tale of Frau Holle (KHM no. 24). Here is an African version of this type of fairy tale (Aath 480).[1]

The Jewelry from the Deep

In an African village lived a wonderfully beautiful girl, more beautiful than all of the other girls around. Naturally all those girls were jealous and hated her and plagued her whenever they could. One day they plotted to play a nasty trick on the girl. They went to the river and buried all of their "finery" in the sand. Then they called the beautiful girl down to the river and told her that they had thrown all of their jewelry in the water because they did not want to be vain, and that she should do this too. The girl was very sad. She did not want to be more conceited than they and wanted to still their jealousy. So she threw her jewelry in the river. As soon as she had done this, they all broke out in peals of laughter, chortling about how completely dumb she was. As they dug out their jewelry they just laughed and laughed.

The poor girl ran along the riverbed and called out: "Dear river, please give me back my jewelry, give me my treasures back please." She ran and ran until she came to a place where the river formed a deep hole. From the depths here in the river she heard a voice call out, "Dive to the bottom and you will find your jewelry." But she did not have the courage to go in. The voice called out again, "Dive to the bottom, for there you will find all your treasures." But she hesitated once more. Then the river called a third time, "Dive to the bottom. Your jewelry lies here."

So the girl mustered up the courage and dove to the bottom of the river. There sat an old woman who was covered in wounds.

> The old woman asked the girl to lick these wounds. Since the woman was obviously in need, the girl did as she was requested. The old woman thanked the girl and said, "I see that you are a merciful child, so here, here is your jewelry." And the old woman gave her even more jewelry to take back up with her. "But now you must hurry back up to the top, because a demon will soon be coming who will eat you." The girl thanked the woman, swam quickly back up to the top, and went home. As the village girls saw the wealth of jewelry that she brought back with her, they wanted to know where it had come from. She told them the whole story. So all of the girls ran right down to that place along the river banks, jumped into the water, and swam down to the old woman. As she asked them to lick her wounds, they called out: "How disgusting . . . who do you think you are? We will never do such a thing." Then the demon came and devoured them all.

This fairy tale was told by Laurens van der Post on November 24, 1996, on an occasion in his honor given by the Research and Training Center for Depth Psychology According to C. G. Jung and M.-L. von Franz in Zürich. Van der Post noted that this is exactly what Jung did. He brought up the treasures out of the depths of the unconscious. Sir Laurens van der Post, who was a friend of Jung's, dedicated his life to fighting racial discrimination, in particular that against ethnic minorities such as the Bushmen, and fought for the preservation of nature (for example, the Kalahari Desert). Marie-Louise von Franz also greatly appreciated him. Although at this meeting the ninety-year-old van der Post depended on two walking sticks, his mind and spirit were clear and alert. When he was requested to say a few words, he told this fairy tale.[2]

The actual origin of this fairy tale is unimportant in regards to the interpretation that I will present. The fairy-tale type Aath 480 is found in an astounding number of variations from Europe to eastern Asia, from Africa to the Americas. We will be seeking the reason why this type of fairy tale is so widespread. Due to the worldwide dispersion and fascination with this motif (a theme that still affects us today), we can deduce that the material is not just a "once upon a time" sort of narrative, but that it is as appropriate as ever. We need to look at it more along the lines of "once upon a time as it was and ever will be," an introductory sentence found in several Eastern European fairy tales. We can assume that a narrative that is so widespread cannot be just simple entertainment. Our feelings speak against such a premise. We also cannot do much with a moralistic approach: "good girls have it good, bad have it bad." Yet, nevertheless, we do feel that—as in most fairy tales—a message lies behind the story. I would thus like to attempt to track down the possible message for us today.

What is the basic structure of this fairy tale? First, with few exceptions, we have two opposing girls, one beautiful and one unattractive. The beautiful one is friendly, modest, helpful, acknowledges the tasks given to her, and tackles the work to be done. The ugly girl avoids tasks, is immodest, impudent, egotistical, greedy, and she wants to get her wealth and riches without making any effort. In the end, the good one is rewarded, the bad punished. Here we encounter two possible patterns of behavior, and then we are given a choice. Is it simply "The beautiful and good have it good; the bad, bad"? Contemporary, emancipated women often have difficulty with the concept of the superficial, dutiful, hard-working little housewife as "Golden Maria" of the Frau Holle cycle seems to be.[3] I can remember myself being not particularly pleased at the time of my engagement when I was given a household book titled *The Diligent Housewife* as a gift. It did not exactly match my image of womanhood. Nevertheless, I somehow could not just totally avoid it. (And the book proved to be very useful.) I do not mean to give praise to the diligent housewife, although I think today this is one part of being a modern woman: "To be in the service of daily matters is to be in the service of life," as the well-known psychologist and author Ingrid Riedel says.

I believe that the interpretation of the Golden Maria figure as an antiquated image of women is too simple and misses the core of this fairy tale. We have to sift here more carefully and consider the actual tasks that the girl was set.

First, we need to take a look at the antagonists of the Frau Holle fairy tale: Frau Holle and her sisters and brothers. Sonja Rüttner-Cova names

Frau Holle "the fallen goddess," and Ingrid Riedel describes her as a goddess who is also known in German-speaking cultures as Frau Hulda and in Scandinavia as Huldre, while as she is known as Perch or "Berchta the Resplendent and Shining" in the European Alps. She resides "down in the valley" or in the "depths of a well" and calls forth the flowers to sprout and the trees to blossom and beckons to the cows to graze. She is the heroine of fountains and springs and in some variations of rivers as well. Yet she is simultaneously a goddess of the heavens who rules over the seasons and causes snow to fall. As children, we wondered how Frau Holle lived at the bottom of a well where there were fields of flowers, trees, and a bread oven and, on the other hand, caused the snow to fall; somehow, she was down here as well as up there in the heavens.

The realm of Frau Holle can be said to be located outside of time and space. It is in the beyond, and she is a goddess. When Golden Maria keeps house for Frau Holle and shakes out her bedsheets, it is not just a simple household task but rather labor in the service of the goddess. And service to the goddess is first and foremost one of "hearing" the call from the bread baked in the oven and the apples ripened on the trees, and then reacting in kind. Ingrid Riedel says it so well: it is to hear the calling of things and to recognize the right moment to act.

What, however, does it actually mean psychologically to be in "the service of the goddess"? Gods, goddesses, demons, and so forth are theological and cultural concepts. The analytical psychology of C. G. Jung uses the word *archetypes* for these highly effective powers and defines these figures as forms of psychic energy that structure, focus, and direct our imagination, precipitating similar images and experiences throughout all cultures in the world. In earlier times, people believed that these psychic energies occurred in the outside world, atop Mount Olympus, in Hades, in springs and in trees. With the onset of Christianity, people began to notice that these powers lived within us. In *Cherubinischer Wandersmann* (1675), Angelus Silesius calls out: "Stop, where are you going? The heaven is within you. If you search for God elsewhere, you will miss him." And in the English language, one differentiates between "sky," the physical outer atmosphere, and the "heavens," a cosmological, metaphysical realm that to a certain extent is also thought to be within. The images of heaven and hell are still used today. They are not to be understood as concrete but rather as symbolic images. When Cupid shoots his arrow, it is a symbol that everyone understands. Our language teems with such images. In politics, heads roll; for businessmen under attack, the issue gets too hot to handle; scientists crack the case; and so forth. Nobody would ever think of taking these expressions literally. The situation is no different in fairy-tale motifs. These motifs are symbolic images of psychic processes; to take them literally seldom makes sense.

Frau Holle is in Jungian thought a symbol of the archetypal image of the goddess, and in particular, the Great Mother, a figure who embodies the mother principle per se. She is that vast source from which all life arises and to which it returns; she is Mother Earth in contradistinction to the Heavenly Spirit of the Father. The experience of the cycles of nature lies well within the parameters of this archetypal image. Here we find the "receptive-containing-protective," then the "creative-fertile-nourishing-and-flourishing," and also the "flooding-overwhelming-destroying-devouring-death-bringing." This archaic image is expressed in a plethora of symbols and mythological figures such as Frau Holle, or the fairy-tale motif of the devil's grandmother, or Baba Yaga, but then also in the symbolism of animals such as the cat, the cow, the bear, and so forth. In antiquity, these animals were attributed to the goddesses. They were probably actual animal goddesses in even earlier cultures. Thus the bear was the animal of Artemis, the sow of Demeter, the cow of Hathor, and so forth. In religious spheres, we find the Great Mother also in the form of the Black Madonnas or the Indian goddess Kali, while in modern dreams we find the Great Mother symbolized by figures such as the grandmother, the Queen Mother, or Mother Teresa. In fairy tales, she is also found represented as special caves, springs, the ocean, forests, and so forth. The source of these various forms of expression is archetypal; she is the archetype of the feminine principle.

In Grimm's "Frau Holle," we find the devouring aspect of the Great Mother in many motifs, for example, in her large teeth or in the shaft of the well into which the two girls jump. In Germany, we find "Holle-ponds" and "Holle-wells" out of which infants are born and which entice them to jump back in again. Springs are sources of life, but they can also be dangerous: one can drown. Frau Holle embodies the very essence of nature and of the elements whose presence calls forth a modest and deferential attitude so that she will not become dangerous.

Look what we have done to our springs, streams, and rivers. They are constricted, straightened, tapped, contaminated, and set to work. Could these be the wounds that have been inflicted on the old woman beneath the river in our African version of the story? Then it is time to be merciful to this goddess of life, to nurse the wounds so that they may heal. Otherwise she will devour us in our hunger for riches like she did the other girls in the village. The wisdom of nature—as Marie-Louise von Franz asserts—consists in her consequence: when land is razed, leached by monocultural farming practices and squeezed out until there is nothing left, then it transforms into desert; when protective forests are felled, then avalanches have free rein; when our bodies are abused, we get ill and thus are forced to look after ourselves more carefully. When many male soldiers fall in war, the birthrate of boys rises. Nature seeks to create a balance and will even employ at times cruel means. In a subtype of the good-and-bad-girl motif, the good girl is exiled to a forest or bathhouse or an old abandoned mill. Here she must share her food with three domestic animals, who then in turn give good advice or help the girl in her need. In a Russian version, the girl must clean a well and tend a pear tree and nurse a sick dog. It always has to do with being kind to nature. The punishment for disobedience is the direct consequence of neglect. For then, when an urgent need arises, there are no relationships to the animals, trees, or springs; no help comes, and the demons do away with the girl.

Frau Holle lives not only in the natural environs that surround us but in the depths of our souls as well. She is the image of instinctive knowledge, and she represents that which is good for us, that which will help heal us, and that which is ripe and needs to be plucked. She is the image of that which must "take the bread out of the oven" when the time is right, that which precipitates snow at the appropriate time. Here she is associated with Chiros, the right moment in time.[4] There are many versions of this type in which the stepdaughter is sent into the forest in winter to gather violets, berries, or apples and there meets the twelve months or the four winds.[5] She is courteous to them and finds praise for each month or for the wind, as each has its task in its appropriate time. (The other daughter, by the way, finds nothing good about any of them.) Here the idea of the right moment in time is particularly clear. The inner knowledge of the right moment is expressed in hunches, intuitions, feelings, body symptoms, dreams, fantasies, and so forth. And here, in the depths of our souls, it is essential to take Frau Holle—our inner nature—seriously. The animals in the previously mentioned fairy tales are images of inner instincts. If we do not care for these, they wither away.

Now, if we turn to the tasks in Frau Holle's realm, we find bread and the oven, both of which are not pure nature on the level of animals, trees, springs, and rivers. Here we find human culture in the background. Such cultural efforts also belong to Frau Holle because culture belongs to human nature in contrast to animal nature. It takes effort to earn our daily bread and to master daily life. This energy is symbolized in the heat of the oven. The oven is, obviously, a typical feminine symbol and is often used in everyday speech when talking about the uterus and womb. Newborn children are sometimes referred to as "fresh out of the oven." In the colloquial dialect of Switzerland, an immature person is described as "not completely baked," while in the Canton of Berne we find the expression "the oven has collapsed," referring to a successfully completed birth. Things "bake" in the oven, and this can also be an inner "psychological" child. Once, while working on a text, I was stuck and did not know how to continue. I then dreamed that I was playing with children during the day, while at night I put them in a red-hot oven (instead of to bed). Basking in the heat in front of the oven, I then spoke with them and wished them, for example, a good night's sleep. Marie-Louise von Franz understood the dream to say that it was not enough for me to dedicate myself playfully to my ideas (that is, "creative children") during the day (that is, consciously), but that these "children" also had to slowly "bake," that is, they needed time to mature in the unconscious and they needed a lot of energy. When we are in Frau Holle's realm and the oven calls to us that the bread is done, is this not an image from our soul telling us that our work is now completed and needs to be taken out into the light of day?

The alchemists also used the image of the oven as a symbol of development and transformation, in their case the transformation of impure metals to gold. They even called these metals in the oven the embryo and emphasized time and again that the gold they were seeking was not ordinary gold but the true philosophical gold. They called their goal the philosopher's stone, the elixir of life, or the *philius philosophorum.* The goal here was an inner psychic process of development and transformation that the alchemists, predecessors of modern chemists, projected onto their materials. The call of the bread could also mean that an inner development, a time of suffering and transformation, was now completed. That which we suffered is now risen, like bread in the oven, and it will provide a nourishment for our souls that we can also share with others.

The apple tree with its ripened apples is also a symbol for the mother. Here the accent lies on fertility and growth. The tree is rooted and stands firm in its place as the seasons change. It blossoms in the spring and puts forth leaves, produces fruit which then ripens during the summer and falls in autumn; the rest and repose of winter concludes the cycle. The apple tree is an image of the fertility of the Great Mother, the duration of which occurs only in cycles. The cyclic transformation of the goddesses is often represented as a feminine trinity, the virgin, the mother, and the death goddess, such as we find in Isis, Artemis, or even in the artwork and beliefs involving the Virgin Mary, who appears as the death goddess in her form as the Pieta. We find the feminine trinity in particular represented in the images of the Black Madonna. We find other examples of this trinity in the Greek Moirai, the three goddesses of fate, or in the Nornen, the three Scandinavian goddesses—past, present, and future—found at the base of the World Tree who also allocate the fate of the individual. The three Moirai are spinners; the first spins the threads of life, the second measures the length of life, the third cuts it off. In the fairy tale of Frau Holle we see this trinity represented in the three activities. The oven correlates to that which is becoming, the apple tree to that which now is, and the shaking of the bed linens and the snow to that which passes on into winter, a passing, however, that for the Great Mother is not final. For she is reborn in spring, often in the gestalt of the daughter, a motif beautifully represented in the Demeter myth. Demeter, the goddess of grains and fertility, has a daughter, Persephone, who is captured and taken into the underworld by Hades. Demeter searches in desperation for her daughter, leaving life on earth to wither away until Zeus decides that Persephone must spend one-third of the year with Hades in the underworld and two-thirds of the year on the surface of the earth with her mother. Persephone, virgin and goddess of death all in one, symbolizes the cycle of vegetation that recedes to the underworld in autumn to be resurrected in spring. Demeter, as mother, is that which endures, and she is, so to speak, the guarantee for the resurrection of her daughter.

It is the spindle, the thread of life, that draws the girl Maria into the depths of the well at the beginning of the tale, and when she emerges she comes back as Golden Maria, announced by the cock, the herald of the dawning of the new day. (Drewermann thus compares her to the sun which, according to conventional association, also descends into the underworld at night to rise again the following morning. This is only an image of the mythos of becoming, being, declining, and rising once again.)

This fairy tale teaches us that descent into the underworld is not in vain, but that desperation, regression, and depression are in the services of renewal. This is true on both large and small scales, in world history as well as in the life of the individual. It is a law of nature. It may comfort us to know that no ending is final but rather the end of a period of growth. No growth continues forever, not even economic expansion, without needing a time of winter, of repose and reflection. Now, if a time of regeneration is to serve to draw forth new strength, if it is to serve to lift up the treasures and fortunes of the unconscious, then it needs to be done with the proper attitude. If we descend into the depths of the soul with Pech Maria's attitude of self-aggrandizement, then we will end in misfortune. Pech Maria also did not descend into the well at the right time. She was not driven by urgency nor was she maltreated by a stepmother. On the contrary, she was a spoiled child.

On the other hand, Golden Maria, who drops her bloodied spindle in the well, represents a situation in life where we are being handled by a stepmother type of constellation, where fate brings us misfortune and suffering (the spindle is an attribute of the Moirai, the goddesses of fate). And the encounter of such crises throws us into the depths of depression. Only when our desperation and suffering reach the very bottom are we ready and able to be trustworthy in an encounter with the unconscious so that the thread of life lost, symbolized here by the spindle, can be found again. Ulla Wittmann emphasizes this point in her interpretation of the fairy tale.

Whoever leaps into the depths of the well cannot reckon that he or she will come up again alive. Yet a genuine sacrifice is unavoidable. Golden Maria sacrifices herself. The girl in the African fairy tale sacrifices her jewelry, that is, that "within her" which is most precious. Here previous life must be sacrificed; one has to let go of what was. Originally this was also the meaning of baptism: to let go of the old forms of life in order that, as a new man or woman, one can begin anew a life related to God. This concept lies at the bottom of all initiation and transition rites: to be separated from daily life, to cast off the past, and to steep oneself in a time of trials and teachings so that the person (oftentimes with a new name and new clothing) can be reintegrated into society. These patterns, which lie at the base of transition and initiation rites, can also be found in the genre of fairy tales employing magical motifs. In contrast to rites, these motifs can be adapted to all transitions in life. Our society has become impoverished in terms of rituals. And we find very few rites regarding the transition into old age. Here fairy tales can fill the gap. They can give us clues in regard to the meaning of life crises.

The stepmother can also be interpreted as the false mother in the sense of an attitude that is determined by others and is not in keeping with one's own nature. Drewermann interprets the stepmother as "mother world." The African fairy tale does this even more clearly. Here, instead of the stepmother and stepsister, we find the village girls. They represent the collective attitude of the society, that is, what one "thinks is right." Anyone who has lived in a village knows what it means when one does not conform to the norms. In a life crisis, one not only feels as if one is being treated by "stepmother Fate," one believes that one is being banned by society, not being taken seriously, maybe being mocked, all just like the girl in the African tale. One finds oneself on the edge; all former values seem to be lost and life energy is washed away like the girl's jewelry in the river.

Returning now to Pech Maria we see that she neither wants to sacrifice anything of her previous life nor does she withstand any of the tests. One is reminded of patients who come to therapy expecting the therapist to write them a prescription to solve their problems. Or one thinks of people who believe that a quick weekend course will free them of their neuroses or of having to make a decision. The transformation and regeneration of the personality requires supreme effort and humble servitude to the goddess.

I was long puzzled by the variations on the Frau Holle story where the girl is asked with whom she wishes to eat and sleep—with the lord and lady or with the cat and dog—or whether she would like to return home in a coach of pitch or that of gold.[6] At first I thought these were simply exaggerated modesty, a form of conventional morality. But as I found similar motifs in non-European and non-Christian versions I had to assume that we are dealing with archetypal motives and a different meaning at bottom.[7]

In a fairy-tale version from Burma, the farmer's daughter is asked by white crows, "Would you like a golden or a silver ladder to climb up to us?" She answers: "I climb no golden and no silver ladders. Give me the ladder that I know from my parents, the ladder made of bamboo." The girl also does not want to sit on golden or silver floor mats but rather one of woven straw. She does not want to eat from golden or silver dishes, but plates of clay and coconut cups. She then receives a ladder, a mat, and dishes all of gold.

I think this modesty has to do with clearly separating oneself from the divine. The white crows from the Burmese version and the "white woman and her husband in the golden castle" in a Swiss version were probably originally gods. To them goes the honor of gold, to them the imperishable and eternal values. Man is but their creation, just like other animals such as the cat or the dog. The earthly man eats from earthly dishes and sleeps on mats of straw. *Quid licet Jovis non licet bovis* ("What seems to be right for Jupiter is not for the ox") was already clear to the ancient Romans. When we descend into the depths of the unconscious, into the distant land of dreams, and are consoled by a dream, or we find an intuitive solution to a problem, or energy that has been lost returns, then the danger is that we identify with this discovery and imagine that we have created the solution (or the dream), we believe that we have pulled ourselves up out of the swamp. In psychology this is called inflation. It has devastating effects. We see this in psychotic people who believe that they are Christ or the mother of God. They have lost their connection to awe and the fear of inner psychic powers that are greater than the ego. In a life crisis, it is essential that one maintains the attitude *Deo concedente,* "if the gods concur." Only when we are open to the unexpected, open to that which the gods or goddesses grant us, only then are we able to perceive new possibilities in our lives. If, like Pech Maria, we already know what Frau Holle should give us, then we have no eye open to something new. One cannot demand to have inner riches. They will only be granted to the person who has an open mind and who is prepared to discover inner resources and inner wealth where it is least expected.

In several versions of this fairy tale the girl must delouse an old woman or comb her hair, and then she is asked to tell what she sees.[8] Pech Maria only sees lice and nits. What else is there to see when one delouses hair? But here one sees an attitude contaminated by bias and partiality that already knows everything there is to be expected and then sees only what it is expecting to see. In these versions, Golden Maria is open to the unexpected. She trusts that hidden in the hair of the wise woman she may also find pearls and jewels along with the lice and nits, and thus she is capable of seeing them. The precious things in the goddess's hair could symbolize the wealth and happiness that come to us with new creative thoughts and ideas. After a life crisis, she enables us to see with different eyes. In another version this theme is even more dramatically represented: the evil stepmother pokes out the eyes of the good girl. But through her ability to laugh roses and weep pearls—to express genuine feelings—not only does the girl's eyesight return (she is able to see the world in a new way) but through a complex series of events, her bridegroom discovers that she is alive after all and succeeds in seeking his loved one. Inner harmony is found again at the wedding ceremony; following ambivalence and doubt, the opposites unite and complement each other.[9]

In Grimm's version of Frau Holle we do not find a wedding symbolizing this form of completion but rather gold; oftentimes it is represented by a golden star on the girl's forehead. Here again the tale does not refer to actual gold but to inner value, inner wealth. As Ms. Sigrid Schmidt informed me, there is another African version in which the girl receives a child as her reward, which for Africans is often the greatest of gifts. A child also implies that the greatest treasure in a new form of development has come to being. After the abyss, life begins anew.

NOTES

1. Aarne-Thompson classification of folktale and fairy-tale motifs; type 480: the kind and the unkind, the bad and the good girl.
2. Van der Post was able to celebrate his ninetieth birthday on December 12, 1996. He died shortly thereafter. The narration of this fairy tale was his gift to the Jungians in Zürich. The version presented here is from the author's memory of the event. A more extensive version can be found under the title "An African Fairy Tale" in R. Hinshaw, ed., *The Rock Rabbit and the Rainbow: Laurens van der Post among Friends* (Einsiedeln: Daimon Verlag, 1998).
3 *Goldmarie* and *Pechmarie,* roughly translated as "Golden Maria" and "Pech Maria" ("Pitch" or "unlucky" Maria), are the names given to two girls by Ludwig Bechstein, early nineteenth-century German historian and author specializing in folk and fairy tales.
4. For example, "Das Waldhaus" (KHM 169), "Vaters Tochter und Mutters Tochter" (Russian fairy tale 10), or "Der Vampire und das Mädchen" (Macedonian fairy tale 25).
5. For example, "Die zwölf Monate" (Slovakian fairy tale from *Märchenpalast*), "Die zwölf Monate" (Greek fairy tale 20), and "Stiefmutter und Stieftochter" (a Croatian fairy tale).
6. "Die zwai Stiefschweschterli" in C. Englert-Faye, *Das Schweizer Märchenbuch* (Basel: Schweizerische Gesellschaft für Volkskunde, 1941) and "Goldig Bethelie und Harzebabi" in Schweizer Vm. Diederichs 1971.
7. For example, from Burma, "Das Dorf der weissen Krähen," or from Brazil, "Das Mädchen, das Palmöl verkaufte."
8. For example, the Italian fairy tale, "Das Wasser im Körbchen" or number 19,

"Der Hecht" in Italo Calvino, *Märchen aus der Toscana;* also, "Die gelbe Kuh," in U. Balschek-Krawczyk and S. Fruh, eds., *Märchen von Müttern und Töchtern* (Frankfurt am Main: Fischer TB, 1993).

9. "Die neidische Schwester" in Otto Betz, *Vom Schicksal, das sich wendet* (München: Kösel, 1987).

BIBLIOGRAPHY

Birkhäuser-Oeri, Sibylle. *Die Mutter im Märchen.* Stuttgart: Bonz, psychologisch gesehen 28/29 (ohne Jahrzahl).

Bolte, J., and Polivka, G. *Anmerkungen zu den KHM der Brüder Grimm,* vol. 1. Hildesheim: Olms, 1982.

Dieckmann, Hans. *Gelebte Märchen.* Hildesheim: Gerstenberg, 1983.

Drewermann, Eugen. *Frau Holle.* Solothurn: Walter, 1994.

Gobrecht, Barbara. "Mädchen: Das gute und das schlechte M." In *Enzyklopädie des Märchens,* vol. 8. Berlin: de Gruyter.

Hilty, Elisa. *Rotkäppchens Schwester.* Bern: Zytglogge, 1996.

Riedel, Ingrid. *Frau Holle.* Zürich: Kreuz, 1995.

Röth, Dieter. *Kleines Typenverzeichnis der europäischen Zauber- und Novellenmärchen.* Hohengehren, 1998.

Rüttner-Cova, Sonja. *Frau Holle, die gestürzte Göttin.* Basel: Sphinx, 1988.

Scherf, Walter. *Das Märchen Lexikon.* München: C. H. Beck, 1995.

von Beit, H. *Symbolik des Märchens,* vol. 1. Bern: Francke, 1952/1967.

von Franz, Marie-Louise. *Psychologische Märcheninterpretation.* München: Kösel, 1986.

———. *Das Weibliche im Märchen.* Waiblingen-Hohenacker: Bonz, 1994.

———. *Archetypische Dimensionen der Seele.* Einsiedeln: Daimon, 1994.

Wittmann, Ulla. *Ich Narr vergass die Zauberdinge.* Interlaken: Ansata, 1987.

VARIATIONS OF AATH 480 MENTIONED IN THE TEXT

Bechstein, Ludwig. *Märchenbuch.* Leipzig, 1857.

Betz, Otto. *Vom Schicksal, das sich wendet.* München: Kösel, 1987.

Blaschek-Krawczyk, U., and Früh, S., eds. *Märchen von Müttern und Töchtern.* Frankfurt am Main: Fischer TB, 1993.

Bošković-Stulli, M., ed. *Kroatische Volksmärchen.* Düsseldorf, 1975.

Calvino, Italo. *Italienische Märchen.* Zürich: Manesse, 1975.

Diederichs, Ulf, ed. *Der Märchenpalast.* München, 1992.

Englert-Faye, C., ed. *Das Schweizer Märchenbuch.* Basel: Schweizerische Gesellschaft für Volkskunde, 1941.

Esche, A., ed. *Märchen der Völker Burmas.* Wiesbaden: Drei Lilien, 1976.

Eschker, W., ed. *Mazedonische Volksmärchen.* Düsseldorf, 1972.

Hinshaw, R., ed. *The Rock Rabbit and the Rainbow: Laurens van der Post among Friends.* Einsiedeln: Daimon, 1998.

Karlinger, F., and G. de Freitas, eds. *MdW Diederichs: Brasilianische Märchen,* Düsseldorf/ Köln, 1972.

Megas, G. A., ed. *Griechische Volksmärchen.* Köln, 1965.

Olesch, R., ed. *Russische Volksmärchen.* Düsseldorf, 1959.

von Rölleke, H., ed. *KHM (Kinder- und Hausmärchen) der Brüder Grimm,* 3 vols., Stuttgart: Reclam, 1980.

Wildhaber, R., and L. Uffer, eds. *Schweizer Volksmärchen.* Düsseldorf, 1971.

Reflections on the "Philosophy" of Marie-Louise von Franz

LUIGI AURIGEMMA

My work in analysis with M.-L. von Franz, which lasted for more than twenty years, naturally influenced every aspect of my life. It could not have been otherwise, for M.-L. von Franz's commitment to those persons who worked with her to untangle the knots in their lives was quite profound, and no aspect of the analysand's personality escaped immersion in the analytical bath that was to reveal the hidden moving forces of his existence. My encounter with M.-L. von Franz was decisive, there where my inner vocation led me to ponder the fundamental questions of the meaning of my life, and of my destiny in death. Of course, I am aware that every thinking human being asks himself these questions at one time or another. But there are some for whom arriving at an answer is of prime importance, or if you will, is the pivotal point of a life. This has been the case for me, and M.-L. von Franz accompanied my questioning and helped me find my answer. Naturally, these questions concerning meaning have always been interwoven with life's events, with the problems of personality and of the capacity for familial and social integration. In this long joint endeavor, I also encountered her own convictions and her deepest certainties, those which inspired her activity as a therapist and her research in areas where, thanks to her vast erudition and her critical acuteness, she made remarkable contributions to analytical psychology. The close proximity in which we worked enables me, I believe, to try to formulate at least some of the fundamental aspects of her "philosophy" and to emphasize its originality.

Let us first be very clear about what I mean when I speak of "philosophy," for it is in no way philosophy according to the rigorous rules of logical thought as they exist in philosophical traditions. Rather, M.-L. von Franz had a vision of the world dictated by internal experiences as intense as they were difficult to formulate, such as the Jungian experience of the Self. Indeed, she never publicly stated her ultimate metaphysical convictions, and sometimes she would make the eloquent and familiar gesture of placing a finger before her lips, suggesting that she preferred to remain silent, like Job in the Bible. Yet what I feel warranted to say on the subject, after so many years of interviews with her, will suffice to expose the essential aspects of her vision of life as well as her hypotheses regarding death and the individual's destiny in death.

M.-L. von Franz's conception of analytical psychology is inextricably tied to that of Jung. They met in 1934 when Jung was already nearly sixty years old, and the very young von Franz was only nineteen. Their relationship would always remain that of teacher to student, but von Franz's very early experience of individuation would soon transform it into a collaboration which only death interrupted more than a quarter century later. It was a very productive collaboration and not only in the form of von Franz's direct participation in the elaboration of the material needed by Jung for his studies, in particular concerning alchemy or, in later decades, synchronicity or the qualities of time, or prime numbers. It was also fruitful in her analyses of fairy tales born of the collective unconscious, and in her study of the dreams of the dying. M.-L. von Franz was instrumental in the spreading of Jungian psychology through her very specific gifts of discourse, of the simplification of language, of dream analysis, and through the broadening of its philosophical horizon. Her participation, profound and polymorphous, in the founding and the elaboration of analytical psychology leads us to consider her work as without a doubt the surest and the most direct approach to Jung's often complex and difficult manner of thinking and to recognize her merit in having been able to express its essential aspects with remarkable scholarship and, at the same time, a pronounced sensitivity to the concreteness of the clinical cases she presented in the simplest manner possible. To this must be added, as I have already suggested, that M.-L. von Franz led some of her followers to find within themselves a particularly tranquil vision of death, which is all the more to her credit. Most importantly, she did this not through an appeal to some sort of faith but by reformulating in her own manner Jung's famous "I don't believe, I know"—that is, by taking her convictions as the occurrence of an internal experience of knowledge, eminently intuitive, of course, but not one of faith. And so I shall try to render briefly the main points of her philosophical teachings and the thread of that which she considered to be her reasonable hopes concerning the afterlife.

From the outset, M.-L. von Franz fully shared Jung's view of Kant's theory of knowledge and understood the reasons formulated by Kant regarding the impossibility of knowing the "thing-in-itself," toward which Jung, in turn, maintained a prudent position of scientific empiricism. But von Franz also saw that the hypothesis of a collective unconscious, based on archetypes filling the ego with knowledge, placed Jung in a quite uncomfortable position between, on the one hand, the ontologism of Hindu metaphysics and Western religions toward which this hypothesis pushed him and, on the other hand, Kantian scientific cautiousness which, on the contrary, tempted him to try to submit all forms of ontologism to psychological interpretation.

In my opinion, it was precisely on this important point that M.-L. von Franz showed her profound originality. Indeed, for her, it is possible to go beyond Kant's demonstration of the paralogism of Anselm of Canterbury's ontological argument formulated in the early eleventh century. "By definition," said Anselm, "God is perfect in all ways. He therefore may not be conceived not to exist." But Kant objected that we may not deduce God's existence from the fact that we can form the idea of His existence, and Jung agreed with Kant. As for M.-L. von Franz, she went further and returned to the core of Anselm's argument, upstream from the point from which Kant had demonstrated its shortcomings. Because, said she, the *Being of Consciousness,* the God of whom Anselm speaks, is not proven by the *intellect* of a subject imprisoned in the duality imposed by the natural world, as Kant had implied, but is experienced within the deepest reaches of psychic reality, it is the very *experience of the Self,* of atman, which *encompasses* the ego in its duality and of which it is the very substance. The subjective moment of consciousness is undeniably real, and consciousness is the alchemists' "stone that is no stone," this image precisely by which they sought to express the undeniable reality of *consciousness which perceives that it is,* that it is *conscious knowingness,* within life but other than life. It is indeed of prime importance to surpass all *Ichhaftigkeit,* all "ego stickiness," for it is only in this way that the subjective side of consciousness that notes its own being is quite *other* than the faculties of human ego, for the most part ephemeral. The veritable individuality which the ontological argument implies as real is in the Self, in atman, and the human ego is its fleeting manifestation in this life. As psychological analysis shows, the confines of ego, the confines of the concrete psyche, are mobile, and analysis provokes continuous displacements as it progressively resolves its conflicts. These reflections lead us to see that prior to the concrete functioning of the ego, it is divine consciousness which, through the infinite succession of its manifestations that tear away more and more profoundly the veil of unconsciousness, becomes ever more conscious of what it is, *absolute knowingness, objectless.* As M.-L. von Franz put it succinctly: "God is Consciousness, with no discursive content."

In these few sentences, I believe that I have expressed the myth of M.-L. von Franz, taking the word *myth* in the compelling sense given to it by Jung of a collective *imaginatio vera* dwelling in the roots of humankind. In a certain way, it is the very ancient myth of final, total liberation, that is, of consciousness being freed from the limits of unconsciousness via the infinite history of nature, *filia Dei.* It is a myth that M.-L. von Franz, and Jung before her, saw as the expression of a "well-founded hope," a means for having recourse to mythopoetic imagination, there where knowledge fails utterly. Indeed, the reality of limits regarding divine consciousness was for von Franz, as it had been for Jung, a deep mystery, the deepest of all. How can one allow for divine imperfection? "And yet," she would say, "when one sees and seeks to understand the reality of all of nature's ardent aspirations towards greater consciousness, the hypothesis of an original and mysterious Unconsciousness *makes much more sense* than the idea of a divine perfection expressing itself in such an imperfect creation." And she added that it is precisely the recognition of the presence of limits at the very roots of creation that gives birth to Jung's idea of a process of evolution whose aim is the reduction of these limits with the hope of eliminating them and of his idea of the expenditures of energy necessary to arrive at the light of consciousness as unique reality. This natural process has led, to the present, in this world, to human life. M.-L. von Franz thought that for every individual soul, this process would continue and reach ever more deeply, through a succession of lives, or to put it more accurately, through innumerable manifestations, and lead to plentitude, to full realization of the conscious Self.

Within this myth, two particularly important points should be emphasized. The first one is the specific angle from which M.-L. von Franz considered psychotherapy. Quite naturally, she considered it foremost as an activity of redress, of reparation, of the lightening of complexes and imbalances, be they from birth or the result of life's traumas or shocks. Yet, at least in the cases of a certain elite, psychological analysis, for von Franz, could lead the process of individuation well beyond that of reparation of weaknesses and shortcomings, to a path of deeper philosophical comprehension, liberating the psyche from its dependence on drive imbalances and the limits of life, leading it to the realization that it does not expire in life, that it is not life alone. Jung expressed the possibility of such an elevated outcome of the process of individuation, affirming that the world of our habitual reality of duality helps us to understand the limitless, by the very fact that through our perception of its limits, it incites a nostalgia for the limitless. It is, for example, in this way that death may be felt not as an *end*, but also as a *goal*, in that it shows the limits of life and thus helps us to understand, to elicit a perception of eternity.

The second point is to remark on the particular light in which

M.-L. von Franz considered the destiny of the individual. Indeed, she rethought and deepened Jung's reflections which perceived subjectivity as an essential part of consciousness. "The Ego is also the Self," she would say, simplifying her thought to an extreme, thereby expressing precisely the *reality* of the ego. Indeed, by stressing the reality of the subject in atman, in the Self, Jung had stressed the closeness between the Self and Taoism's golden flower. And this confirmed his conviction that the moments in which the psyche is most open to the Self, most conscious of the Self, *are timeless,* and that consequently the individual psyche can escape the limits of life and of death and go beyond them in some way incomprehensible to us. Jung expressed these convictions in private and shared them with his closest followers. But in the end, they remain like the golden bird in the wooden cage of an old fairy tale von Franz analyzed; that is, at the very limits of what can be understood.

M.-L. von Franz was every bit as careful in her publications. But in interviews, she was freer in expressing her convictions, sustained as they were by her solid and logical mind, far from the reassuring illusions and naiveties of traditional religious beliefs. As was her habit, she used simple language, direct and rich in images that covered her reflections and her most serious convictions: "In death, I shall join all of my other selves." Or, "In death, we shall have eternity and ubiquity." Yet if she often repeated that "something must remain after death," she was quick to add, "but it is so difficult to figure out!" For she was well aware of all of the dangers of anthropomorphism. In fact, beyond all of her familiar and simplifying expressions, she sought to express her most profound inner certainties, that is, that "something" of an individual consciousness *remains* after death *insofar as,* during life, this consciousness expanded its *state of awareness* and deepened it, "compressing" itself throughout its manifestations until the end of time while maintaining its *unique singularity* that, in life as we know it, is carried by individual egos. She lived, in this manner, her profound religiousness; her sense of the divine, which was constantly present and needed no institutional frame, expressed itself rather in the wonder and the joy she felt as she listened to a dream or other message arising from the unconscious depths of her analysand. All of her followers with whom she shared these convictions most certainly drew from them a broader vision of their personal destiny, greater courage in the face of life's difficulties and of their own death, a heightened sense of responsibility, as well as the joy of feeling within themselves, at least in moments of grace, the *certainty of a reality of consciousness unlimited by space and time, thus rooted in eternity.*

M.-L. von Franz held these convictions until the end of her life, exposing them again in 1984 in her work *On Dreams and Death: A Jungian Interpretation* (1986, 1998), which was her final attempt to express her idea of a "purified Ego"—Jung had spoken of a "superior Ego"—underlying the fleeting ego of this life, and which, in a manner and to an extent we cannot know, *remains* beyond death, manifesting itself in time and in space in other forms, ever more differentiated and ever more conscious.

In these notes, I have tried to summarize the main intuitions and reflections of M.-L. von Franz regarding life and man's ultimate destiny in death. These intuitions and reflections, we must remember, were in no way mere personal speculations but rather were nourished and verified by a daily rapport with deep interior sources, that is, her own dreams and those of others or by other manifestations of the unconscious such as phenomena of synchronicity and other equally irrational means and ways. These few notes also show the great seriousness of a life lived totally in the new world of analytical psychology and stress both the high level of her scientific creativity and her devotion to her patients, her capacity for compassion for their suffering, as well as her art of interpreting the language of the unconscious. This art was greatly enhanced by her innate gift of intuition but also by the richness of all of the references coming from her vast knowledge of the contents of the collective unconscious.

All of this would be enough to make M.-L. von Franz an exceptional scientific figure, and yet she was much more than this. It is with this "much more" that I would like to conclude these pages, in grateful recognition. Indeed, for those who were lucky enough to work with her, M.-L. von Franz was a guide, a reassuring companion, passionate and yet balanced, often gay and sometimes even funny, patient and relentlessly positive. For these reasons and more, she was a beautiful example of humanity and remains quite alive in each of us as an essential part of himself.

Individuation in the Spirit of Love

DIETER BAUMANN

To begin with, I would like to thank Dr. Emmanuel ("Manolis") Kennedy-Xypolitas for his invitation to write a contribution in honor of Marie-Louise von Franz.[1] More than five years have gone by since her death. At her funeral, Dr. Anne Maguire delivered her "valedictory address" by which she bade farewell to the deceased whom we had just lost, and in which she expressed in warm and profound words the feelings and thoughts this loss had left her with. In doing so, I dare say she spoke not only out of her own heart, but also out of the hearts of many of us; certainly out of mine.

The designation "valedictory address" chosen by Dr. Maguire, a word that until then I had never heard before, somehow struck me and remained in my memory. "Vale" means "fare thee well" and used to be put at the end of a letter addressed to a friend when Latin was still the international language between educated people. If I am not mistaken, "vale" means "stay in good health," "thrive," "prosper." Bidding farewell to a deceased person seems to me, therefore, to have a double meaning. On one hand, one wishes her good luck for her voyage into the mystery of the unknown beyond. The gifts the Egyptians used to present to the dead to accompany and sustain them on their journey are an example of this. On the other hand, accepting, alone and in company of others, the sadness about a beloved person who has died, bewailing her by celebrating her memory, will also have an effect on the mourner. If the person who departed from one has dedicated her life to her *individuation in the spirit of love,* the mourner will be encouraged in his decision and effort to assume the same task in his own stead. His mourning will acquire a positive meaning that will cheer him up in his own enterprise.

Marie-Louise von Franz herself is an example in case. Her faithfulness to C. G. Jung, during his life and after, enabled her to carry on his opus, not by imitating it, but by dedicating herself to her own creativity in a spirit akin to, and shared with, him. Thereby, she also gave strength to the hidden or invisible church, an expression, she told me, chosen by St. Augustine to account for the kinship a human being who is dedicated to the relation with the Self feels when he or she meets a person who does the same in his or her own life. The feeling of relatedness goes beyond any outer label, such as for instance "Jungian."[2] It seems to me that we are here in the presence of two paradoxes: one being the fact that if somebody is really himself he is really "social," i.e. in relation with the community (rather than somebody who just wants to play a role); the other, that linkage and faithfulness to another being does not block one's independence, on the contrary. Quite unjustly, Marie-Louise von Franz was sometimes misunderstood, or even accused of, being an "orthodox Jungian." "Orthodox" means "with the right opinion or belief." How is such a "right opinion," let alone "right belief," at all possible, if we know that everything is an unfathomable mystery? Jung was a searcher, an explorer, a seeker and finder whose endeavor it was to formulate as accurately as possible what he discovered on the way of his life, in order to communicate it to, and share it with, his prospective reader. But as far as I can tell, he never allowed himself to become infatuated with what he had discovered, nor to succumb to the temptation to transform it into a closed scientific system. Others have tried to do so and have missed the point. For C. G. Jung went on wondering all his life. In no way did

Marie-Louise von Franz transform his discoveries and descriptions into a dogma, but, so it seems to me, she went on searching on her own, in her own creative way, thereby allowing what Jung had discovered as buds to blossom into flowers, which in turn have become fruits and new seeds. Jung's work can be compared with a growing tree, or with the growing branch of a tree: a sort of genealogical tree of the spirit of mankind, which is also a tree of knowledge, the objective knowledge granted to us by the Unconscious. In my opinion it is C. G. Jung's invaluable merit, as well as Marie-Louise von Franz's, to have opened for us the access to the objective knowledge of the psyche by translating most important elements of it to us in terms of our age.

Thus when Emmanuel ("Manolis") Kennedy asked me for a contribution to this book in remembrance of, and honor to, Marie-Louise von Franz, his request was for something personal, if possible. At first I felt embarrassed and at a loss. This feeling hasn't left me since. All that really matters was, and still is, of such a personal nature that it needs to be protected by silence. Therefore, the considerations which I should like to share with the reader will of necessity be more allusive than revealing.

My gratitude to Marie-Louise von Franz implies, among many other aspects, the fact that she, like C. G. Jung, had a deep respect for the secrets I told her, as well as for those I did not. She herself expressed[3] that to a true relation belongs the respect for the other being's difference, including what you cannot understand in him, instead of labeling it with psychological "explanations," often for classifying purposes which disregard the individuality of an individual.

This attitude seems to me to be an expression of the mystery of Eros, on which the feeling of tact is based. There are things that can only grow and eventually blossom under the veil of silence and the seal of secrecy, lest they be nipped in the bud. As the *Turba philosophorum* puts it: *Et vas fortiter cooperite, ne flos fugiat* ("and close the vase [i.e., the retort] well, so that the flower cannot escape"). In my younger years I was sometimes, in a naïve way, not secretive enough, a lesson of patience I had to learn since, and am still learning. It can happen that a person inadvertently tells you a secret which he should keep to himself inside. I mean the very things of the kind that C. G. Jung could only write in his *Memories, Dreams, Reflections* after having promised, and seen to it, that they be published only after his death. For they probably belonged to his myth.

If, then, such an unwitting disclosure happens—for instance, in an analytic situation—a lot depends on the attitude and the awareness of the listener to whom the person entrusts his secret. Since the communication comes from the depths, the listener may become fascinated and curious. This can be extremely dangerous, as for instance in certain "group" psychologies and events, especially if there is little or no respect for a person's inner life; the participants may even be encouraged, or encourage themselves mutually, to betray their innermost secrets, as if they were for public use. If there is but little awareness of this problem, or even none at all, and if there is no distinction between the things that can be told and those that cannot, the result is often a psychological strip tease with disastrous consequences, such as a real loss of soul. If, however, the listener has also an inner life and is in a conscious and committed relation with his own center, he will react adequately—i.e., with bashfulness and respect, or even forget what has been told to him. This kind of oblivion seems to be an instinctive reaction from nature, protective for both persons. One may even have to go so far as to pretend not to have noticed the *tremendum* of the revelation. It seems to me that this is expressed in many legends and fairy tales, in which certain questions may absolutely not be asked, for instance about the origin of one's mate, especially if he or she is of a suprahuman origin (above in heaven or in the depths of the water or below in the earth) and has a numinous character.

I am grateful to Marie-Louise von Franz for having granted to me this respectful and related attitude. I dare say it was possible because she was fully dedicated to her own creative process of individuation.

In a sense, creativity is the endeavor to disclose and to hide the secret at the same time, by giving it a more general form that enables one to express it indirectly, by way of similes, amplifications, and the like: *ignotum per ignotius,* as the alchemists would say, in C. G. Jung's observation, i.e., expressing "the unknown through the (still) more unknown." The more unknown, paradoxically, is an explanation, or revelation, or an experience of sudden illumination or enlightenment. Strange as it may appear at first sight, by suggesting still more darkness, the idea that the *ignotius*, "the more unknown," may be an explanation for the *ignotus*, "the (less) unknown," can be a terrible disappointment for an ego who has the idea that understanding something means possessing it with or through the intellect. But if the ego, with its limited consciousness, experience and knowledge, is aware of that limitation and of being part of an unfathomable, limitless[4] and ineffable whole which is at the same time the center of the psyche,[5] it may be an experience of revelation of this mystery of the whole through the channel of the *ignotius*, "the more unknown," by which a piece of the objective psyche may be transmitted to the ego as such, as a whole, and not only to its intellect or any other partial aspect of it.

Marie-Louise von Franz, quoting Jung, if I remember well, once said to me that the introverted person can only enter into a true relation with other people via the *détour* of doing creative work. By her example and her heartening trust, she encouraged me to do so. With her, this respect and esteem for the other person's uniqueness was accompanied by a great trust and a warm feeling, which encouraged me to seek and follow my own way through and around the obstacles of life.

These considerations bring me to a very crucial and delicate point. As Marie-Louise von Franz remarked, Logos has more to do with causality, as well as with clearly defined intention and realization of it; conversely, Eros has more to do with the relation with the *unus mundus* and with synchronicity—where two or more events come together and thereby enter into a relation with one another—with receiving and bearing, undergoing, rather than being active for a goal to be reached.

The idea of striving towards a goal, as it has been developed in the West, may be symbolized by an arrow. It has created a form of thinking which makes utter precision possible, and given rise to our technological civilization and barbarity. Usually it tries to pinpoint single causes, and (unconsciously and often uncritically) thinks that the secret or the explanation is to be found in the simplest, or possibly the smallest, particle, say of matter or energy, or in one single cause etc. (However, the recent concepts of field, potentiality, concomitance etc., come already nearer to synchronicity.)

Naturally, by my school education, I was, with my way of thinking, as biased as most of those who strive for scientific intellectual knowledge. When I had the privilege to hear my grandfather, Carl Gustav Jung, speak about synchronicity at the Psychological Club of Zürich around 1950, his discoveries were most enlightening for me. I also remember the lively part Marie-Louise von Franz took in the discussion, in the course of which the physicist Wolfgang Pauli advocated a common language for both physics and complex (=analytical) psychology.

All this was an almost revolutionary revelation to me. At my young age (in my early twenties), I assumed that to understand something meant to find out its cause and to "possess" it with the intellect, which I also assumed unconsciously to be above life at large. Therefore I found C. G. Jung's method of collecting associations and surrounding, say, a symbol in a dream, with related material from religion and folklore etc., that is to say, with amplifications, on the one hand quite appealing, on the other hand very unsatisfactory for the intellect (in the sense of understanding). However, when later in my life I wanted to understand a dream, a myth etc., I tried, and still do so, to apply this method of amplification. I saw that it helped people, myself included, to understand therewith expressions of the unconscious, and admired C. G. Jung, Marie-Louise von Franz and many others for their wide, deep and pertinent knowledge of the symbols. In the course of time, I observed that certain amplifications act as revelations which make things "click" with understanding in a mysterious way and help to express the meaning of something. This corresponds to explaining *ignotum per ignotius.*

Such an event of sudden understanding is a *cognitio matutina.*[6] At the same time, it is an experience of being linked with, and belonging to, mankind, and of receiving a share of its experience and wisdom, i.e. of partaking of what Jung has called the objective psyche.

Often this happened and was granted to me when Marie-Louise von Franz interpreted one of my dreams and contributed her amplifications to their understanding. Only now do I realize that they were gifts from love, and it dawns upon me that the amplificatory method is an act of generosity of feeling. (I think that a good teacher is one who hands over his knowledge as a gift.) It has do to with Eros, because in it we put things together as gifts.

In this context, it seems to me to be emblematic or significant, that the last lecture Marie-Louise von Franz gave in public bore the title and dealt with: "The Rehabilitation, by C. G. Jung, of the Feeling Function in our civilization."[7] I think this rehabilitation is exactly the thing she did herself. As a student she worked daily four hours, during eight years, so she told me, on a book about fairy tales, which was subsequently published by Hedwig von Beit in three volumes.[8] Although being in her right, she renounced to insist upon being her being mentioned as the main author, or even to file a lawsuit. But that meant facing a possible threat with slander against Jung. He being ill at the time, she wanted to protect him from the trouble and from being hurt, which would probably have resulted. Resigning her right is in my opinion an act of love. Fortunately, she could, later on, draw from this reservoir, in which by her hard work she had accumulated a bulk of knowledge and wisdom—for instance for her many lectures in which she interpreted fairy tales. Those three volumes on the symbolism of fairy tales have remained not only a fountain of references, but above all a *source of wisdom*. No wonder C. G. Jung called her "a little genius," an understatement only he could allow himself to make (personal communication). The interpretation of fairy tales she offers in her lectures are relative to her original work, enriched and enlivened by her subsequent life-experience, including the one she continued to acquire in her work as an analyst.

In her essay about the inferior function, Marie-Louise von Franz relates and explains that you can more or less educate the first three functions of orientation by using your will.[9] The fourth, so-called inferior function (which it is only in as far as its weak and difficult accessibility for the ego is concerned) comes, however, from the unconscious and the Self. One cannot guide it at will, but one has to stoop and bow down to it with a religious attitude, for it is numinous, being closely related to, or even fused with, the unconscious and the Self. Marie-Louise von Franz is herself an example and a model for this attitude: Being a "thinking type," she took the time, the trouble and the pain to bend down towards her feeling and to expose herself to it, to receive the message it conveyed to her. Her works bear witness to this attitude of hers, through which she put her extraordinary, if not to say ingenious, capacity of thinking at the service of feeling. However complicated and subtle her thinking is—if we consider for instance her book *Number and Time*—it never degenerates into mere intellectualism, but vibrates with feeling that comes from the depths. I dare say that it is an expression of the *anima mundi,* by which, as she once put it, we are in relation with mankind and all our fellow creatures, the animals, the plants and all the elements in both their material and spiritual aspects.

Was it this deep feeling of participation which made her say, some months after the Chernobyl catastrophe, that this was the revenge of matter on us for our not considering matter as life?[10] On this occasion I had to admit that I had been thinking till then with the widespread prejudice that life only starts, or should start with, say, the virus, the amoeba, the syncytium, or with organic chemistry.[11] This definition is completely arbitrary, for there is no reason why the revolution of the planets around their sun, or of the electrons around the nucleus of the atom, the sunshine, the flow of water, should not be considered as life. Maybe the shadow of objectivity is to reduce a living being to a thing, with the assumption that things don't live. Maybe that is why in certain situations we prefer to say "cattle" instead of "cows" or "troops" instead of "human beings risking their lives and dying serving as soldiers." In our minds, we bereave individual beings (in an even much larger and more general sense than one limited to just human individuals, for whom, however, these considerations also hold fully) of their right to live by converting them mentally into lifeless "things" or objects. This is already a murder and often used as a pretext for "justifying" killing. Regarding somebody as being just an example of a category has more to do with benumbing and freezing the moral pain inflicted by conscience than with anything else.

So, looking at reality, both with one's eyes and one's heart, is a cross which, so it seems, has to be borne by one whose lot and decision it is to strive after his or her own yet unknown meaning. Bearing the conflict between thinking and feeling is one aspect of this process of individuation and keeps both sides alive, and prevents one from the identification with either. It helps one to become precise and humane. It makes one also think of Marie-Louise von Franz's great love for the animals. She loved them as her friends.

For achieving this paradoxical task through the painful way of her individuation, which is to carry one's own cross, and for helping me, like many people, partake of this task, I feel the deepest gratitude for Marie-Louise von Franz. Considering how much she had to suffer, how bravely she did it, and how gallantly she fought not to be discouraged by it, one should have wished her a more merciful old age. Her love, her work, and her example, along with her deep commitment to the search for meaning, are of such a nature as to encourage the individual on his or her lifelong quest and endeavor to be and become himself or herself. She did it in the spirit of Love.

NOTES

1. As well as for his invaluable patience and sense of humor during the realization of this project. My thanks go also to Dr. David Eldred for his very precious help and his enlightening suggestions.
2. C. G. Jung said once that fortunately he was not a Jungian, but Jung himself! He was not especially fond of people who were just "followers," but was pleased, he told Marie-Louise von Franz, if his work could stimulate somebody else toward his or her own creativity.
3. In her essay and last public lecture on "The Rehabilitation, by C. G. Jung, of the Feeling Function in our Civilization." In *Beiträge zur Jung'schen Psychologie: Festschrift zum 75. Geburtstag von Marie-Louise von Franz.* Edited by José Zavala, Raphael Monzo and Gianni Ruska. Victor Orenga, editor. Valencia, 1990, p. 32. (The lecture is in German.)
4. According to Anaximander, the ´Απειρον (the "limitless," "infinite") is "the root of all beings." Cf. Diels, *Fragmente der Vorsokratiker,* 7th edition (Berlin: Anaximandros, 1954), A9, A10, A13 (*infnitas naturae),* etc. (passim); B1, B2, B3.
5. "Deus est circulus, cuius centrum est ubique, cuius peripheria vero nusquam." Matthias Baumgartner *(Die Philosophie des Alanus de Insulis)* ascribes this sentence to the *liber Hermetis* or *liber Tresmegisti,* Cod. par. 6319 and Cod. Vatic. 3060 (communication from Dr. Emmanuel Kennedy).
6. A term used by St. Augustine and quoted by Jung in his essay on "The Spirit of Mer-

curius" (1948), in *CW,* vol. 13 (Princeton, N.J.: Princeton University Press, 1967), pars. 299ff. The *cognitio matutina* ("morning knowledge") corresponds to the *scientia Creatoris.* The other kind of knowledge or consciousness is the *cognitio vespertina* ("evening knowledge") and corresponds to the *scientia creaturae.* As St. Augustine (*The City of God,* XI, vii) puts it: "For the knowledge of the creature, in comparison with the knowledge of the Creator, is but a twilight; and so it dawns and breaks into morning when the creature is drawn to the love and praise of the Creator. Nor is it even darkened, save when the Creator is abandoned by the love of the creature." C. G. Jung (ibid., par. 299n): "If we equate *cognitio* with consciousness, then Augustine's thought would suggest that the merely human and natural consciousness gradually darkens, as at nightfall. But just as evening gives birth to morning, so from the darkness arises a new light, the *stella matutina,* which is at once the evening and the morning star—Lucifer, the light-bringer." It seems that the *cognitio matutina* means the experience of knowledge and understanding in the blessed moment it happens; whereas the *cognitio vespertina* is the result of imitation, repetition, dogmatization, conceptualization, polishing etc., until it has become a mere formula which is used by man as if he were its Creator. C. G. Jung (ibid., par. 304): "It seems to me that Augustine apprehended a great truth, namely that every spiritual truth gradually turns into something material, becoming no more than a tool in the hand of man. In consequence, man can hardly avoid seeing himself as a knower, yes, as a creator, with boundless possibilities at his command. The alchemist was basically this sort of a person, but less so than modern man. An alchemist could still pray: 'Purge the horrible darkness of our mind' *(horridas nostrae mentis purga tenebras)* but modern man is already so darkened that nothing beyond the light of his own intellect illuminates his world." "Occasus Christi, passio Christi." That is surely why such strange things are happening to our much lauded civilization, more like a *Götterdämmerung* (= twilight of the gods) than any normal twilight."

7. Published in J. F. Zavala, G. Ruska, and R. Monzo, eds., *Beiträge zur Jung'schen Pyschologie. Festschrift zum 75. Geburtstag von Marie-Louise von Franz* [Contributions to Jungian Psychology. Festschrift for the 75th Birthday of Marie-Louise von Franz] (Valencia: Victor Orenga, Editores, S.L., 1980).
8. Personal communication. See Hedwig von Beit, *Symbolik des Märchens,* vol. 1; *Gegensatz und Erneurung im Märchen,* vol. 2; *Index,* vol. 3 (Bern: Franke Verlag, 1986).
9. Cf. James Hillman/Marie-Louise von Franz: *Lectures on Jung's Typology* (Texas: Spring Publications, 1971).
10. In a meeting arranged by Ruth and Gianni Ruska in the summer of 1986 at the Hotel Sonne in Küsnacht, with Marie-Louise von Franz and the Tai-chi master Chungliang Al Huang as special guests, to discuss with a group of privileged friends.
11. Syncytium: a multinucleate mass of protoplasm resulting from a fusion of cells.

Reflections on von Franz's Work with Number Archetypes

CHARLES R. CARD

Marie-Louise von Franz has traced the beginning of her involvement with number archetypes to a day about two years before the death of C. G. Jung when he handed her a small slip of paper upon which he had begun to gather notes about the mathematical characteristics of the first five integers. He said to her, "I am too old to be able to write this now, so I hand it over to you."[1] At the time she did not know whether he intended for her to pursue his study of number archetypes, or if he simply wanted her to hand it over to someone whom she might meet that would be suitable for such a project. After Jung's death she preferred to assume the latter because she felt incapable of doing it herself. However, as a long interval passed without the appearance of anyone to take up the task, she was "bitten" by her conscience and subsequently entered into a long and intensive period of research and writing that culminated in the publication in 1970 of her treatise on number archetypes, *Zahl und Zeit* (*Number and Time*).

As indicated by the subtitle of this work—"Reflections Leading toward a Unification of Depth Psychology and Physics"—von Franz's intention with *Number and Time* was to continue to explore the ideas that had grown out of the collaboration of Jung with the Nobel laureate quantum physicist, Wolfgang Pauli. Von Franz was, despite her reticence, well positioned to take on this task, for she had worked closely with both Jung and Pauli during the decade of their collaboration—helping each by translating passages from alchemical texts and working with Pauli to explore the symbolism of his dreams and visions that were related to his intellectual quest. In the course of this collaboration, which in its most active phase spanned the years from 1946 to 1954, Jung and Pauli arrived at a set of propositions about the nature of reality that mark a fundamental departure from the tenets of the worldview of modern science that has prevailed since Descartes. Jung and Pauli came to hold that the realm of mind, *psyche,* and the realm of matter, *physis,* are complementary aspects of the same transcendental reality, the *unus mundus.* They held that archetypes act as the fundamental patterns of behavior whose various representations characterize all processes, whether mental or physical. In the realm of *psyche,* archetypes organize images and ideas; in the realm of *physis,* they organize the structure and transformations of matter and energy and account for acausal orderedness, as well. Furthermore, archetypes acting simultaneously in the realms of both *psyche* and *physis* were held to account for instances of synchronistic phenomena. From this perspective, Pauli advanced the possibility of the development of a "psycho-physically neutral" language based on archetypal representations and made an attempt to formulate a lexicon for such a language.

Jung and Pauli were not able to advance further beyond the hypothesis comprised of these bold propositions. In two letters written by Jung to Pauli in May and October of 1953, Jung expressed his interest in pursuing the archetypal nature of simple whole numbers. To Pauli he explained that,

> My dreams and my intuition have both referred me to natural numbers. . . . I therefore believe that from the psychological point of view at

> least, the sought-after borderland between physics and psychology lies in the secret of the number. . . . Thus, I believe that there is more to be gained by examining more closely what the two fields have in common, and it seems to me that it is here that the mysterious nature of numbers is the most obvious thing for forming a foundation for both physics and psychology.[2]

Jung hoped that he could spark an interest in Pauli to take up the investigation of number archetypes, but Pauli was not inclined to do this. In a letter written by Pauli to Jung in late December of 1953, he asked to postpone his response to Jung with regard to number archetypes.[3] In fact, Pauli never did correspond further with Jung about number archetypes. However, Pauli did formulate a partial response to Jung in his essay, "Naturwissenschaftliche und erkenntnistheoretische Aspekte der Ideen vom Unbewussten," written in celebration of Jung's eightieth birthday, where he expressed his interest in exploring the archetypal ideas that form the basis of mathematics, particularly the idea in arithmetic of an infinite series of integers and the idea in geometry of the continuum. By late 1954, with what were to be only a few years remaining in each man's life, the collaboration of Jung and Pauli effectively came to an end.

Starting from Jung's initial hints, von Franz investigated number archetypes as dynamical ordering factors active both in psyche and in matter. In *Number and Time*, she examined aspects of number and numeration drawn from a wide variety of cultures both ancient and modern, primitive and technologically advanced. She discussed in particular detail the qualitative aspects of the structure of the number archetypes that give rise to the first four integers. As well, she investigated the dynamical aspects of the number archetypes and their relationship to physical and psychic energy, and she discussed historical and mathematical models of the *unus mundus* and the role of number archetypes in synchronistic phenomena.

From her investigation of number archetypes, von Franz concluded that the primarily collective quantitative aspects of number that preoccupy Western number theory are complemented by individual qualitative aspects. To illustrate these aspects of number, she cited examples of the treatment of numbers in ancient Chinese number systems and concluded that the Chinese did not use numbers as quantitative sets but as emblems or symbols: "Numbers thus serve chiefly to make visible the circumstantial individual aspects of the cosmic unity or whole."[4] Chinese numbers also contained an essential relation with time: "In China, numbers signify organizations which vary in time, or transient 'ensembles' of inner and outer factors within the world-totality."[5]

Common to both Western and ancient Chinese approaches to numbers, however, is the use of numbers in establishing regularity and order. Jung had stated that "[number] may well be the most primitive element of order in the human mind . . . thus we define number psychologically as an archetype of order which has become conscious."[6] As with all archetypes, the number archetypes have an inherent dynamical quality—that is, they represent abstract patterns of rhythmical behavior. Von Franz held that:

> The archetypes primarily represent dynamical units of psychic energy. In preconscious processes they assimilate representational material originating in the phenomenal world to specific images and models, so that they become introspectively perceptible as "psychic" happenings.[7]

In *Number and Time,* the *quaternio* of archetypes that underlie the first four integers are discussed in particular detail. Summarizing their archetypal behavior, von Franz explained that,

> Numbers then become typical psychological patterns of motion about which we can make the following statements: One comprises wholeness, two divides, repeats and engenders symmetries, three centers the symmetries and initiates linear succession, four acts as a stabilizer by turning back to the one as well as bringing forth observables by creating boundaries, and so on.[8]

Von Franz postulated that representations of this *quaternio* provide the dynamical patterns that underlie all processes of perception and symbol formation in the psyche and account for the structure and transformation of matter and energy in the physical world:

> Natural numbers appear to represent the typical universally recurring, common motion patterns of both psychic and physical energy. Because these motion patterns (numbers) are identical for both forms of energy, the human mind can, on the whole, grasp the phenomena of the outer world. This means that the motion patterns engender "thought and structure models" in man's psyche, which can be applied to physical phenomena and achieve relative congruence. The existence of such numerical nature constants in the outer world, on the one hand, and in the preconscious psyche, on the other (e.g., in the quaternary structures of the "psychic center," the triadic structure of dynamic processes, the dualistic structure of threshold phenomena, and so forth) is probably what finally makes all conscious knowledge of nature possible.[9]

The dynamical behavior of the number archetypes, in particular the *quaternio,* is thus held to characterize all physical processes and all mental acts of perception and symbolic representation. Thus, the number archetypes are thought to be universal aspects of symbol formation. Consequently, as von Franz has pointed out, the number archetypes should provide the means to construct what Pauli had called a language that is "neutral" with respect to psycho-physical distinction. Such a language, as yet undeveloped, would offer an archetypally invariant basis upon which representations of all physical and mental processes could be established.

The cluster of propositions that grew out of the collaboration of Jung and Pauli constituted a hypothesis about the role of archetypes in the structuring of reality. Through her research into number archetypes, von Franz has significantly clarified and extended the archetypal hypothesis of Jung and Pauli such that it may be restated as follows:

> All mental and physical phenomena are complementary aspects of the same unitary, transcendental reality. At the basis of all physical and mental phenomena there exist certain fundamental dynamical forms or pat-

> terns of behavior called number archetypes. Any specific process, physical or mental, is a particular representation of certain of these archetypes. In particular, the number archetypes provide the basis for all possible symbolic expression. Therefore, it is possible that a psycho-physically neutral language constructed from abstract symbolic representations of the number archetypes may provide highly unified, although not unique, descriptions of all mental or physical phenomena.

Von Franz was not satisfied with *Number and Time;* she called it "a rather unreadable book" and regretted that it had failed to communicate and provoke discussion of its central tenets among mathematicians and physicists. With it, she had tried to take Jung's initial hints somewhat further and to show that a "real, absolute isomorphism is present" between representations of the number archetypes as they appear in the psyche and in the physical world. She said, "I was able to take this up to the number four. Then it became too complicated, and at that point I also hit my head on the ceiling," just as Jung, too, had hit his head on the ceiling prior to turning the project over to her.[10]

Number and Time unquestionably leads the reader through forbidding terrain; it assumes extensive knowledge of Jungian psychology, as well as knowledge of major developments and issues in twentieth-century physics and mathematics. It is an attempt to create a discourse between the areas of depth psychology and physics, with the intent of working toward their ultimate unification—a task that can only be seen as Herculean. Presently there are two factors that have helped to improve the accessibility of *Number and Time.* The first is the publication in 1992 of von Franz's *Psyche and Matter*, a collection of twelve of her essays and lectures which clarify and amplify much of the content of *Number and Time* and as such comprises a suitable companion volume to it. The second factor is the emergence in the past two decades of a growing interest in the collaboration of Jung and Pauli, including the publication of their correspondence and much valuable secondary source material. From the vantage point offered by these works, it is now possible to reassess the importance of *Number and Time.* By developing and refining the central ideas of the Jung-Pauli collaboration, it points, through its examination of the number archetypes, to the possibility of finding a way by which Pauli's psycho-physically neutral language might be obtained. Should this be achieved, it could become the means for the development of a post-Cartesian archetypal science in which a unified inquiry into the nature of mind and matter could take place. If this is so, then von Franz's most obscure work would easily become her most important.

I first encountered Marie-Louise von Franz's work in 1974 when, during a period of convalescence with a hip broken by a bad fall, I read her essay "Science and the Unconscious," the conclusion to *Man and His Symbols.* Apart from Jung himself, no one has had a greater influence on the reshaping of my view of the world than Marie-Louise von Franz.

I did not discover *Number and Time* until 1979, when, as sometimes happens, the book literally jumped from the library shelf to my hand. It took two years and three readings before I felt that I understood what she had written. Shortly afterward I began to gather my thoughts in the form of an essay that I entitled, "An Inquiry into the Role of Archetypes in Physics." In September 1985, with considerable temerity, I decided to send a draft of the essay to von Franz. A few months later I received a reply that astounded me! In a short letter dated December 10, 1985, von Franz wrote, "I have now read your inquiry into the role of Archetypes and it gave me great pleasure. Actually, it is the very first paper which gives a really intelligent reaction to my Number book. Nobody noticed that I am proposing a new paradigma."

Prior to my contact with von Franz in 1985, I had felt quite alone with these strange, wonderous ideas that left me to suspect that perhaps I was howling at the moon. Von Franz's assurance that I had understood her correctly was immensely encouraging to me. Then, in the months and years that followed, there began to appear works by other physicists—David Peat, Kalvero Laurikainen, Charles Enz, Hans Primas, Herbert van Erkelens, and others—that explored synchronicity, acausal orderedness, quantum nonlocality, Pauli's philosophical thought and his relationship with Jung, and so on, in books, journal articles, and conference proceedings. Happily, this arcane and largely unknown area of thought was being opened for a wider public discussion.

I met with Marie-Louise von Franz only once. On August 5, 1992, while on the way to a conference at Helsinki that concerned Pauli's philosophical thought, I was able to spend an hour with her at her summer residence at Bollingen. We sat by the hearth of a large stone fireplace, talking and sharing peach pie and tea. Although necessarily brief, my memories of our visit remain vivid.

In the months that followed my visit with von Franz, I had several dreams that I sent to her. In the first, which was dreamed shortly after I had completed the final published version of my Helsinki paper, I experienced childbirth. The labor comes upon me suddenly; I move to a squatting position, and my field of view is simply a clean expanse of red linoleum floor. After some contractions, the baby emerges without difficulty, and it and I are healthy and at peace.

In the second dream, I find myself in the presence of an attractive young woman whom I think I recognize as one of my students. In her care is a beautiful young child. She smiles at me but says nothing. The look on her face, however, implies that this is our child. At first I am shocked and incredulous, but the gentle insistence of her gaze confirms that this is true. During the day following this dream I took a walk at lunchtime to the nearby beach. On the way I began to think about this dream and to actively imagine who this young woman with this baby might be. After a while I came to realize that this young woman with the curly hair and strong full face was Marie-Louise von Franz. Finally, in a brief dream fragment, just before sending these dreams to von Franz, I am given a birth certificate for the baby, as though to authenticate the birth.

At the time of these dreams, I did not know what this child was. Ten years later it is still not clear to me. It is my hope that someday adequate representations of the *quaternio* might be found on which a psychophysically neutral language could be based. Its formulation is a terribly hard problem, because it involves, as Jung put it, "the same 2,000-year-old one: How does one get from Three to Four?"[11] But more than ever, there are hints from disparate fields such as quantum physics, neurophysiology, nonlinear dynamics, and cognitive studies of mathematics that suggest that this approach may be fruitful.

NOTES

1. M.-L. von Franz, *Number and Time* (Evanston, Ill.: Northwestern University Press, 1974), p. ix.
2. C. A.-Meier, ed., *Atom and Archetype: The Pauli/Jung Letters 1932–1958* (Princeton, N.J.: Princeton University Press, 2001), letter 64J.
3. Ibid., letter 66P.
4. Von Franz, *Number and Time,* p. 41.
5. Ibid., pp. 41–2.
6. Ibid., p. 45.
7. Ibid., p. 155.
8. Ibid., p. 74.
9. Ibid., pp. 166–7.
10. M.-L. von Franz, *Psyche and Matter* (Boston: Shambhala, 1992), p. 37.
11. Meier, letter 64J.

Color and the Imagination

FEDERICO DE LUCA COMANDINI

Active imagination is a subtle and difficult aspect of analytical psychology, and one hardly known at all outside of specifically Jungian circles. We could say that in many ways it goes right to the core of the therapeutic project proposed by Jung and takes us well beyond the interpretative stance which the ego generally tends to assume. Active imagination brings us face to face, in a dialogical way, with those important questions and aspects of psychic life that we might say belong to the realm of the spirit. They are questions that take us beyond the disciplines of philosophy or of religion or of psychology itself, questions at times so fundamental as to defy any attempts at locating their exact origin or circumscribing the fields to which they belong. In terms of psychotherapy, this method represents an important resource for dealing with the whole question of the conclusion of analysis, a moment in which the need to establish a link between all that has been acquired and consolidated in the analytical setting as such and a responsible way of dealing with everyday life calls for a very personal resolution. This imaginative method as Jung outlined it fosters a form of independence from analysis itself which naturally can be carried forward as long as analyst and analysand feel the need to further examine and consolidate aspects of the personality. It is a truly original and creative way of facing the thorny question of the resolution of the transference. One is often reluctant to let go of the protected psychic space of the analytical encounter for fear of the routine reality outside, but the use of the imagination suggested by Jung can transform that space into a truly imaginative space, one in which each person feels and is faithful to his or her own personal way of meeting the unconscious. In this way we can indeed go beyond analysis without having to give something up—we can rather be enriched and not sacrifice psyche to our sense of reality.

The whole idea of *cure,* which is of great importance within the context of any emergency situation, is ultimately as psychologically poor as is the medical model itself. Failure to grasp much of the imaginal richness of psychic life is often due to the lamentable and arrogant autoreferentiality of psychotherapy which tends to see everything in terms of the patient/analyst encounter and never tires of applying the "therapeutic metaphor." In this way psychotherapy fails to create anything which goes beyond itself; it forgets that it is after all only the prototype of an *opus* that is more far-reaching and that each individual is called upon to develop. If psychotherapy is not able to see *beyond itself,* then the patient, upon leaving the consulting room for that last time, will be left in the dark. If nothing else, active imagination is a way to continue taking care of oneself.

Naturally, active imagination comes into play at what we might call an advanced phase of analysis, a stage in which any symptoms blocking the freedom of the individual have been removed, where a reasonable level of adaptation to life has been reached, and where the individual has acquired greater consciousness and flexibility in meeting unconscious phenomena. Let us try to imagine such a situation—an analysis that might be defined as "successful." If the individual continues to feel a sort of psychological tension, what sense is there in proposing the same paradigms over and over again? If we presume that the work is finished, then the desire on the part of a patient who wants to continue in his or her psychological search will be seen as a form of neurosis. But perhaps, in such a situation, all we are doing is attributing to the patient a fault which we cannot see in ourselves—if we have nothing else to offer or to propose and hurry him or her out of the consulting room, then it is the patient who risks losing a sense of psyche while the analyst (who may already have lost his!) remains glued to the chair. It is not enough to simply be wiser at the end of an analytical experience, we need to be able to open the way to other goals and perspectives. Jung saw those goals and perspectives in the creative development of one's own symbols, and indeed we ourselves will only be credible and trustworthy to the extent that we attend to this personal creative work of our own.

Now we need to shift our point of view, to move from an analytical (or better, synthetic) standpoint and try to imagine a close encounter between the position of consciousness and the figures and images of the psyche. We need to imagine an intermediate space between consciousness and the unconscious where the task at hand is the elaboration of a personal synthesis that comprises what remains of the will power of a consciousness differentiated by the experience of analysis and what remains of our unconsciousness, something we are rooted in despite all of our efforts, education, and good manners. Jung reminds us that it is ridiculous to think that the *smaller* can somehow contain the *greater*, or that the ego can somehow manage and direct the unconscious. As we all know, the unconscious from the Jungian point of view has a vastness and expansiveness, a collective nature, which cannot be reduced to what has simply been repressed by the individual. If analysis has thoroughly sifted through the complexes of an individual, then he or she will have access to the dimension of the archetypes, to those further possibilities that resonate in the deepest humanity of each one of us. The spirit in which we encounter the unconscious will then be a much different one—it will no longer be a spirit fired by the idea of conquest but rather by the feeling of relationship with that unconscious root that is for every ego, the source of inspiration and instinctual connection with nature itself.

It is interesting to juxtapose for a moment the symbolism of colors, especially as developed by Lüscher, and Jung's vision of psychological types, which provides us with an overview of the main functions of consciousness and the way they are organized in the personality of an individual. The familiar arrangement of these typical modes of operation of consciousness along the four arms of a cross is helpful. What Jung calls the rational functions will be found in opposition to one another at the extremities of one axis while the irrational functions will occupy the ends of the other axis. What Jung suggests here is the existence of four possible ways of functioning for consciousness, but needless to say his is an indication that upon further examination reveals eight or even sixteen modalities.

What Jung terms *rational* functions, that is, thinking and feeling, are mutually exclusive ways of establishing order, of providing a rationale, of ordering reality in a reasonable way and while the former of these (thinking) will make use of concepts and will investigate the meaning of things, the latter (feeling) will be concerned with the question of value and the validity of things, of whether they are acceptable or unacceptable. The *irrational* functions, on the other hand, are concerned with reality as it is or as it presents itself; intuition could be described as the function concerned with possibilities and with the future development of a situation while sensation, linked to the here and now, is concerned with concrete reality.

If we place this vision of psychological functions side by side with the theory of colors, we find that the color blue has many affinities with thinking while red can be seen as the color of feeling. Yellow, which is a quick and solar color and which (as sulfur) expresses the possibility of transformation and future development, can naturally be seen as being related to intuition while green, the color of balance and equilibrium is related to sensation, that is, to the direct perception of things as they are.

The coordinates of active imagination are different insofar as the ego does not identify with any one function to the exclusion of others nor does it utilize any sort of grid in evaluating situations as the theory of colors might do. It operates on a level different from the one where we find the hierarchy of values and colors, different from the one occupied by an ego set on interpreting with the aid of its chosen function(s). As we said before, all of this implies the presence of an ego that has been tested, has shown that it possesses the necessary psychological and analytical capabilities, and has integrated the riches of the work of discrimination and differentiation carried out thus far. This new level is different from the one where the ego is center stage with its aims of expanding and conquering new territory. What comes into play here is a personal and individual level of encounter with the unconscious where an evenly weighted dialogue between the two parts can take place. We might even call it a sort of wakeful dreaming carried out not by just anyone, but by a person who at this point is able to avoid slipping completely into the unconscious. Naturally this calls for a profound trust in one's own inner life—trust that grows out of the interplay of consciousness and the unconscious which together produce a new ethical stance that goes beyond the ethical systems our civilization has to offer and that takes us beyond the various ideologies which claim to interpret the unconscious objectively. These are yet again the pitfalls of a civilization based on ego whereas what the imaginative approach offers is a chance to elaborate a new attitude—one that allows us to continually interpret life with all its problems together with the unconscious. The real "problem" with the unconscious, with the instincts, and with Nature itself is really the problem of finding an agreement, a plane on which both sides can interact in accord.

Let us now look at some examples of active imagination in which color comes into play. The examples I shall cite are relatively simple ones that do not require any further case material or theoretical framework and obviously do not pretend to be exhaustive treatments of the patients' psychological situations. The first example comes from the experiences of a thirty-five-year-old man (whom we shall call S) who has a government position in a department of social services. He had come into analysis because of a disturbing form of anxiety and frequent mood swings. He tended to seek refuge in the use of substances such as alcohol and, at times, cannabis. We might call this tendency to let himself be overwhelmed by the unconscious hysteroid. There did not appear to be, however, anything in the situation that was particularly threatening. In a relatively short period of time the analytical work produced appreciable results—S's symptoms were greatly reduced as his ability to reflect on the causes of his problems increased (his level of social adaptation was already good). Three or four years into the analysis, S had a particularly significant dream: he was in his childhood home together with a young woman of whom he was especially fond. On looking at her face, S was struck by its intense expression and by a ray of green light that emerged from it. The entire atmosphere of the house was different and the dreamer noticed how his parents' bedroom had been modified by the effect of this ray. The doors of the wardrobe and the walls of the room were covered in splendid frescoes of great artistic value which he had never seen before. He was unable to describe the subject of the frescoes in detail but had been struck by images of nature and vegetation motifs.

At that time S was already familiar with active imagination and used it from time to time. But even though this dream possessed a numinous quality, it did not spontaneously lead to an imaginative encounter. The thread of the active imagination continued as before, with meetings and dialogues involving an unknown female figure who was a sort of inspirational muse or anima figure for him. But roughly a year later, S was struck by an intense feeling of loneliness and was no longer able to contact his feminine guide. He began a descent into the dark, accepting what was an unavoidable loss of orientation. The experience was as intense as it was paradoxical for him, for while the feeling of being lost oppressed and worried him, he had no desire to find the way. This loss of orientation had fallen upon him so heavily as to eliminate any impulse on the part of the ego to overcome it. Naturally, a moment of this sort can be dangerous but it was evident that it marked a decisive change in his life. He recognized that acceptance of this state and a serious confrontation with it could be a real initiation experience. In any case, it was clear to him that the situation had to be lived as it was.

What captures our attention in this example is the darkness into which S descends: it is an intense, pulsating darkness, with an unusual aura around it. It is somehow close to a sort of very dark blue with all of the traditional associations that color arouses (deep reflection, depression, and so on). But the characteristics that emerge with the greatest force are the pulsating nature of the darkness and the intense aura surrounding it. During an experience of active imagination, S later found himself in a passageway and even though he was in no hurry to get out of this situation, he slipped through a sort of hatch and ended up in an underground area which was similar to a wide corridor with green walls. A series of impressions rapidly came to him, as though he were in the belly of a ship or in the basement of a hospital, in an operating room or the maternity delivery room. After getting his bearings once again, the faint light enabled him to see a door which he opens. He then finds himself bathed in a strange sort of green light (remember the ray of light from his dream!); this light is almost material and yet there is something about it that cannot be felt. It is as intense and as pulsating as the darkness, but it is light. A number of other things happen during this experience of imagination, including encounters with new figures, but in any case the experience emerged as a watershed compared to what S had experienced previously. He even suspended active imagination completely for some time, as if this intense psychic event had reached a high point and required time to sink in. At the same time, in an almost imperceptible way, a new spirit of initiative was taking shape in S, as if that light had given him a renewed sense of participation in life. S had stopped looking for solutions to the task of living and this gave a new sense and meaning to his actions; S had not actually sought any of this himself.

Unlike the work which is done on dreams, experiences of active imagination recounted in analysis are generally not interpreted by the analyst. All of the conscious and unconscious elements of the personality contribute to the creation of something that is absolutely individual, and any sort of interpretation, even if done with the best of intentions, would be a form of interference. I shall limit myself here to some personal impressions aroused by S's experience. Following his active imagination, he spoke of a feeling of psychic freedom and of a new reason for his actions. He also mentioned a sort of separation and distance from the gut involvement he had always felt in the things around him. Even though S was gifted with an excellent dialectic, he seemed content to accept these sensations without trying to define or explain them any further. S's point of view had gone well beyond the task of adaptation to the world, and through the experience of analysis he was able once again to find a sort of introverted centering—what he was living now was an experience of transcendence that did not imply a renunciation of the world but rather the discovery of a new psychological motivation in what he lived. He was no longer dependent on concrete goals but was wiser and more free—his was the attitude of a consciousness that had been freed from an identification with the ego.

In the months and years to come, S noticed in the context of various forms of imaginative experiences (dreams, active imagination, unusual perceptions connected with synchronistic events) a green light or phenomena closely resembling it. These always coincided with important moments in his life, moments that were in some way transformative, as if the ray of light had left its mark and this mark was the point of reference for the experience of transcendence.

It is interesting to notice that among the various experiences of active imagination that analysands have recounted to me in analysis, there is yet another one which includes the motif of points of light. The patient in question was a woman, L, of about thirty years of age, who was nearing the end of her analysis. She taught music in an important conservatory and was also an accomplished concert performer, known in both national and international circles. The problems that had brought L into analysis had been resolved, and during an experience of active imagination that L was already involved in, she suddenly saw a series of points of light which seemed to indicate a pathway. With a certain amount of trepidation, she let herself be guided and even though she came up against various complications, she continued following these sparks which eventually led her to a tall blazing fire in the midst of a clearing. The fire seemed to be animated by an unusual light similar to a bright shade of red. Yet L emphasized that "that fire could not really be described as being red; it was something that went beyond any other sort of experience." On moving closer to the blaze, L noticed that in the midst of the tongues of fire there was a dancing salamander, an element which was linked to a childhood memory of a story she had been told years before by her father about Benvenuto Cellini and which was emblematic of the suffered and difficult relationship this Renaissance artist had had with his own father. In time, L found herself up against a similar difficulty. Her father complex was indeed the most problematic aspect of her psychological biography and during her analysis it had been amply dealt with; but it was L herself who was able to find the definitive creative resolution to the problem in the wake of the experience of the points of light. I shall say no more about what this creative solution entailed, both out of discretion and in order to respect the agreement reached with L herself. I should rather like to move on to yet another moving story of active imagination before summing up.

V was a thirty-three-year-old man who was blind due to complications connected with the diabetes he had had since infancy. When he came into analysis he had lost his sight five or six years earlier. He was afflicted by a particularly powerful and destructive mother complex that was further complicated by the state of dependence he found himself in. He had isolated himself more and more because of a series of odd restrictions imposed on him, subsequent transgressive behavior and inevitable feelings of guilt. The various rituals surrounding the administration of insulin, attempts to conceal his illness out of shame, and finally his loss of sight had closed him off from others and from the world. Considering the social position of his family, they should have had greater psychological sensitivity and understanding than they did in fact show toward V. When I met him, he was totally enveloped by his mother, who was as generous in nursing him as she was oppressive in managing his life. V had been brought to the brink of desperation by attacks of anxiety related to the fear of impotence on the one hand and compensatory obsessive fantasies on the other. His was a state of enraged passivity, and the inappropriate ways in which his anger tended to explode inevitably backfired on him, making things even worse. What V called his daydreams, that is, his fantasies, were naturally filled with anguish and yet they were a sort of foreshadowing of the resources that he would subsequently discover and develop through active imagination. At this time, these fantasies were compensations enacted by the ego, fantasies of empowerment that grew out of his fears of impotence: he imagined himself a race car driver or a daring airplane pilot. Normally in analysis, such an idealizing use of fantasy needs to be analyzed and overcome, but this delicate situation called for caution since the fantasies acted as the forces which kept a shimmer of vitality alive in V. They were the only thing keeping him afloat, and it would have been wrong to deprive him of them immediately. It was also possible to catch a glimpse here of an aptitude which, aimed in the correct direction, would give V opportunities for development: such an accomplished race car driver would be able to maneuver in a way others would not! During his second year of analysis, V had a dream which struck him considerably.

He was walking along a wall of red brick, and he could see and yet couldn't see, a sort of paradox that appeared often in his dreams (and while I haven't enough case material at hand to be certain of this, I presume this paradox must be a sort of constant in the dreams of people who have lost their sight). In so far as he cannot see, V trips over a man who is lying on the ground and loses his balance. He is about to fall, but the man he tripped over supports him to avoid this from happening. The man, who turns out to be blind as well, but unlike V was born so, then asks V to help him get up. This may have been stimulated by the fact that as one of the results of analysis, V had begun taking part in the activities of an association for the blind; he now had relationships with people sharing his own condition—something he had spurned previously. Now in the dream, V and the other man mutually support one another and continue walking along the wall.

V then carried on with the dream through active imagination. To tell the truth, it was somewhat of a "dare" to suggest active imagination to a person who had not yet worked through many aspects of his psychological situation in analysis, and I didn't know if he would be up to a confrontation with the shadow. At the same time, I felt relatively certain about the quality of the relationship between us (something unknown to him up until that moment in his life) and trusted in the intuition (in the light of the direction the dream seemed to take) that here was an opportunity that needed to be grasped.

Up until then I had simply listened to the fantasies that V recounted and had neither encouraged him nor criticized him. Now I decided to go further and to explain to him the steps which would change and correct the perspective of his approach. V took these suggestions enthusiastically, encouraged by the unexpected interest I was showing in his favorite activity. Following my suggestions, V took the dream as his starting point, and as he gradually found his own individual style, the seriousness with which he proceeded (so different from the bombastic tone of his fantasies) gave me the impression of great genuineness right from the beginning. I prefer not to go into any further detail; suffice it to say that this experience of imagination continued for several months with various additions to the initial theme.

At the beginning, V's attitude toward his partner in the dialogue was one of evident distrust; the response of the man was to joke with V and to prod him ironically into taking a more courageous stance. A sense of humor and of irony were at the same time emerging as powerful characteristics of V's own personality, qualities that previously had been buried beneath the bad-tempered and angry disposition in which he was trapped. What I consider the second phase of this experience is extremely interesting from a psychological point of view. The man who is V's partner in this dialogue and who was, as you will remember, born blind, asks V to describe to him the many forms he has never been able to see. In particular he asks V about colors and wants to know what yellow is, what green is, what red is, and so forth. I can still remember the chills that ran down my spine as I listened, eyes closed, to V recount this experience. And while the definitions that he strove to provide were well-constructed, there was also a definite quality of pathos in them. Just what is color for someone who has never seen it? The other man continued to answer ironically, insisting that something was missing in what V had to say. Little by little, V's distrust turned into a feeling of companionship.

During the third phase of this experience, now that the relationship between V and his dialogue partner was one of free and mutual exchange, the man revealed something to V. The content of his revelation was this: above and beyond all the definitions V might try to provide him with, the one thing that still escaped him was the light, because things have a special aura around them. Those terms *light* and *aura,* which we have already seen in other examples, here reach a level of intensity that is, to say the least, moving. The two continued their conversation, and all of a sudden that wall of red brick, which had previously seemed to be endless, did in fact come to an end and what opened up beyond it was a wide and luminous vista with its own special light. V recounted it with a smile on his face and now for him, too, there seemed to be no words to describe the situation. The analogy with the ray of green light and with the red of the fire is powerful, for also in these cases there was an aura which seemed to be without color and which turned into points of light.

Sadly, V was to die just a few years later, but much of the effort and heaviness he had felt in facing up to life had been alleviated by this experience. His attitude to life changed and little by little he was able to reach out and take the satisfactions that he had deprived himself of before. In a sense, the daring pilot and the race car driver finally had his day! He is very much alive even today in my own feelings.

The wide open perspective of active imagination, as we said earlier, does not lead to the sort of growth the ego can boast about or feel proud of. It sidesteps completely our Western (and Christian) penchant for ethical perfection in the hopes of integrating every manifestation of oneself into the ego. The naïve and arrogant nature of such a project are completely foreign to this approach. What real sense does it make to define ourselves as being rational or irrational, feeling-oriented or thinking-oriented, intuitive, or realistic only then to try to assimilate the opposite in order to be better? With active imagination we approach a level of psychic reality where the opposites "have it out between themselves" as it were, where they self-regulate themselves either through affinity or divergence, and all of this within a confrontation between peers in which the point of view of the ego and the complexes of the unconscious are of equal weight and value. Psychology can thus take us toward a sort of awareness that is far different from the enlightened rationalistic one we have been stuck in for far too long. How can we ever hope, in this world so torn apart and suffering, to find a true spirit of dialogue if we don't envision the possibility of change within the psyche of the individual person? Only those who are able to avoid totally identifying with their own will and desire (without completely renouncing these) will be able to accept as their traveling companion their own personal internal diversity and then recognize and accept, in a balanced way, the diversity of others.

Active imagination does not call for a weak ego, but rather for one which is strong enough to show the determination that a sense of adaptation to reality requires; but at the same time, it calls for an ego that is open and ready to share a sort of common destiny with the figures of the unconscious. These figures, the "twin brothers and sisters" of the figures that fill the dreams we analyze in therapy, will thus be able to actively participate in the elaboration of a wider and more inclusive ethical stance. In the final analysis, what counts is that the "close encounter" of active imagination really take place so that the notion of consciousness that has been handed down to us might open up and accept a dynamic lived out together with the unconscious. This, I think, is what the experience of active imagination can give us, and those who venture into this territory hoping to find something else will no doubt be disappointed. Perhaps it is best to put aside the classifications we are used to using; if active imagination and its new plane in the psychological life of the individual are to be our new point of view on things, then we needn't ask if one is a sensation type, or a feeling, thinking, or intuitive type, just as we needn't ask if things are yellow, red, blue, or green. The colors and the psychological functions that correspond to them are gateways more than anything else. Some people enter by the yellow door, others use the red, blue, or green one, and this gives the life of the individual and the way the ego of that individual has functioned its particular hue. But once we have gone over that threshold, it no longer makes sense to continue doing psychology in those same terms. We might even say that the typology itself and the whole symbolism of the colors do not go beyond that threshold. They will remain useful in the everyday management of our affairs and none of us would want to be without them, but they do not have a place as such within this new psychological habitat. Along the path that takes us beyond the threshold of ego consciousness, a path marked out by the imaginal, what really prevails is the experience of psychic wholeness. Perhaps this is the reason that the stories of active imagination cited above speak of an aura of light that is at the base of every color.

In the context of active imagination, color itself becomes the depository of the light of transcendence. Each color conveys something of what the individual was, something of his or her own style of life and personal story, the way the hues of an old photograph give shading and texture to the image—but now they become aspects of light that indicate and guide us to the transcendent where the oppositions that are the fruit of an identification with the ego can be overcome. In certain moments, our own lives will glow with that special light or aura and the various colors which this will have for each one of us will speak of the specific gateway each of us tended to use, or of the function that tended to predominate in each person's life. Beyond that gateway, none of this matters anymore.

The psychological experience of transcendence allows us to move into another dimension where the color of the personality, like the color of one's skin or one's religious affiliation or cultural background, all give way to a greater reality where the archetypal restlessness of the human spirit encounters the *lumen naturae* so jealously guarded within the psyche.

Marie-Louise von Franz

A Model of Devotion to the Spiritual World

NIKOLAS DORBARAKIS

When I read for the first time in my life Marie-Louise von Franz's books, I was greatly impressed by the emphasis she gave to the inner world. However, that wasn't the only feature in her writings that lured me so much; it was mostly her concise and direct way of conveying her faith in this inner world. At times, certain passages from her books gave me the sense that whatever she described was simply taking action inside me. They gradually aroused my interest in this world on a practical level as well. In due time, I began to contemplate initially about myself and then about the others and ultimately about the world.

Von Franz's clarity and the depth of her writings were even present when she referred to meanings difficult to grasp, which made me think that her mature and terse words regarding grave issues in life stemmed from an intense and experienced way with the magical world of the unconscious.

Through her books, I soon came to realize to what extent we may lose our sense of orientation chasing chimeras, how much we get detached from our inner world when we are confined to the nets of power games that seem to acquire a greater and greater dimension in our contemporary world.

In our days, contemporary man gives all his care to material values; as a result, he has become extremely preoccupied with consuming things, trying, through his increasingly spendthrift habits, to find a deeper meaning in his life. What is more, he is so very much attached to those activities, that is to say, "material values," that in the long run he has come to think that the whole issue of his existence is absolutely and exclusively in relation to his material prosperity. That is always the case with one who has suspended or lost touch with the inner world and the ability to view things symbolically and become connected with his cultural roots. Consequently, the man who has distanced himself so much from those traditional values desperately seeks a value in his life, being nothing else but the emphasis on objects or material values or assuming a domineering position in life in the sense that he seeks to impose his powerful attitudes on others.

In every man's life, the necessity of the existence of values is great, since whatever those values might be, they constitute his visible axis which guides his movements and advances his moral satisfaction along with his status in society. Consequently, his existence acquires the meaning he is looking for, "la raison d'être." However, when those values are exclusively placed upon external objects of natural character or upon conquering a certain social status, then a definite need arises to possess, to show off, or to impose those objects or attitudes as the most important things in one's world. When contact with one's cultural heritage is absent, when communication with the symbolic form of language has been distorted or lost, and when ignorance of the archetypal world prevails, including lack of affinity with the wealth of legends, fairy tales, and mythology, then certainly those values have been projected and placed upon external natural objects or upon acquiring a certain social status; as a result, a whole world, our inner world is underestimated, despised, ignored.

In our contemporary societies, the emphasis is mainly on the conscious aspect of life, and the treasure that is contained in the depth of our existence seems to have been fully ignored. We mainly focus on what seems to be tangible, and in our hard efforts to make it extremely valuable, almost a guide or an image of orientation that will have the power to keep away the lurking chaos, it is being idealized or deified. The center of the conscious part of our life becomes our "ego," and so it instantaneously has been enriched with more value than that which it deserves. It has been idealized, or even deified, making the contemporary extraverted man ambitious and obsessed with material values, extremely selfish, arrogant, and almost identical with the archetype of God, wishing strongly to impose his own thoughts, moods, and attitudes on others without an option, with no alternative, without respecting the will of others with whom he has contact, social or of any other form, regarding in an audacious way the inner world—this archetypal source of wealth—as being material expendable (excrement to avoid, using a more offensive term), which stands as an obstacle in his completion of his egocentric plans.

Attitudes of the kind that ignore the "inner world" and despise nature constitute a grave form of hubris (*ὕβρις*), and they lead to inflation which soon leads to one's fall, as a form of compensation. When the inner world has not been given its due care and attention, then the unconscious intrudes in its efforts to restore things back to normal, that is to say, in the measure of human dimensions. This invasion becomes feasible either through nightmares or psychosomatic symptoms, or weird and unexpected negative forms of behavior, sometimes even through psychotic manifestations. It intrudes dynamically, as it always happens when one shuts the door on something that forms part of his existence. And that should always be there since its presence restores a man's real dimensions, reminding him of what he has left out of his life in his effort to attain perfection instead of integrity. All the above mentioned problems which may arise constitute nothing else but efforts to remind one that he ought to return to his real size and restore a very important aspect of himself. Every effort of that kind seems to manifest an intention of "curing" essentially an abnormal attitude of a man who moves toward one direction only, taking no consideration of the entity of his existence, and even in this weird way, it is leading him to this specific struggle to embrace and include this neglected aspect of himself, which is vital for his completion; the agon (*ἀγών*) itself is his personal human life with a full meaning, his own individuation.

Movements that are characterized by one-sided attitudes, and consequently intense elements of absolute stance, are easily recognized by the emphasis they place on the conscious part of life, on the ego, on matter, ambition, showing off, and power. On the contrary, movements that take into consideration the other side, that is to say, that pay attention to the inner factor, the inner world, the world of the unconscious, shift their center from their ego to the self which functions as a magnet that attracts, gives a sense of orientation, a sense of meaning to every known or unknown element of the total life of a man. And only the fact itself that this new center is being assessed and taken into consideration makes a man stand in awe before God and nature, an unprecedented feeling of satisfaction, certainty, independence, and autonomy, whereas at the same time it fills his heart with optimism, poetry, and respect for his very existence and for the existence of his fellow men. An element of this kind carries all the familiar features of modesty of human measure, of democracy, of brotherhood, and of mental sanity. All these might be love, or perhaps the very essence of it.

Upon reading *Shadow and Evil in Fairy Tales* and *The Feminine in Fairy Tales,* I became conscious of the great emphasis Marie-Louise von Franz laid on the world of fairy tales, in the vivid and terse way she depicted the psychology of the heroes in every fairy tale, giving at the same time lucid interpretations regarding the plot and the actions in every story; her in-depth analysis triggered my mood to deal with and see correspondingly, under a different perspective this time from the one I had so far, Greek mythology, analyzing its main characters through Marie-Louise von Franz's deep analytical angle. By bringing those mythological figures into the proscenium, I longed to see them under the spectrum of analytical psychology, being deeply influenced by her clear and direct way. Since I am Greek myself, Greek mythology was and still remains a challenge for me. Greatly influenced by Marie-Louise von Franz, today, the heroes of mythology, those mythological figures, constitute the main and essential theme of my lectures and my psychotherapeutical sessions with my patients.

Archetypal material is to be found in abundance in Greek mythology, which in its turn directs anyone who decides to delve into it to solutions regarding immediate issues of one's daily life along with issues which contain a higher meaning. Being in touch with mythology inevitably leads one gradually to archetypal issues. Legends, myths, and fairy tales, like dreams, perform an astonishing deed: they reunite man with the deep world of the unconscious, giving him thus the chance to set himself free from his stance in the world of his conscious life and ego.

Greek myths—like all other myths—carry within them archetypal material that expresses a deep and invaluable psychological truth, which can be applied to daily human issues. Any form of touch with the content and the innermost meaning of a myth has a therapeutical value and influence. All those figures who hold the main part in Greek mythology or in the ancient Greek tragedies written so long ago by Euripides, Aeschylus, and Sophocles or in the Homeric epics do exert a cathartic form of influence, under the right spectrum of identification, on human soul. They invariably constitute certain reference points, when one experiences similar conditions, since they have the ability to define somehow through their plot the final outcome.

To illustrate the above mentioned I would simply refer to a woman who, while she has certain capabilities, never resorts to them or exploits them but, for the love of an ambitious man, sacrifices everything for him. She is bound to bear the fate of Medea, the famous witch who possessed the craft of magic and who had excessive power like her aunt Circe; she expended it all on her love for Jason and finally, deeply mortified, she destroyed what they had created together: their children. Correspondingly, one should think of a similar outcome for oneself when, under the state of his lofty aspirations, he neglects the innate and powerful emotions for the sake of his selfish tasks. And that will be the time when that neglected side will become his downfall or will ruin him by invading his life and knocking down everything he has so far built and has been so proud of.

Another case worth mentioning is that of a man who strongly wishes to be in affinity with his soul, in this innermost depth of himself, very close to his faithful Penelope and his Ithaca, in that case one's own anima, and who then ought to know that this will be a difficult journey full of obstacles and winding rough paths. He will have to combat weird and unseen creatures, lust, and lofty aspirations very much like the way his distant ancestor, the shrewd and cunning Odysseus, had to go through. He will be drowned, a total shipwreck, unless he acts with prudence under the vigilant eyes of the goddess of wisdom, Athena; he should also comply with the rules of his unconscious down there in the depths of himself where reigns Poseidon, the god of the sea, who frequently turns it into stormy weather, and rough waves prevail upon this difficult voyage when one ignores his terms.

Aesop's fables are full of animals as the main heroes, those creatures who know nature better than anybody else and guide one who refers to them to contemplate or brood over the issues of his life, providing him with solutions, namely, either what to do or what to avoid.

If one observes carefully the content of the myths or of the fairy tales, one will soon find out that they hide in their plots numerous and great truths which can be fully applied to his daily life, since the issues they tackle are always eternal and up to date. Within man's unconscious, these archetypal ideas are in reality a form, an inherited material, a legacy of models and thoughts. However, contemporary man seems to have lost contact with his inner nature. Myths and fairy tales offer him one more chance to be reunited with it. Decoding their deepest meanings, one can approach the archetypal material and feel its therapeutical value, which is nothing else but one's own awakening and consequently a realization of one's own task and condition. At the same time, they instruct one accordingly and reveal the outcome of one's attitude. Marie-Louise von Franz's work on myths and fairy tales remains invaluable.

Myths reunite man with this deeper world of the collective unconscious, with this priceless wisdom of mankind. And if man can tune in to that inner voice and become aware that he himself simply happens to be the carrier of those messages and their strength and that he is not the one who possesses that manna, then he should be able to reap most of the benefits of the collective unconscious and lead himself to the right path for a real development of his own personality. The meticulous work regarding the interpretation of myths is the means Marie-Louise von Franz employs, in order to initiate us into the deep world of the collective unconscious.

On studying Marie-Louise von Franz's work, I came to a closer understanding of many parts of C. G. Jung's writings, since her comprehensive and lucid way of pinpointing most aspects of his work made me even more sensitive to analytical psychology. In a tangible form I experienced a direct way of explanations that really astonished me and was deeply touching, while at the same time being in personal Jungian analysis under the auspicious eye of her faithful and bosom friend (Emmanuel Kennedy), who also was one of her closest coworkers, I was initiated into the depths of the psychology of the unconscious.

Then it so happened that on a sunny spring evening, I found myself a guest in von Franz's house in Küsnacht. The content of her books and the rumors I had heard about her had turned her figure into a living legend for me. I thought of her as being a wise woman, tall, chubby, kind, respectable, helpful, speaking in a deep voice words of wisdom; a figure that contained a number of elements of the Great Mother.

Full of anxiety, I crossed the threshold of her doorstep. I tried to conceal most of my feelings regarding what was happening around me, a thing which made me feel even more embarrassed. She herself was sitting on a chair situated next to a table with a nice vase full of beautiful colorful flowers. It turned out that she was short and of a thin build. She was dressed in a beautiful blue lady's suit and her gray hair was neatly combed. Behind her glasses, I could observe her eyes, which made me feel that they hid inside them a great deal of knowledge and wisdom. I sat next to her after she had given me a warm welcome. She could sense my embarrassment, and she soon told me in a voice that had nothing to do with what I had so far imagined: "I have heard that you've got your own Bollingen." I was flabbergasted, for she greatly astonished me by starting our communication with this statement. With Bollingen, she designated her own personal space, her tower in the homonymous village in Switzerland. She used to spend lots of time there, getting in touch with her inner world and, as a result, acquiring full consciousness of herself with which she subsequently infused her written work, offering it to us to quench our thirst. With her remark, she stated what was of great importance to her. I automatically thought of C. G. Jung, who felt likewise whenever he was in his tower in Bollingen: "At Bollingen I am in the midst of my true life, I am most deeply myself. . . ." I felt somehow at once in a similar way. And then I viewed my own personal place up the mountain Pindos under a different perspective, as if the place itself had acquired another dimension so far unnoticed by me. It dawned on me then that there I was bound to *create.* This phrase of hers urged me to an even deeper soul-searching and made me pay even more attention to the unconscious, to the "stone." As we were conversing on various issues, suddenly silence prevailed and it lasted for some time. Then Marie-Louise von Franz broke this silence in her smooth voice: "There comes Hermes in this room"! I thought of turning my head round to see who the gentleman with that ancient Greek name was. However, I was so absorbed in our conversation, and mainly in that deep silence, that I completely lacked the energy to do so. At that moment, I sensed in the depths of my soul the presence of Hermes as a thoroughly personal state, the way she did too, a presence rising from a deep human mental communication.

Marie-Louise von Franz's attitude and words made me see simply, on a personal and practical level, the meaning that mythology had in my life and its application to life and human relationships. It is as if everything seems to preexist in the depths of ourselves. Up to a certain measure we are able to feel, we participate in those great events of life which seem to be taking place within us, we become modest silent spectators and abide by the greatness of that inner world, without losing touch with the external one, viewing it under a different angle. This process is therapeutic.

The same atmosphere reigned in my subsequent meetings with Marie-Louise von Franz in her house in Küsnacht and in her tower in Bollingen. Every time I left her venues, I was spellbound and a full man, having fully formed my concept about her existence: she was a simple, an ordinary human being, thoroughly dedicated to "Bollingen," to the inner world, and at the same time a woman showing unparalleled respect to cultural heritage which she seemed to apply everywhere. If respect or allegiance to "Bollingen" and to cultural legacy through the symbolic language defines what we call spirituality, then her contribution to it is beyond assessment. To a simple question of mine, she would often answer by citing a fairy tale or a myth, and then I would have nothing to say. In my silence, I experienced the truth inside me.

If one asked me to describe Marie-Louise von Franz in a few words, I would simply say: "a model of devotion to the spiritual world."

I recall now one of our meetings, as we were conversing on a comment of hers on one of my dreams, in which she appeared as one of the main figures. I told her what she meant to me. Then she reached out for my hand and she held it for a few moments. Ever since that approach, this warm handshake has been etched deeply inside me, as if it were a tacit agreement under the form of a silent contract, a holy vow that I would never forget the touch and the devotion I ought to have toward the Greek cultural heritage and the "Bollingen". . . the "stone."

Tao

JEAN-PIERRE DUPORT-ROZAN

Nel giallo della rosa sempiterna che si dilata e diroba e redole odor di lode al sol che sempre verna, mi trasse Beatrice. . . . [1]

DANTE ALIGHIERI

Toward the end of the 1970s, Jorge Luis Borges dictated a short story entitled "The Rose of Paracelsus."[2] In this text, the alchemist Paracelsus is more or less presented as Rembrandt's *Philosopher in Meditation,* a painting which can be seen at the Louvre. The furnace is cold and the retorts are covered with dust; here we are in front of the "abstractor of the quint-essence" rather than the alchemist.

> Down in his laboratory, to which the two rooms of the cellar had been given over, Paracelsus prayed to his God, his undetermined God—any God—to send him a disciple. . . . Night had expunged the dusty retorts and the furnace when there came a knock at his door. Sleepily he got up, climbed the short spiral staircase, and opened one side of the double door. A stranger stepped inside. . . . The master was the first to speak: —I recall faces from the West and faces from the East, he said, not without a certain formality, yet yours I do not recall.

At this point the disciple to be proposed a deal: he would become the master's disciple provided the former brought a rose back from ashes.

> I wish to see with my own eyes the annihilation and resurrection of the rose. . . . —There is still some fire here, said Paracelsus, pointing toward the hearth. If you cast this rose into the embers, you would believe that it has been consumed, and that its ashes are real. I tell you that the rose is eternal, and that only its appearances may change. At a word from me, you would see it again.

After trying vainly to persuade him to take his word for it, Paracelsus threw the rose into the flames and he added: "All the physicians and the pharmacists in Basel say I am a fraud. Perhaps they are right. There are the ashes that were the rose, and that shall be the rose no more." At these words, deeming Paracelsus a charlatan from now on, the young man went out, not without picking up again the gifts he had brought with him. And Borges concluded: "Paracelsus was then alone. Before putting out the lamp and returning to his weary chair, he poured the delicate fistful of ashes from one hand into the concave other, and he whispered a single word. The rose appeared again."

In this brief narrative, Paracelsus, often shown as some thaumaturgic physician smacking of heresy yet otherwise known as the "Luther of medicine," fades away behind the sage. He launches into a reflection which takes place on several levels, and it is obvious that the main point lies in the difference between believing and knowing. What does the visitor want indeed? He wants to watch a miracle before getting involved, because believing is obviously not enough for him. This is the bench scientist's, the expert's, approach, who pursuing knowledge demands a piece of evidence, and what a piece since it is nothing less than seeing a rose rising from its ashes!

Each of us readily acknowledges that the seeds of destruction lie within what exists: should a glass fall on a tiled floor, the odds are that it is going to break apart. There seems to be quite a world of difference between saying so and admitting the opposite, that is, that from within the fracture, even from within nothingness, existence might spring out.

However, some day something must have started out of nothing, *ex nihilo*, and as Paracelsus answers the question: "What is it you would do to bring it back again?" Borges has him say: "I use other instruments. . . .

I am speaking of that instrument used by the deity to create the heavens and the earth." Here a hierarchy is introduced. Indeed Paracelsus emphasizes the necessity of seeing the creation as the elemental principle: thus, the rose will have to be brought again according to the procedures that are those of all that has been created out of nothing. Here is the image of a discontinuity generating life, that is, a continuity arising from a fracture, from nothingness. And as far as life is concerned—one's own life—each of us does know that the continuity of one's existence is only secured because the discontinuity it contains while channeling it brings it out again every other second. So we experience the peculiar discontinuity underlying each of our heartbeats, each of our breaths—everything that preserves the basic rhythm of life within us. And when the last rupture prevails, continuity—the continuity of the electroencephalogram, of the electrocardiogram—stands for death: then external continuity has swept into the field where vital regulation occurred and preserved life on the basis of controlled discontinuities.

Learning and knowing obviously imply that he who wants to learn or know should first be alive, that is, channel the biological rhythms his life depends on. The hierarchy alluded to by Borges in this short story is precisely that of life, which stands first with regard to discourse, thought, or any individual activity. In a more learned manner we might say that the way of regulation, characterized by fractures wrapped up in a continuity, is ontologically antecedent to the way of the *logos.* For Leibniz to be able to speak of music as a "mathematics of the soul when the soul is not aware that it is counting," it was necessary that his own biological regulations keep his body and soul together so that his personal integrity should be manifest while such thought could be expressed.[3]

In other words the continuity-discontinuity dyad underpins and generates the determinism-chance dyad, which is expressed through the logos. What would music be without its rests, without fractures or discontinuities? Only the fracture with what precedes and what follows the sound gives the latter its color and identity, and without the discontinuity lying between letters, lines, and words, this very text under our eyes would amount to very little.

The logos concept, inherent to any living demonstration and covering many meanings, all of them related to the Indo-European root *leg*, involves the sense of "to gather, to choose, to pluck."[4] This classical Greek term is used concerning the most basic piece of information as well as in the sense of discourse, speech in general: rhetoric, dialectics, or still in a mathematical sense where reason amounts to logic as well, for instance in the form of an equation, as it amounts to verbal deduction in the vernacular. In either case the function of the logos is to break down a situation—however complex—into a unique expression that summarizes it, but such a function, proper to the logos, is always secondary with regard to the fracture the individual's continuity regulates and constrains.

It seems that Zeno of Elea was the first who emphasized that the way of the logos necessarily required the way of the regulation preceding it, without the latter depending on the one that followed it. Aristotle saw Zeno as the father of dialectics. The dialectician is the one who invalidates the argument his interlocutor proposes by showing it ineluctably leads to a contradiction. Zeno is known for the four paradoxes he stated: according to the first of them, Achilles will never reach his goal although it stands at a finite distance which, by dichotomy, is sent away to infinity. The second one, known as Achilles and the Tortoise, is the most famous and, using the same argument about infinity, it shows that Achilles will never catch the tortoise, which started before he did. Of a different nature, the third paradox consists for Zeno in concluding that a flying arrow can only be at rest. The argument uses the fact that at any period of time the arrow occupies a space equal to itself, and that motion is impossible because a period of time has no parts (if there was motion, the arrow would occupy a position during a part of a period of time and another one during another part of the same period of time). As regards the last paradox, far less known and much disputed, the Stadium, it is based on an inconsistency leading to the same conclusion as the third one. Now, what seems remarkable is that the first two paradoxes damage the continuity of space and time, whereas the last two say the opposite, namely that space and time cannot be discontinuous. Therefore space could not be composed of sizeless and divided corpuscles, and time of divided and lengthless periods.[5] In this way, Zeno tells us that for the logos the continuity-discontinuity aporia, that is, the way of regulation, is founding: the way of the logos is generated by the way of regulation according to a necessary condition. Indeed, the collapse of any individual's biological regulations brings about the collapse of his logos, while nothing can be concluded a priori from the opposite.

In his "Alchemy of the Word," Rimbaud seems to show that he is speaking of the way of regulation when he says: "J'écrivais des silences, des nuits, je notais l'inexprimable. Je fixais des vertiges,"[6] or when he writes:

> Je l'ai retrouvée
> Quoi?—L'éternité.
> C'est la mer
> Mêlée au soleil[7]

as though he were describing a continuous and discontinuous merging oxymoron.

The science we know, which is the main metamorphosis of the way of the logos and whose main goal, as René Thom mentions it, is "to reduce the arbitrary of description," is built on determinism.[8] Inherent to it, predictability is also its specific hallmark. To Aristotle, the sublunar world—unlike the sky where everything is quite foreseeable—is subjected to chance. Likewise, for Epictetus, in this world "of existing things some are in our power, others not in our power."[9] In mathematics, as early as the sixteenth century, the quite fundamental notion of function held all that is not in our power, while the variable stands precisely for what is in our power. It was up to Pierre-Simon Laplace to provide a definition of universal determinism. He did so in a remarkable phrase, famous from then on: "We must now consider the present state of the universe as the result of its previous state, and as the cause of the one that is going to follow. Given for one instant an intelligence which would comprehend all the forces by which nature is animated and the respective situation of the beings who compose it—an intelligence sufficiently vast to submit those data to analysis—it would embrace in the same formula the movements of the greatest bodies of the universe and those of the lightest atoms; for it, nothing would be uncertain and the future, as the past, would be present before its eyes."[10] In our days, the driving force behind science is there, and the recent French "dispute about determinism" bears witness to it.[11]

Beyond determinism, the discontinuity, the rupture, the singularity are more and more part of the scientific landscape, and the most various formalisms try to express their impact, to convey their meaning. But such meaningful fractures are also manifest in artistic expression. In his painting *The Madonna of Port-Lligat,* and even more so in his first version of it, Salvador Dali makes discontinuity play a part in every way on the painting and, in the first version, the fracture goes as far as splitting Gala's image—as if she had been chopped. This characteristic, indicated by the irruption of nothingness, is striking when we compare Dali's work with Piero della Francesca's *Madonna and Child with Saints* (Montefeltro Altarpiece) at the Brera Gallery in Milano, which inspired Dali. Piero della Francesca's painting shows the duke of Montefeltro kneeling before the Virgin and the baby Jesus. In both paintings, an apse appears in the background; it is in the shape of a scallop, and an egg is hanging from it by a thread. But in Dali's painting the apse is cut up into several well-delimited and symmetrical pieces, and both the scallop and the hanging egg are in the intercalary void on top of the vault. Fracture can be seen everywhere and obviously conveys the singularity of the discontinuity in what was formerly dedicated to the regularity of the geometrical continuity; it is as though the latter contained within itself the discontinuity Dali made obvious five centuries later.

As to the way of regulation, François Jullien expresses precisely in those terms the concept of the Tao in "a philosophical interpretation of the *I Ching.*" He writes in his preface: "Of all the books the various civilizations can have produced, or dreamt, the *I Ching,* or *Classic of Change* (that is, the *Book of Changes*) might well be the most peculiar. Not so much because of the message it is supposed to convey than, first of all, in the way it is composed. . . . It is not made with words first, but only with two signs, the simplest that exist: a continuous and discontinuous stroke, unbroken or broken,—and—," and he adds further on: "Here is a 'book' which, in its principle, does not aim at conveying a meaning. . . .

Yet, what looks, as such, to make a book so little, was used as a basic work by all civilizations."[12]

What is the Tao then? Trying to answer the question is useless. About Lao Tzu's *Tao te Ching,* Claude Larre, translating Tao by "Voie," adapted the first four lines in this way:

> Voie qu'on énonce
> N'est pas la voie.
> Nom qu'on prononce
> N'est pas le nom.[13]

Similarly, Etiemble regards a poem entitled "La roué" as an illustration of the notion of Tao:

> Les dieux font tourner une roué:
> Ces vieux enfants jouent au cerceau.
> L'abeille y tourney avec les plantes
> Et l'hirondelle avec les cieux.
> Les morts ont perdu la jante;
> Les vivants n'en voient plus l'essieu.[14]

Through the continuity-discontinuity dyad the Tao seems to emerge as an unusual demonstration of the regulating principle of the universe, as the way of an absolute reality, like an epiphany and an epithalamium. The poet who says:

> Et le temps a pose
> Sa mains sur son épaule, et se laisse aveugle
> Conduire sous la voûte des nombres purs,[15]

also speaks of the Tao, as does Rainer Maria Rilke: "Wolle die Wandlung. O sei für die Flamme begeistert."[16] The way of the logos, stemming from the way of regulation, makes it possible to escape from the fascination of things; naming something, pondering over what is, over the absence of nothing, is standing back and trying to escape from the spellbinding enchantment which lives within us. To be able to recognize oneself in the reflected image the mirror of Nature reflects to each of us is, of course, the first condition to escape such a fascination.

In this connection, Marie-Louise von Franz relates this anecdote about a Scottish shepherd:

> An old Scottish shepherd who lived a secluded life found a pocket mirror one day which a tourist had lost. He had never seen such a thing before. Time after time he looked at it, was amazed, shook his head, then took it home with him. His wife watched with increasing jealousy as, time and again, he furtively drew something out of his pocket, looked at it, smiled, put it back. When he was away one day, she quickly took the mirror out of his coat pocket. Looking at it, she cried, "Aha! So *this* is the old witch he is running after now!"[17]

NOTES

1. "In the yellow of the Rose Eternal / That spreads, and multiplies, and breathes an odour / Of praise into the ever-vernal Sun, / Me Beatrice drew-on. . . ." *Divina Comedia,* "Paradise," translated by Henry Wadsworth Longfellow, XXX, 1. 124–127.
2. In *The Book of Sand and Shakespeare's Memory,* translated and with an afterword by Andrew Hurley (Penguin Books, 1998).
3. Quoted by G. Steiner in Roger-Pol Droit, *La compagnie des contemporains* (Paris: Odile Jacob, 2002), p. 259.
4. This root can be found in particular in the word *intelligence.*
5. This commentary about Zeno's four paradoxes is from Nicholas Falletta, *Le livre des paradoxes* (Paris: Belfond, 1997), p. 109; translation: *The Paradoxicon* (New York: Doubleday, 1983).
6. "I turned silences and nights into words. What was unutterable, I wrote down. I made the whirling world stand still," in *A Season in Hell,* translated by Paul Schmidt (New York: HarperCollins, 1976).
7. "It has been found again. / What? Eternity. / It is the sea mingled / With the sun," in *Arthur Rimbaud, Collected Poems,* translated by Olivier Bernard (London: Penguin Classics, 1997).
8. See Thom's definition: "On peut affirmer qu'expliquer scientifiquement un certain nombre de phénomènes, c'est—autant que faire se peut—réduire l'arbitraire de la de-

scription des dits phénomènes," in "L'espace et les signes," *Semiotica* 29: 3/4 (1980), p. 206.

9. *Manual of Epictetus.*
10. P. S. Laplace, *A Philosophical Essay of Probabilities,* translated by F. W. Truscott and F. L. Emory (New York: Dover Publications, 1951); translation of *Essai philosophique sur les probabilitiés* (Paris: Christian Bourgois, 1986), pp. 32–33.
11. See Krysztof Pomian, ed., *La querelle du déterminisme* (Paris: Le Débat/Gallimard, 1990).
12. François Jullien, *Figures de l'immanence* (Le livre de poche, 1995), pp. 7–8.
13. *Dao De Jing. Le livre de la Voie et de la Vertu,* traduction et présentation de Claude Larre (Paris: Desclée de Brouwer, 1977), p. 17 (literally: "The way that is spoken of / Is not the way. / The name that can be named / Is not the name").
14. "The gods make a wheel turn: / these old children are playing with a hoop. / Over there the bee's turning over with the plants / and the swallow with heaven. / As a result the dead have lost the rim; / the living no longer see its axle," in *Philosophes taoïstes* (Paris: Gallimard, Bibliothèque de la Pléiade, 1980), p. xlviii. This poem is by the French poet and translator André Gâteau (d. 1997).
15. "And time has placed / Its hand upon his shoulder, and lets itself / Be blindly led beneath the vault of numbers," in Yves Bonnefoy, *In the Shadow's Light,* translated by John Naughton (Chicago: The University of Chicago Press, 1991); translation of *Ce qui fut sans lumière* (Paris: Mercure de France, 1987).
16. "Will transformation. Oh, be inspired by the flame," in *Die: Sonette an Orpheus, Zweiter Teil XII;* translated by Stephen Mitchell, *Sonnets to Orpheus* (Boston: Shambhala, 1993).
17. In *Dreams* (Boston: Shambhala, 1998), p. 15.

The Song of Exile

> Only vitrification makes verification possible;
> yet there is more truth in movement
> than in the petrified detail.

The child is a unique book
devoured by a goat
which breaks him
into black petrified details where from now on
the delicate world of a musing and resolute being dwells:
murder and suicide by mutual consent
like a divine wedding of nostalgia and beyond.
Debt of hatred and
debt of love.
Dark theme of an opus
the whole reality conspires to
in the incipient movement.

Then time embraces death
and sets the flow against such exiles:
the meaning lies in the coincidence.
The child walled up in the man
by the constance of the oscillation connecting them
is first of all a woman, captive of her hopelessness:
a vague drift
in the perception
of deceitful evidence.
From her prison, committed to her own denial,

with her fists
she
hits
the man
anchored in his certainties,
and begets movement.

Towards an inaccessible land
where she only recognizes his absence of spirit:
ruthless wandering
of a consciousness
chilled to nothingness.
Death cannot answer
and the child cannot change anything.
Standing there indestructible,
spiteful for ever
from the dark and lightning desire,
the son,
who does not listen to what is,
the living child speaks to his dead father.
Between them silence.

A shift
adrift
and, against a background of disaster,
the man confronts a stranger:
the Outsider.
Pure emotion
shaking and creating
a rustling silence,
a clearness trapped by shadows;
a nothingness is shown in transparency.
Fearful, uneasy,
staggering and swaying
from chaos to horror,

enduring the agony and dizzy spells of insanity,
he questions his memory
and discards the motionless detail verified
for an absence that shines.
The infinite fault of a populated distance
looms in the present:
and meaning stemmed from the Other.

Jean-Pierre Duport-Rozan

December 22, 2002

Encounter in the Unconscious

ANDREA DYKES

Dear Dr. Emmanuel Kennedy,

I hope this small tribute to Marie-Louise von Franz will be acceptable for your Festschrift. Although I have many very meaningful and enjoyable memories of her in reality, yet these two dreams, where we met not in this world but in the Unconscious, still remain the most important of them all.

Sincerely yours,
Andrea Dykes

I think the best way in which I can add my tribute to Marie-Louise von Franz is by telling two dreams I had of her during my analysis (not with her). I had been bowled over by her first lecture on "The Dreams and Visions of Niklaus von der Flue," the very first lecture I attended at the Institute; afterward someone said to me: "Now don't go imagining all the lectures here will be like these." How right she was! I did not know

Marie-Louise at all at that time, but I think the Unconscious immediately responded to her inner value. That night I dreamt:

> *I was in a big shaft in the ground with Dr. von Franz, she was explaining something to do with words and language (something which has always fascinated me). But she spoke very softly, not with the ringing tones I had heard in the previous day's lecture, and I could hardly hear what she said, which greatly distressed me.*
>
> *Then we came up out of the shaft into Bellevueplatz. There Dr. von Franz pointed out a black stake, several feet high, sticking out of the ground and told me it dated from ancient Egyptian times, it was the first statue of the first Man and God. Next she pointed up into the branches of two trees. I saw that a branch from one tree had been taken across and joined to the trunk of the other tree so that they made an unbroken living arch. I was very impressed and felt I was in the presence of something holy. Dr. von Franz confirmed this, telling me that the very earliest ancient Egyptians had joined those trees, and that they, the arch, and the space it enclosed* were *in very fact the God. This because they had been united. But the most sacred of all was the empty space enclosed by the trees, just because it was empty. I thought to myself, "Yes. Of course one cannot try and visualize or impute anything to God."*

Of course, I found her hard to understand; I was by no means ready then to understand all the implications of the dream, but in the unconscious I had recognized her profound spiritual side, which in actual fact fitted so comfortably with her everyday life, as was typified by our coming up into the everydayness of Bellevueplatz and finding there the holy emptiness. On considering the dream at the time I felt, rather uncomfortably, that the black stake could also be the stake at which unfortunates used to be burnt. It did indeed symbolize the later suffering which is a part of any genuine spiritual quest.

A year later I dreamt:

> *I was standing on the grass verge of a country mountain road. Marlus drew my attention to a large equal-armed slate cross lying on the*

> *ground. She explained that in some sense the cross was* me *and I was the cross. I was profoundly moved and realized it referred to something beyond the ego. I then looked down at a lower level and saw a pool full of fish. They were swimming around in an apparently aimless manner; then suddenly they all formed into a close circle, shoulder to shoulder with their heads pointing inward. In the center thus formed was an absolutely symmetrical circle of still, clear, empty water.*

Slate is a sombre stone but makes excellent and durable roofing.

Decades later, when she was already suffering from her final illness, she said something about crosses. I said: "You gave me a cross once" and told her the dream. She shook my hand and thanked me for telling her.

The empty space in the arch of the first dream and the still, clear water of the second both refer to the enormous importance of the Unmanifest behind and beyond all aspects of the Manifest.

Like all the really deeply serious people I have ever known, Marlus was blessed with a wonderful sense of humor and ability to enjoy the small as well as the great things of life. I have never laughed more than I did when staying with her in her Bollingen Tower.

In all the dreams I ever had of her, Marie-Louise von Franz was very much a Self figure for me.

Having Had the Honor . . .

DAVID ELDRED

Having had the honor of working on the translations and the editing of several of the contributions to this Festschrift, one sees how clearly the spirit of Marie-Louise von Franz lives on. Many of these essays share astute and loving observations of Marie-Louise von Franz, several focus on the quintessence of this woman's lifework lived in devotion and fidelity to the psyche and the utterances of the soul, and still others relate their own creative endeavors offering interpretations of personal dreams and experiences. Many share their thoughts and observations with such depth, insight, and acuity that I can hardly add anything new at all. Can one say it better than: "It is for us, as well as for the world, an immeasurable piece of providence and good fortune that a woman like Marie-Louise von Franz lived, and that we were able to meet her" (see Gotthilf Isler's eulogy, p. 63). Or: "through the painful way of her individuation . . . and for helping me, like many people, partake of this task, I feel the deepest gratitude. . . . Her love, her work, and her example, along with her deep commitment to the search for meaning, are of such a nature as to encourage the individual on his or her lifelong quest and endeavor to be and become himself or herself" (see Dieter Baumann's contribution, p. 175). Or: "I was touched by her spirit in such a way that I could feel her warmth, her humor, and her wisdom. She accompanied me as an inner friend, and I held inner conversations with her, asked her questions—what she would do?—and so forth" (see Vreni Suter's contribution, p. 523).

I would thus like to limit myself to two anecdotes and then conclude with a few dreams that Marie-Louise von Franz related to me, dreams which are, in a way, complementary to those related by others in this Festschrift.

The first anecdote goes back to 1980 when I was doing an internship at the State Hospital of Lucerne with terminally ill cancer patients, gathering their dreams in preparation for a dissertation on the psychodynamics of the dying process. Marie-Louise von Franz had agreed to be my mentor for this work, and after about a year of collecting dreams, I prepared my first attempt at an analysis and interpretation. I had delivered the first one hundred and fifty pages of my dissertation to Marie-Louise von Franz a few weeks before, and I was now sitting among the stacks of books and papers, an elegant Buddha, sundry other figures, plants, and stones in her library, awaiting my hour.

But before this anecdote is told, I must say that I had pretty much forgotten this incident until I read the words of José Zavala, who said that he never failed to be astounded how often Marie-Louise von Franz could explain, elucidate, and capture an entire life process with such a brevity of words. Words simple and natural, penetrating the depths and hitting the mark. Words that not only harbored striking wisdom, but vibrated with vigor out of which one could draw the very substance of life. I bring his thoughts here not only because they render so poignantly the very essence of Marie-Louise von Franz's insight and manner, but because this anecdote is about how she was able to "explain it poignantly" without any words at all.

On that sweltering day in June 1980 I took my seat in the cool, shaded room amidst the surfeit of books in her library and nervously waited—suspended between my hopes for enthusiastic, positive support and my linen shirt languoring ever more with perspiration. The door handle moved slowly down from three o'clock to six . . . and Marie-Louise von

Franz entered the room carrying my carefully bound manuscript. As she crossed the room, she remarked that she had read my entire work. She positioned herself in her chair, set the manuscript to her right on a side table, and remained still. Something was probably up: she had not yet sought my eyes. Then she picked up my dissertation with her right hand . . . and . . . slipped it silently into the wastepaper basket by her chair. She looked over to me silently, shrugged her shoulders, and gave me a bit of an apologetic smile, the kind one gets from a friend when you have just lost the vote for a seat on the student council in high school. It was me who then spoke, asking hopefully: "You're suggesting that I start again?" She offered no word of criticism or harshness but simply answered with: "Go to the source material on death and dying in the literature of cultural anthropology; then study the Egyptians, the Etruscans, and the Romans for example; research the Native Americans in the eighteenth and nineteenth centuries; there is some important stuff in Borneo and Indonesia; flesh out your amplifications. The material from your patients is a gold mine and the spirit behind your work is genuine; it is just that your analysis is in the air. Go to the source on death customs, rituals, and beliefs, and your work will then naturally take a very different turn."

During the next twelve months, I discovered the symbolism of death, mourning, and funerary rites. I buried myself in the stacks of several libraries in Switzerland and added the New York Public Library and the Library of Congress on a trip to Washington, D.C. These libraries were a refuge, the material the solace and sustenance for a soul confined for thirty years in the shallows of rationalist reductionist thought. Looking back, she was of course completely right in regards to the content of my analysis. Nevertheless, she had apparently seen enough to value the part of me that—beneath all the interpretative foolishness and inflation of my first attempt—was thirsting for deeper answers. And her challenge was the most beautiful *votum* of trust and belief that I have ever received from a teacher. Such a vote of confidence from the mind and the heart of this woman changed the lives of many people forever.

Many years later, my partner and I spent several summers and an autumn or two with Marie-Louise von Franz in her tower in Bollingen.

Marie-Louise had such a deep love of nature and such a simple, natural integrity that, much to the befuddlement of many people, she spent quite a few months a year living in this tower by a frog and yellow lily pond where there was no electricity or gas, only an outhouse with a sack of lime and a shovel, cold water in an old stone fountain in the living room-kitchen, and a large fireplace that you could pretty much step into. She was an avid naturalist who never cut a tree for the firewood she needed but searched the woods, gathering the fallen branches, and she cut all her firewood by hand. Nothing was done with electric tools or apparatus. No plugs for laptops. Morning coffee, lunch, tea, and dinner, the dishwater, the heating, everything revolved around her fireplace.

During the weeks we spent with her, we loved to prepare "grand meals" at night. Rack of lamb, roast turkey, grilled jumbo shrimps, broccoli béarnaise, salmon ravioli, fried potatoes, squash, corn, and so forth, with menu cards presenting the dishes with outlandish names and an occasional Brunello del Montalcino or an Edward the VIII given to her by friends. She would tell wonderful stories of Barbara Hannah, C. G. Jung, Franz Ricklin, her father, and many others. Humorous anecdotes, sad and tragic stories, of victories and defeats, loves and disappointments in friendships, all brimming with life. Memories of sitting on a bench on top of a mountain pass with Barbara Hannah and C. G. Jung in the very last years of his life, where Jung said to them: "Look carefully around, take in the grasses, the trees below, the stones at our feet, the flowers, the ringing bells of the cows. Since we sat down on this bench, the world has ever so slightly changed; it can never go back. When I am gone, come back in your minds to this bench . . . we will sit here, together, for eternity."

I spent the entire day preparing food, the fire, firewood, the coffee and teas. Guests at four in the afternoon, new guests at the table in the evening. And at night, after a cognac to toast the meal and the friends, she would bring out her Sprüngli chocolates, given to her by one dear soul or another. (During one entire season, she convinced me that the little green cakes were filled with marzipan, which she knew that I did not like, thus she kindly gave me first choice and, as a favor to me, took those all upon herself. At the very last meal, she revealed that she had rooked me for three weeks: the green ones turned out to be filled with the finest of dark chocolate, and she broke out into cackles of laughter while I only grumbled something about being gullible. She commented that she had counted on my conviction that she was an elderly lady, honorable and fair, when, in fact, dark chocolate was simply her favorite. It happened to be mine too. And this she knew.)

But this is not the anecdote I set out to tell. Rather, one day in October we had packed our bags and were preparing to depart from Bollingen. The "changing of the guard" was necessary. Marie-Louise was then dependent on caretakers and friends so that she could stay in her tower, and she wanted to spend one more week of autumn there. It was still just the three of us, for the new woman had not yet arrived for the coming week. I had said goodbye and finished packing the car while my partner was upstairs sharing a few words of farewell. It was a joy to lean up against the car and do nothing more than take in the slight chill and dampness of the Sunday morning breeze coming out of the forest. My mind wondered to the school class off in the distance, chattering away as they came toward me through the woods. I saw no one and thought little about them. At the edge of the pond, I wondered how much deeper the dry spell might drain the basin before winter, looked about for a frog or fire salamander . . . and that class of children was still chattering away coming toward me with no one yet in sight. I distracted myself a few more times—my partner was taking an awfully long time—checked the oil, nudged the tires, and still the children's chatter with no one in sight. Wondering where all these kids were, I decided to go over to the little ridge in the woods and look down. But just as I began my walk, I passed a large oak and suddenly realized that all of the chatter was coming from up in the tree. The branches of the tree were trembling with hundreds upon hundreds of quail fluttering and chirping and hopping around among themselves, a whirling mesmerizing flurry of voices and wings. I had seen maybe one or two quail in Bollingen in my life, nothing like this. The quail must have gathered there to prepare for their flight south. It was one of the moments in life where one stands alone in front of a wondrous marvel of nature. I went up and told Marie-Louise about the quail in her oak tree. She asked to be helped to sit up in bed and requested that I open the window, and she listened with reverence and joy to what she said was "the song of resurrection. . . . Quails had been the birds of resurrection for the Egyptians."

In her final years Marie-Louise occasionally shared with me some of the more difficult dreams that she had had. Maybe this was because I had spent many years working with severely ill and dying adults and children. Maybe she shared them with other people as well. But I would like to include three dreams that she told me in the last months of her life, dreams that are painful, fearful, certainly not easy, but I bring them here because they are a natural side of the heaviness of individuation and the agony of the death process, because they were very much natural to Marie-Louise, and because they are beautifully complemented and balanced by dreams mentioned by others in this Festschrift. These dreams were told to me in the last six to nine months before her death. She made little ado about them but recounted them openly and was relieved in a sense to share them.

Despite her enthusiasm for life, she suffered moments of severe doubt. With a mind like hers, she was quite adept at dissecting the entire philosophical foundations of her work and Jung's, leaving herself exposed to the brutality of worldviews that momentarily shatter psychology and theology or scatter the theories of the natural sciences and the evolution of consciousness to the wind. And doubt she did. She was the type of scholar who certainly put herself and her work in question.

The first dream I would like to relate occurred possibly nine months or even longer before her death. She had been in very difficult physical condition for years and a part of her would have liked to have been able to go. In this dream:

> *She was climbing a mountain. The ascent was anything but easy, the path treacherous and long. But she was determined to reach the summit. And with arduous, exhausting work she slowly approached the top of the ridge with joy for she was so looking forward to what was on the other side. Finally she arrived . . . and over beyond the mountain was a vast nuclear wasteland. She woke up in shock.*

She commented that the dream threw her back into the search within for her own spirit and soul, and, like everyone else, she had fallen prey to the temptation of setting one's values and aspirations in the peaks of the outer world.

The next dream I would like to relate occurred a couple of months before her death.

> *She was out in the universe, in sheer darkness, and suddenly coming towards her was a smallish black dog. She was filled with terror, for she knew that this dog was pure evil. She awoke in fear.*

I think such a dream is, first of all, simply a rendition of a truth. The more one chooses to face evil—or even challenge it for what it is—the darker it directly shows its face. I also think that it is the natural opposite of the love and joy of other dreams, an opposite that she often said we must integrate in order to live life on this earth to its fullest. As other authors have noted, Marie-Louise von Franz was very clear that—from our point of view—nature, and even God, could at times be fierce and grueling. Such an encounter with evil would certainly be a "natural" confrontation as one attempts to fully complete one's life. She herself was not terribly upset about having had the dream, but the fear of that degree of evil made her shudder.

A third dream is beautifully complemented by the dream of the household caretaker who dreamt that she came down the stairs in Marie-Louise von Franz's home and there stood C. G. Jung in the hallway, who she then let in to visit Marie-Louise (see the end of Gotthilf Isler's eulogy, p. 62). In her own dream, which occurred a few months earlier, she dreamt that:

> *She had met Jung. He had come to her, and she was so happy to see him. She thought, now is the time, he has come to meet me. But he looked at her sternly and said that she could not come with him. And he turned and walked harshly away. Her heart was broken. The loneliness unbearable.*

It was apparently still not yet the time (see Gotthilf Isler's rendition of Marie-Louise von Franz's dream at Bahnhof Enge). The agony of this dream, however, found its catharsis in the caretaker's dream just weeks prior to her death.

"Getting old is certainly not for pansies" she once told me, and Marie-Louise von Franz experienced all sides—the opposites pulling her at times to the brink—while other dreams show the abundance and completion of her life. It was her honesty, clarity, and courage that gave so many people the strength to venture an attempt to carry their own fates and form their own destinies.

In closing I would like to share a poem written for her and shared with her, a poem which was inspired by her courage, her integrity, her grasp of the psyche and spirit, and by the love in this woman's heart.

I Will Hold You, Marlus

(to my mentor, Marie-Louise von Franz)

I will hold you Marlus
as the scepter of Isis
to drive back the succubus,
with her ratty black tresses
her eyes void, devouring.

I will hold you, Marlus
as the staff of Asclepius
to repel the putrifying forces
and rout the hideous steeds
of my imagination.

As a wanderer
(dessicated, bewildered, bleak,
beneath Kalahari sun)
I will hold you as my hands
hold cool waters

lifted high,
dripping,
quickening
my uncertain face.

Beneath the crowns of beech and oak
fluttering with the voiceless flurry
of flock upon flock of quail,
I will hold you, Marlus
as the witness
holds the moment.

At your hands I have learned of uprightness
of loyalty and truth
of unrelenting conviction.
I have learned of other ways and sacred books.
I have learned of fear
I have stared into the heinous maw of the Fenris Wolf
with his grisly eye
sparkling from a rabid light.
And I have clutched this light in my skinless hands
and seen his reflection
behind my face.
And I know you too have seen,
for his face you once described.
You have filled me with courage
and I have looked,
and begun to see
and I am still withstanding.

I will hold you, Marlus
as the sailor
holds the sextant for his captain
as they rail against the midnight
beneath del Fuego storm.

I will hold you
as the novice holds the crystal-quartz;
the devotee
an ancient Coptic text;
From you I have learned to raise my eyes while kneeling
although at this time in my life I am no one to question
so I keep my eyes to the floor.

I wish I could have held you
as a man
holds a woman
whose destiny is lifted
at Mithraic chambers of the fidel.
But instead,
yours was a destiny
of austerities of the heart;
and solitudes.

May you take me as an honor guard,
think of me once as friend,
know that in this season,
a'fore these chambers,
in this crypt beneath the midriffs,
I stand here for you
little to give,
late in life.

I will hold you Marlus
in the cavity behind my ribs.
I will walk you to your gate
and lay my hand upon your shoulder
as we stand among the yellow lilies of your pond.
And before you turn away,
a twinkling in your eye,
a military gesture of farewell,

a one-gun salute
I will already miss you terribly.

I will hold you, Marlus
in hopes.
I will stand here at your pond with you forever.
And ask that you might think of me
When my time comes to approach my gate.

I will hold you, Marlus
as a man holds the ring
removed from his loved one's finger.
He reads the inscription one last time,
and lays it in the palm of his hand.

I will hold you, Marlus
as a man holds back his tears.

Bridging the Gap Between Physics and Depth Psychology

HERBERT VAN ERKELENS

When I started to study physics, mathematics, and astronomy, I was only seventeen years old and a great admirer of Albert Einstein, the man who created relativity theory. But after three months of study, I became interested in Jungian psychology. What impressed me in particular was the vision of the "world clock" published by Carl Gustav Jung in *Psychology and Alchemy*. Through that vision I learned that physics alone would never lead me to the secret of the cosmos. I understood that dreams and visions constitute a more personal way of getting into contact with the mysterious center where the Self and the cosmos meet.

For more than a year, I felt torn between physics and depth psychology. Why should I put energy into a study that could not satisfy the deeper needs of my soul? But I saw no alternative. In the end I grew angry with God. Why did He let me suffer? I fell on my knees and told Him that He would not succeed in breaking me into two. Then I felt a lot better. I even cherished the hope that depth psychology would no longer bother me.

The next day I entered an antiquarian bookshop and found the book *Zahl und Zeit* (*Number and Time*) by Marie-Louise von Franz. According to the subtitle, the book was an attempt to bring depth psychology and physics closer together. I was stupefied. I had not expected that God would react so quickly. But I knew now that I was saved. Somewhere in Switzerland there lived a depth psychologist who believed that depth psychology and physics could be unified. I adopted her as my second mother, read her book *Zahl und Zeit* several times, and continued my study in physics.

In May 1984, I took my doctor's degree in theoretical physics at the University of Amsterdam. I left this academic specialty in order to concentrate on the relationship of modern physics and depth psychology. Around this time, I found another hero: the famous theoretical physicist Wolfgang Pauli. Einstein had considered him as his spiritual son who would solve the remaining problems in physics. But I knew that Pauli had been the neurotic scientist whose dreams Jung had published in *Psychology and Alchemy*. Hence, I expected that he had lived a religious life following the demands of the unconscious. But there was no biography of Pauli available to support this supposition.

At the beginning of 1988, the Free University in Amsterdam asked me to start an investigation into the relationship of modern physics and religion. I decided to start this project by doing some research in the private life of Pauli. In this connection Dr. Carl Alfred Meier advised me to contact Marie-Louise von Franz! That was really surprising. I had not expected to meet her personally. I knew she had Parkinson's disease, and I did not want to bother her too much with my effort to unify depth psychology and physics. But because of Pauli I decided to visit her. My father made a small painting for her, because he knew how much she meant to me.

The encounter on July 1, 1988, lasted one hour. In the first half of the interview, von Franz destroyed my image of Pauli as a serious, spiritual seeker. According to her, he had always avoided an encounter with the numinous. When things got hot, he just ran away. First I could not believe this. But von Franz insisted. Pauli had never realized the symmetries in his own vision of the world clock. He had not led a life that could have bridged the gap between modern physics, depth psychology, and religion.

Within thirty minutes, the goddess and the hero of my life had shrunk into ordinary human beings. Von Franz was full of rancor, which I did not understand at that time, and Pauli fell from his pedestal by having been a coward in religious affairs. During the rest of the encounter, I asked von Franz about her present interests, and finally I gave her the painting by my father, a still life showing stones and a beautiful thistle. From a stubborn woman von Franz suddenly turned into a child who had received an unexpected present. She began to radiate happiness and said: "This is a mandala in forms of nature."

It took me quite a long time to digest this first encounter with von Franz. She had advised me to study the letters Pauli had sent her between 1948 and 1956. These letters were to be found in the archives of the *Eidgenössische Technische Hochschule* (ETH) in Zürich. When I started to study these letters, I discovered that the unconscious had sent Pauli many dreams about a possible unification of physics and depth psychology. Pauli had even found the meeting point between quantum physics and depth psychology. It was a mathematical symbol that constituted the heart of quantum physics and at the same time meant to Pauli his relationship with the spirit of the unconscious. During an active imagination, a Chinese lady, clearly a personification of the anima, had taken this symbol as a ring from her finger and let it float in the air. The lady called it "the ring i." In mathematics, *i* denotes the imaginary unit or square root of minus one.

Thanks to this Chinese lady, I had found the symbol that could heal the split in my own soul! But why had von Franz not published the ring i in her book *Zahl und Zeit*? In February 1990, I had a dream about a meeting which focused on the relationship of physics and depth psychology. In the dream, I told a man that von Franz had no understanding of mathematics. A stranger said: "It is curious that quantum physics can be connected with introspection."

A week later, I attended a seminar in Germany about quantum physics and depth psychology. On that occasion, I met the Swiss Jungian analyst, Eva Wertenschlag-Birkhäuser, who showed an interest in the later dreams of Pauli. I sent her those dreams, and we began interpreting them. Since Marie-Louise von Franz had been a friend of Eva's parents, she could easily arrange for me a second encounter with the woman who meant so much to me.

We decided to visit von Franz together, and we took with us some dreams of Pauli we did not understand. It was on a Wednesday in February, and I didn't feel well because of some problems that had arisen in my struggle with the unconscious. But von Franz was in good spirits. She first commented on a couple of dreams from my student days. Next I read aloud the dreams of Pauli. She had no problem analyzing them. But then I showed her a dream in which the imaginary unit played a decisive role. The dream, published now in an appendix to the Pauli/Jung letters, proceeds in seven steps. During the last three steps, four eggs transform into mathematical formulas from which the ring i arises as symbol of the One.

Von Franz stared at the seven steps. She first said: "This is the axiom of Maria Prophetissa." Then she continued: "But that is impossible." To our surprise, von Franz did not understand the dream. She could not follow that an alchemical axiom could be expressed in symbols of modern mathematics. She said: "The ring i cannot be a symbol of the unconscious. You can calculate with the imaginary unit and with the unconscious you cannot." I have never understood this argument, since the whole of mathematics rests on an archetypal foundation. Even though you can calculate with the ring i, it still remains a symbol of the Self.

Later I understood that Pauli had hurt von Franz very much. He had never taken her remarks seriously. In an interview meant for the Dutch television, she said: "I sometimes made scenes, when I thought Pauli was really on the wrong track. Then he just made joking remarks that I looked prettier the more I was angry. He didn't take my remarks seriously. I banged on the table and said: 'I mean it seriously. It is a dangerous point.' But he just scoffed at it. He had a patriarchal outlook on women. Women were pleasant things to play with, but not something to take seriously. That really was one of the difficulties."

Finally, we showed von Franz the vision by Pauli in which he had to perform a square dance with various personifications of the unconscious, among them the Chinese lady. Von Franz had published part of this vision in *Zahl und Zeit,* so we knew that it meant something to her. Immediately, she started telling us that the union of opposites can never be a static thing: "Sometimes you are in harmony with the anima, at other times you're not. Hence life is a dance where you meet the inner partner and then part again."

The strange thing was that I had heard these words before. Many years earlier I had practiced Israeli folk dancing. I still remembered a particular dance that helped me to get married. The explanations the teacher had given with respect to this dance were in complete agreement with what von Franz was telling me. I had always had difficulties in my relationship with the anima. But now at least I began to understand why.

Three years later, when I was writing my book *Wolfgang Pauli und der Geist der Materie* (*Wolfgang Pauli and the Spirit of Matter*), I sent von Franz my own interpretation of the square dance of Pauli. I had analyzed this dance mathematically with the help of a book on chemistry and crystal permutation groups. In reply, I received a letter in which von Franz only remarked that the whole thing had cost me a lot of effort. I was quite angry because of this remark. So I decided to find a better explanation of the dance, a more psychological one.

This time, I incorporated what I had learned from von Franz herself, namely, that you have to sacrifice the ego in order to contact the Self. I wrote a wholly new chapter in which I looked only at the psychological meaning of Pauli's mathematical dreams. I did precisely what Pauli had failed to do, to connect dreams with his personal situation and to try to understand them from this subjective perspective. Finally I had understood the game, and the next letter from von Franz was a flattering one.

By adopting Marie-Louise von Franz as my second mother, I became one of her spiritual sons. But sons have to leave their mothers. A week before she died, I had a dream in which I left the mountain cottage where students were studying the work of von Franz. Outside, I was not alone. Von Franz herself was watching me. That stimulated me to walk into nature and to admire the many flowers which opened because a refreshing rain had bathed their buds. When I walked further out of sight of von Franz, I saw that big animals were approaching me. They were startled by human interventions in nature. I could not hide myself. There were only some birches in the neighborhood. I decided to confront the animals. I gripped the trunk of a big elephant in order to make friends with him. At that moment, an intense feeling streamed through me. I had made contact with the natural world more directly than ever before.

REFERENCES

van Erkelens, Herbert, ed. "Wolfgang Pauli, the Feminine and the Perils of the Modern World. An interview with Marie-Louise von Franz by Hein Stufkens and Philip Engelen, IKON-television, Küsnacht, November 1990," *Yearbook of the Dutch Interdisciplinary Society for Analytical Psychology,* vol. 13 (1997), pp. 67–75.

———. "Wolfgang Pauli and the Chinese *Anima* Figure," *Eranos. The Magic of the Tortoise,* vol. 68 (Ascona: The Eranos Foundation, 1999).

———. *Wolfgang Pauli und der Geist der Materie,* edited by Thomas Arzt in collaboration with Eva Wertenschlag-Birkhäuser, Charles P. Enz, and Bernward Thiel. Würzburg: Verlag Königshausen and Neumann, 2002.

A Memory of Marie-Louise von Franz

GUIDO FERRARI

A good number of years have gone by since I first met Marie-Louise von Franz in Davos, at the World Congress of the International Association of Transpersonal Psychology (1983). I was there as a journalist but also as a film director in the hope of making a documentary on this meeting for the Italian language channel of the Swiss television. Many famous people were present at this event and many of these were destined to grow even more famous in the years to come. The Dalai Lama, who had not as yet been awarded the Nobel Peace Prize, was there with a large group of monks. His was indeed a mysterious and fascinating presence to which we were not yet accustomed and his talk on love and compassion held the attention of the thousands of people who followed it there in the auditorium with great feeling. I also recall the talk given by a Jesuit, Father Enomya Lassalle, on the question of Zen meditation applied to Christianity—a bold topic for those times. The Swiss psychiatrist Elisabeth Kübler-Ross spoke about the phases of death, also an unexplored subject at the time, while Stanislav Grof described the experiences of his patients, obtained through holotropic breathing that took the place of LSD use; these included extraordinary experiences of communion with all things, encounters with mysterious beings, recollections of past, even ancient, experiences and of past lives and intrauterine happenings. These, too, were experiences nearly unknown at the time. The ethnologist Michael Harner spoke about shamanism and the techniques of ecstasy he had studied and experienced with the Indios in Amazonia. Among the other names that stick in my mind because of their fascinating talks are those of anthropologist and psychiatrist Claudio Naranjo, the Sufi teacher Irina Tweedi, Buddhist meditation master Jack Kornfield, Zen master Baker Roshi, and the master of Kundalini yoga, Gopi Krishna. It was for me as well as for many others an extremely important moment in which I discovered many things and found confirmation of intuitions I had come to through my reading and encounters. It was a moment in which I experienced an expansion of consciousness and faced up to new questions. It was, in short, a turning point.

I recall especially well the opening address delivered by Marie-Louise von Franz, an honor bestowed on her as an international recognition of her research as well as a courtesy extended to the country hosting the congress. Small but with a strong and assured voice, and without making any concessions to the usual protocol of such a formal occasion, she began talking straight away about the inner quest of the Swiss saint, Niklaus von Flüe. It was for me a real eye-opener. I knew the usual things one learns in school about Niklaus but I was fascinated by his story and by Marie-Louise von Franz's ability to follow his process of individuation as it unfolded in the visions that the saint communicated to his confessor. It was a difficult path indeed, but one which turned a farmer and a soldier into a truly enlightened man. The religious spirit of Niklaus came to life and took on meaning for our countries and for our times. The talk had a special resonance in me and deeply touched my heart. An enthusiastic round of applause followed von Franz's exposition, and it was evident that I was not the only one who had been touched by it. I later met her in the atrium and complimented her on her work. I recall spontaneously adding, "so there is no need for us to go all the way to the Himalayas, we actually have our own guru!" She smiled, amused by the remark, and since she didn't know me, I introduced myself to her. I told her straight away without thinking that as a television journalist I wanted to recount the story of Niklaus that she had explained to us, but to an even wider audience. She seemed interested and added that we could talk it over together. Since we were staying in the same hotel, she gave me an appointment to meet in the hotel bar later that same afternoon. It was only then that I realized just what I had done! Perhaps I was going to have the opportunity to work with the famous Marie-Louise von Franz on a subject which was extraordinary. Fear and enthusiasm both welled up within me, along with a sense of determination.

Our meeting turned out to be very pleasant indeed. It was true that Marie-Louise von Franz was famous, a person with an immense amount of knowledge and depth, but she was also modest, direct, and down to earth. No doubt it was back then that an image started forming within me—the image of a housewife dedicated with care, diligence, and feeling to the large and small things of life. This is the image with which I was to dream of her on several occasions.

I explained to her just how a documentary on Niklaus might be organized: she would comment on the visions of the saint and I would have actors reenact the scenes in the actual places where the saint had lived. I could see that she liked the project, and the following morning when she came down to breakfast, she gestured to me calling me over to her table. Smiling and obviously amused by the whole matter, she said that she had already thought of the "libretto" of the documentary, in other words, the screenplay. She assured me that as soon as she got home to Küsnacht, she would type it up and send it off to me—something which she did in fact do just a few days later.

In preparation for the actual filming, I went to Küsnacht twice, and I asked von Franz to explain some of the visions which, despite the comments she had already sent me, still weren't clear to me. And of course I ended up talking about myself, involved in an exchange with Brother Klaus and with this famous analyst. Spontaneously, memories and reflections that I had never dared relate to anyone arose freely in my mind because I felt at ease and understood, without there being any sort of judgment. What struck me more than anything else was the freshness with which she dealt with my questions, avoiding any sort of prefabricated answers. She was really *there* and totally available. The experience was like looking at myself in a clean mirror or like seeing myself just as I am in a natural light. The image that comes to me now is that of an Alpine lake in which the sun, the blue sky, but also gray clouds heavy with rain or snow, are all reflected, a lake in which the reflections of the clear blue light of the sky, the violent flashes of lightning bolts, the tremulous light of the stars, and the linen-white luminosity of the moon can all be seen.

I spoke with her about the beauty of the places where Niklaus had lived and told her about the local theater company, which staged the life of the saint every year and which would collaborate in the making of this documentary. I told her that the valley had remained intact and that I would not have been surprised to see Niklaus there in his hermitage or to run into him as he walked along the banks of the nearby river, absorbed in meditation. I had started imagining the actual filming of the scenes.

Von Franz confessed that she, too, had been struck by these places when, on Jung's advice, she had gone to visit them. Since the door of the hermitage was unfortunately closed when she got there, she tried to peer through an opening in the wall only to see a little red devil there in the dark, who said, "so let's hear what you have to say." She explained that this was a challenge that she had to take up as it was also an invitation to delve into the question of Niklaus; she took up the challenge with great commitment, and it resulted in her famous book on the saint's visions. The fact that she had seen fit to share these things with me gave me great pleasure, as mutual trust is an essential ingredient in the relationship between the two parties involved in an interview.

So amazingly precise was von Franz's exposition that we were able to film her entire commentary on the visions of Niklaus in just two mornings, and nothing needed to be repeated, though from time to time she asked if we might take a short break. Even though her illness had already begun to affect her facial expression and stiffen her body, her eyes were glowing with life and her tone of voice along with the generous movements of her hands gave special emphasis to various moments in the saint's life; one of these, for example, was related to the sensation he had when he was young of being unworthy, without realizing that he was already on the path of his inner quest. This had been a source of great suffering for him, and von Franz seemed saddened by it as though the saint had been right there with her or had been one of her analysands. I recall how, during one of our breaks, she shook her head and said that nowadays Niklaus would be diagnosed as a neurotic because everything is so cut and dried today. But Niklaus, she added, was very introverted—that was his path.

I certainly would not attempt to summarize the contents of that interview; it deserves to be seen in its entirety in the documentary broadcast by the Italian language and the German language channels of Swiss television in 1987 to mark the five hundredth anniversary of the death of the saint. It can be purchased from the Stiftung für Jung'sche Psychologie, and the complete text of the interview was also published in the journal *Jungiana,* vol. 9 (2000). What I want to do is to reminisce about that very special meeting I had with this great scholar and try to pass on the feelings I had then and which are still alive in me today; I feel that by doing this I am doing something important and helpful for myself as well.

I can't help remembering how heartily von Franz laughed as she recounted how Niklaus, on his way to Alsace, met a farmer who told him to go back home, adding that the Swiss were not very well liked because they were, after all, mercenaries. She then went on to point out that once he was home, the saint's children found him sick and delirious, but the community did not turn him out as a madman but rather realized that he was deeply committed to his inner quest and helped him. It was obvious how moved she was as she spoke of the suffering Niklaus had had to endure. She was also very amused when she told the story of how a high-ranking churchman, in the hopes of exposing the saint's fasting as a hoax, paid a visit to his hermitage. Niklaus caught the prelate completely off guard by telling him that he had been lying regarding the real value of the wines he kept in his cellar. Niklaus had literally looked into his soul and the prelate, blushing with embarrassment, fled from the hermitage. The words of von Franz brought Niklaus to life in such a concrete and human way that I felt he was right there praying, crying, and laughing in the consulting room in Küsnacht beneath the quiet eyes of the great Buddha and in the reassuring presence of the old dog who, after being present during so many analytical hours, probably would not have been surprised to pick up his scent.

When he was old, after so many efforts and trials, Niklaus was called upon to face up to his most difficult test—that of the experience of the dark God, an experience that had shattered many others on their inner quests. Niklaus acted as Job had—he submitted and threw himself down, trying not to lose his grounding in reality. From that moment on, he used a mandala as an aid to meditation in order to find his own center once again, and in the solitude of his hermitage he sought to reconcile good and evil, to unite the opposites. Those who came to visit him could not help but notice that his expression had changed. Here von Franz stopped, and from the tone of her voice and the expression on her face I could see how deeply absorbed in the saint's drama she really was. We had reached Niklaus's last great vision, that of the spring from which welled up the water of life and the water of knowledge, which despite their suffering and because of selfishness, the people back then virtually ignored, just as we today persist in ignoring it. With this vision Niklaus had reached the deepest center of his soul and he was at peace. He died a few years later, in 1487. I was deeply moved and my heart was filled with love as Marie-Louise von Franz affectionately commented on this vision: it was a moment I shall never forget.

Niklaus was responsible for a number of miraculous cures after his death, and I asked von Franz for an explanation of this. What I really wanted to know was whether she believed that the saint's immortal soul had been at work here. She told me that she did but that she couldn't prove it, adding, "Anyone who doesn't want to believe it is free not to." I admired her courage at that moment, and I would like to try and be equally courageous by recounting an incident that happened to me during the shooting of the documentary. I was in my hotel room, drawing up the list of my expenses that I planned to submit when I realized that I had mislaid a restaurant receipt. I have to admit that I thought that I could be reimbursed just the same by adding the amount of the restaurant bill to the other items in my expense account. When I was about to go out of the hotel room, I suddenly could no longer find my wallet. I looked for it everywhere but to no avail and then went down to the reception desk to see if anyone had found it but no one had. I then went back up to my room and started searching for it again. Out of the blue, I heard a low, almost hoarse voice say to me in old German that I was really something! and that I should look inside myself. Almost automatically I checked my jacket pocket again, and lo and behold, the wallet was there! Needless to say, I was really taken aback and was then able to honestly and correctly complete my list of expenses! For years I never breathed a word of this to anyone, until I met up with Marie-Louise von Franz once again at an international conference in Germany. During a pause, I plucked up the courage to talk to her about it. She was most amused by the story and said that there had obviously been a dematerialization and then a materialization. Unfortunately, I didn't have the courage to ask her if she thought the voice had been the voice of Niklaus. She no doubt would have replied, "Anyone who doesn't want to believe it is free not to." She also added that my neglect in filling out my expense account list was not really such a serious matter—something which reconciled me again with myself.

Since we are on the topic of the paranormal, I should add that the shooting of the film went smoothly and that the weather was clement the entire time. The working atmosphere among those involved in the filming was excellent, and everyone, in an almost magical way, just seemed to be at the right place at the right time.

The way in which I found the person to play the part of Niklaus himself is most interesting. I had only just arrived at Sachseln to reconnoiter the area when I saw a tall, thin, elderly, ascetic-looking man with white hair and beard walking along the road, and I immediately thought that he was the one to play the part of Niklaus. A short time later a local sculptor who was helping me get acquainted with the people of the area introduced me to that very gentleman, saying that he was the right person for the role. When I got to know him, I realized that he fit the role perfectly, not only from a physical point of view but also in terms of his sensitivity and closeness to the saint. He told me that after his retirement he had moved to Sachseln because in a military retreat during the Russian campaign he had taken a vow to stay near Niklaus if the saint would help him. He had no trouble donning an old tunic and kneeling down in prayer in front of the cameras.

When the documentary had been edited and mounted, I invited von Franz to Lugano for a screening of it. She had given me a totally free hand and had not taken part herself in the actual filming of the scenes. I had, however, sent her the text of the documentary, which she had sent back to me with a few corrections pencilled in, along with just one comment written in her shaky hand, which had given me great pleasure: "Sehr gut." She arrived in Lugano accompanied by Emmanuel Kennedy, then a young student of hers and today a psychotherapist himself; he graciously acted as her "bodyguard." The screening of the film was uneventful with the exception of a moment near the end of the documentary when von Franz was obviously deeply moved—it was the scene in which the elderly Niklaus, with outstretched arms, kneels in prayer before the setting sun. The scene then darkens to indicate his death only to brighten again to show a series of beautiful votive offerings.

Later, during our lunch at a grotto in Montagnola, as we sat beneath the old chestnut trees, von Franz brought up that last scene of the saint's death, complimenting me on how beautiful it was and asking who the actor was. A few months later, when the documentary had already been circulated, she told me that the actor had contacted her and that he was a very special person indeed. She told me that she had received letters of appreciation from a good number of viewers, and that she, a Protestant herself, was particularly delighted to have received a note from the mother superior of a convent of cloistered nuns near Sachseln.

During our lunch near Lugano, I asked her about her views on life after death; she told me about her recently published book, *On Dreams and Death,* in which she analyzes a number of dreams of dying people that seem to show that the soul itself gives indications that life continues beyond death. I told her of my own experiences with Elisabeth Kübler-Ross and of the stories I had gathered from people who had lived through a death experience. The documentary on Niklaus had led us to discuss the difficult topic of death, and von Franz examined various aspects of it, moving from the culture of ancient Egypt, through alchemy, and on to shamanism. It was a brief lesson delivered with clarity, simplicity, serenity, and a sense of hope. That evening, we met again for dinner out on the terrace of our Montagnola hotel, enjoying the beautiful view over the lake.

Subsequently, I paid Marie-Louise von Franz a few visits at her home in Küsnacht. I had grown very fond of her. Each time, I could see how her illness was progressing and so my visits were brief, at times no more than a quick greeting. She was perfectly lucid and managed to tell me that she was working on Arabic alchemy. Whenever I went abroad on business, I never failed to send her a postcard. The work we had done together on the life of Niklaus had been a special privilege for me; I had felt that the love of a greater presence had been at work.

When I think of Marie-Louise von Franz today, I think of her as a wise, simple, modest person who truly knew how to nourish life—this must surely be the reason why each time I dream of her, she appears as a cook bent over a stove, intent on preparing a meal.

A Reminiscence

GILDA FRANTZ

It was the mid-fifties. The Los Angeles group was just forming a professional society. It all began in the forties when James and Hilde Kirsch came over from war-torn England, followed by Max Zeller. James Kirsch had already had a hand in starting the Zürich group, the London group, and probably one in Palestine as well.

It was a very creative time in Los Angeles. My husband, Kieffer E. Frantz, M.D., had recently become the medical director of a low-fee clinic that opened its doors in 1952. It was the first analytical psychology clinic of its kind anywhere in the world to offer low-fee analysis (and low fee in those days might mean a dollar a session with James, Hilde, or Max Zeller, all analysts who had worked with Jung). Kieffer was its director from its inception until his death in 1975, and in his honor, it now bears his name.

Los Angeles had a very small but dynamic Jungian community of which the Analytical Psychology Club was the nucleus, which was made evident by the APC being actively involved in bringing analysts from Zürich to lecture here. Many members who didn't go to Zürich could experience the work of Swiss analysts, or analysts who lived in Zürich and who were close to Jung. Many people in Los Angeles were encouraged to go to Zürich to study, including my husband, who came back with stories of the lectures and life there. The Club had an education fund, probably initiated by James and Hilde Kirsch, for the express purpose of importing analysts such as Marie-Louise von Franz, Barbara Hannah, Rivkah Schärf, C. A. Meier, and Heinrich Fiertz, as well as Dora Kalff, to recall just a few. Later, analysts Esther Harding and Eleanor Bertine and Edward Edinger came from New York. Hilde Kirsch and James Kirsch always opened their home to these visitors from abroad, and some of the visiting analysts saw analysands for a few sessions. This was while they were conducting seminars and lecturing.

The 1950s were quite conventional in many ways. Jung's attempt to wrest individuals from collective thinking comes to mind. Men wore ties and jackets to meetings and women all seemed to dress alike. Not so the Jungian community. While the founders were European and had that sensibility, there was a feeling of openness to that which was nonrational, and it was very exciting. Although I enthusiastically went into analysis not long after I married Kieffer, I had less than a handful of years of analysis, which consisted mainly of dealing with ego development and bolstering a lack of confidence. I was pregnant with my second child, Marlene, when I met Marie-Louise von Franz, and it was one of the most important meetings of my life, then and now.

Dr. von Franz was here to lecture, brought to Los Angeles by the above mentioned Analytical Psychology Club, and my husband and I had come to a reception to honor her and Miss Hannah. If memory serves correctly, the APC arranged an authentic Native American dinner in her honor. Her wit and humor bubbled through and during the evening, especially when someone said something to the effect that while the food no doubt was authentic, it also possessed very little flavor! Which was the truth. We all laughed as it was in good humor, and she laughed loudest.

I was in my late twenties and she in her late thirties when we met. I was immediately drawn to her. She was so *alive,* so animated, articulate, exciting and brilliant, and she had a playful side and was exciting to be around. She told me that she had suffered a deep betrayal recently, about her life work being published by her collaborator Hedwig von Beit without crediting von Franz for writing it, but even so she exuded a vitality that was rich.

We found out that she and Miss Hannah were planning a little holiday in "Indian country" in a couple of days, and Marlus (which she encouraged us to call her) was eager to go horseback riding to really experience the Old West that she had read about and seen in the movies of her childhood. I think they were going to Montana or Wyoming. She had a long-held romantic notion about the West and could hardly wait to experience it. "It's not a good idea to ride on a Western saddle in a dress," I warned tactfully when I learned that dresses and blouses and skirts were all she had packed, and even though I am no horsewoman, I said I would lend her a pair of my own blue denim jeans so she could enjoy playing cowboys and Indians! She happily accepted. She returned them the next time she came to California to lecture, neatly laundered, folded and pressed.

Another favorite story involves a letter I sent when I was editor of the APC's monthly newsletter. I wrote to invite her to come visit Los Angeles again and lecture to the club on any subject she chose. By return mail, I received a simple white envelope with no return address and within it was a plain piece of white paper, very thin, on which she had written in her tiny script: *Dear Mrs. Frantz: I am sitting on three eggs. When they are hatched I will come to Los Angeles. (signed) Marie Louise von Franz.*

Of course, the three eggs were her first three books, and when she finished she was indeed true to her word and she did come. What struck me at the time of receiving her letter was her simplicity and lack of persona. I couldn't imagine that such a famous woman would have stationary without any imprint of her name or status. Now that I am an old lady, (and I do have letterhead stationary), whenever I write a friend a note on plain paper I think of Marie-Louise and smile. I understand it better now than I did then. She was utterly unpretentious. And I loved that about her.

Another great time was when she was invited in 1978 to lecture at the Panarion lectures in Los Angeles. My beloved husband had died three years before, and I was a new analyst (I had been in the training program before his death). The painter Sam Francis gave a dinner party at his home and invited some of the speakers, and I was fortunate to be a guest along with many others to honor Marie-Louise. We were seated next to one another, and I told her of an interesting event in my life that had just occurred. My daughter Marlene, with whom I was pregnant when von Franz and I first met in the fifties, excitedly had told me about a house that was for sale, which happened to be almost around the corner from Sam Francis's house. Marlene was coordinating the Panarion conference that summer and attending a class in Hindu mythology taught by Dr. Kees Bolle, a student and colleague of Mircea Elliade, at the University of California-Los Angeles. Before class, Dr. Bolle confided that he was selling his house. She wasn't thinking of the house as being for me, but thought it would be perfect for her uncle. The moment I heard about this house, I felt a shiver go through my body, and I went to the I Ching and asked what the meaning was of this possibility. The coins came up with the hexagram 24, which is Return. I went with my brother to see the house the day after tossing the coins, and I loved it. He didn't. I told this to Marie-Louise and she said, "Of course you must buy this house. This denotes the Self, that you are completing one phase of your life and beginning again." I had already impulsively told Dr. Bolle I would take the house, but Marlus's response sealed it in my mind. After dinner, I drove her past the house on the way to her hotel and showed her a small restaurant a block away. "Ah," she said, "that little restaurant will be like a mother to you, and after work you will be able to get hot soup and bread there." And like in a fairy tale, I did buy the house and live there still, and the restaurant did feed and nourish me after a long day of analytical work for many years until the owner retired.

Marie-Louise is very much a part of this house and my life professionally and personally. A book I turn to again and again is her *Creation Myths*. I am always confident of finding some wisdom, some story, that will help me or someone in my practice. Often before giving a lecture, I dream of Marie-Louise, and she is an encouraging figure in my dreams, always compensating for my inferior thinking. When I had the idea to dedicate an entire issue of *Psychological Perspectives* to her in honor of her major contribution to analytical psychology, due to her death it became a memorial issue instead. For the title, I used a quote from the letter of a young man who hadn't known her but had corresponded with her. In this letter, I read that she told him to "concentrate the heart" when he sought advice as to what to do about his writing. I titled the issue *Concentrate the Heart* in her memory. And now, as I write these words, I feel a contraction in my heart and know that if I can concentrate the heart, there is wisdom there and love there and creativity there.

One of my favorite memories happened toward the end of her life. A book came out, written by a long-ago analysand with whom she had worked, which kindly mentioned me in the introduction. Unfortunately, the publisher misspelled my name, and it was printed as Gilda von Franz! Of course, it was a typo, as the author knew my name, but I felt enchanted when I saw it. I made a copy of the page and sent it to Marie-Louise with a short note saying I had always wanted to be a part of her family. By return mail came a note from her, written in someone else's hand: "Dear Sister" was the salutation, and she thanked me for making her laugh. She signed it herself in her dear tiny, now shaky, handwriting. What a precious woman she was.

I know that when the film *Matter of Heart* came out, some people commented that in some scenes her fingernails were very dirty. I loved her dirty fingernails. I knew that during the filming she had carried wood into the house, cooked over a sooty fireplace, and had been digging in the earth. I loved that she cared about what she was doing and not about how it looked. She once remarked to me when she was in Los Angeles that she thought she looked like a potato sack in the dress she was wearing. She didn't, but by then she had a mature figure and seemed suddenly self-conscious. She didn't look like a sack, but she was a woman, a genius, who spent more time with the soul than with primping. She always looked quite beautiful to me. There will never be another woman like her, and it is my loss and the world's loss.

I have read and heard a great deal about how she planned her own funeral and reception and music. None of this is out of character for a woman who was elegant, beautiful, and imaginative as she. Facing death she used her imagination and creativity about the Beyond and the end of life. In other words, she died as she had lived.

How fortunate I have been to have known her. We were not friends in the usual, casual sense, like having coffee and sharing secrets, but she was certainly a spiritual inspiration for me, and I feel extremely loyal to her, and if that isn't a friendship, I don't know what is.

Marie-Louise von Franz as Thesis Advisor

ROBERTO GAMBINI

My decision to enroll at the C. G. Jung Institute back in 1978 was a crucial change in my life. I needed to find a new profession, as my total being refused to go on doing the things I had been previously prepared to do. I had studied law and social sciences in my hometown, São Paulo, and had earned a master's degree at the University of Chicago. I thought I was a scholar, so I had started a career at a very good university that had just been founded, and I also worked as a sociologist in public service.

It was a painful depression that made me seek Jungian analysis back in 1974. My analyst had spent some time in Zürich, and he was one of the first to offer that kind of work among us. During my years in Chicago, I found Jung's *Memories, Dreams, Reflections* and knew, even before reading it, that my whole outlook on the world, the mind, and the psyche would change as I absorbed his ideas. In the sequence, I found *Man and His Symbols,* and this time I was caught by Marie-Louise von Franz's article. I immediately felt a vivid attraction to her way of thinking and went after her books, published by Spring, starting with *Shadow and*

Evil in Fairy Tales, followed by many others. Although I obviously had to read and study sociology and political science for my work, all had become dull and only Jungian books, especially hers, were of interest to me.

Quite unexpectedly, after three years of analysis, it dawned on me that my true vocation was to be a therapist. This discovery was to me like a revelation, like a bubble of meaning that had made its way from the bottom of a lake to the surface. I was then faced with a difficult situation: either I had to start again from the beginning and enter a psychology undergraduate course, or I could go back to the United States, where I had been a Ph.D. candidate, and try to qualify by writing a thesis in some neighboring field, or I could do something radical and join the Zürich Institute, which was actually the only place in the world that would open its doors to somebody in my situation.

Dr. Adolf Guggenbühl-Craig visited São Paulo in 1977 to set the official basis for a newly founded Jungian Society that was seeking recognition. But it accepted only psychiatrists and psychologists, and not somebody with my curriculum. He must have been aware of that limitation, and I suspect he did something on my behalf after I wrote to the Institute seeking admission.

When my wife, our little *dachshund,* and I disembarked in Zürich, I already had an appointment with my analyst-to-be, Dr. Heinrich Karl Fierz, and a deep hope that Dr. von Franz would agree to be my thesis advisor. This is the story I briefly want to tell here, because I think it deserves to be shared.

First of all, it is important to note that, unlike most of the students who start their training at the Institute, I had from the beginning a very clear idea of the research I wanted to do and the kind of thesis I expected to write. The reason for this was twofold: on the one side, as I had given up my American Ph.D., I had to put forward a certain amount of creative energy that had not been allowed to flow within the rigid boundaries of an academic format. And as I definitely had Jungian psychology under my skin, it was imperative that I try to bring it together with my prior education in the social sciences, like merging the waters of two rivers in the same bed (this was already an influence of Jung's task before he found his own field of action, as I had read in his *Memories*). The second reason for my having a written research project was that I needed financial support to be able to spend almost four years in Zürich, and this I luckily obtained from a research foundation in my country which reluctantly approved my unorthodox project. I had put such enormous energy into it that I succeeded in convincing its scientific board of advisors that this unheard-of Jung Institute was after all a serious place of study and research.

A short time after my training and analysis started, I wrote to Dr. von Franz explaining to her the situation and asking if she would agree to be my advisor. She gave me an appointment in Lindenbergstrasse, a few houses down the street from where Dr. Fierz lived. I then felt that my real intellectual work would start.

I collected my research project and the Brazilian books I wanted to show her in a Migros paper bag—I remember every detail. While we began to talk in her library, Laura, her boxer, felt so attracted to the three thick volumes of the sixteenth-century Jesuit letters that I had laid on the carpet that she could not avoid chewing a corner of one the volumes. Perhaps Dr. von Franz took that as a sign. She, too, was interested in my idea that the early missionaries who went to Brazil to convert the Indians to Catholicism were projecting the Christian shadow onto them, to summarize my project in one line. She immediately got the point. I said I would select from Jung's *Collected Works* all the passages in which Jung wrote about projection, which alone would take a long time. She said I should read his letters, too. Then I would read another four hundred letters written by the Jesuits from 1549 to about 1560, collecting all the passages in which they portrayed the Indians, in order to analyze them using Jung's concept of projection. Then I would read Jung's seminar on the Spiritual Exercises of Ignatius Loyola, for which written permission by a member of the Jung family was required. Next I would study the history of the Company of Jesus, and in the end I had to shape a style of thinking and writing that would bring together Jungian psychology, history, and anthropology.

She agreed; I felt relieved. She believed in me. I was not alone, my intuitions made sense. If the great Marie-Louise von Franz had not dismissed them as nonsense, I could now seriously believe in myself. I lost no time and immediately started to work.

Only much later I learned that she had just finished her fundamental work on projection, *Projection and Recollection in Jungian Psychology: Reflections of the Soul.* At that time, it was already being translated into English by William H. Kennedy, but she made no mention of it. She made me go all the way, reading most of the volumes of the *Collected Works*, Jung's letters and seminars, until I finally came to my own understanding of what projection was—and to do so, I had to plunge into Jung's work and that is how I really learned something. At the Institute, there was not a comparable demand to read systematically his work, so this is how my training took off.

We had made an agreement that I would send her a copy of each finished chapter. As I had a research plan, I just followed it, step by step. I was anxious to hear her comments on my first paper, dealing with projection, because I had to go back to neurology and Freud, the different perspective adopted by Jung, and the basic points he made: that projection simply happens, that it is the way the psyche works, that it is not the ego that makes it, since an unconscious content projects itself, that there are four stages of projection, and so on. I expected that she would summon me to an appointment in which she would make corrections and suggestions and reveal to me some hidden secrets of Jung's theory. But instead, she sent me a laconic letter: "Dear Mr. Gambini, I have read your paper. It is OK. Go ahead. Marie-Louise von Franz."

Was she not interested? Or had I done something reasonable? "It is OK," she had said. So I went on. For the next two years, I plunged into the material, following my plan, which I did not change during the whole research. So a pattern of relationship developed between us. Each time I would send her a new chapter, she would reply with exactly the same letter. I have kept all of them. "It is OK. Go ahead." Nothing else. Maybe she was too busy. Maybe I did not deserve more. In my experience at the University of Chicago, my master's advisor always gave me a hard time, he was never satisfied, he wanted me to do something different from what I had in mind, we quarreled, he made me read books that added nothing to what I was pursuing, he wanted me to be his disciple and spread his ideas. Before that, at the University of São Paulo, I had followed many friends doing their dissertations and had become aware of a pattern of relationship between advisor and candidate, in which the first tries to mold the student's mind to be a continuation or a by-product of his or her teacher. I had seen how these relationships are building blocks of the academic power structure, as in a feudal system, each professor creating a court of followers. I had always abhorred this way of growing outwardly at the cost of sacrificing one's free thinking and was happy that Dr. von Franz was not following that pattern. But on the other hand, I was left with a "go ahead" and ignored what pattern, if any, she was following.

When the time came—exactly when my wife was giving birth to our daughter (our son was born when I began working)—I finished my "Projection and Conversion of Souls—A Psychological Study of Indians and Jesuits in Sixteenth-century Brazil." Dr. von Franz approved it and two experts, Mr. John Hill and Dr. José Zavala, were invited for the final exam. As we sat by a window overlooking the lake in the newly opened Küsnacht Institute, my advisor opened the session by complaining that I had sent her a very bad photocopy and that I had to pay more attention to the feeling function. She made brief strong comments and left, because she had other obligations, leaving the three of us to discuss the thesis. She said my work had its importance, because white civilization had to come to terms with its destructive shadow. I left without knowing if I had been approved or not. Later, I learned that I had been successful, and shortly after, having fulfilled all requirements, I was granted my diploma.

Shortly before returning to Brazil to start my new life, I made an appointment with Dr. von Franz to bid her farewell and pay my bill. When I mentioned it, she said: "You can give me 150 Swiss francs." I had expected her to charge me much more than that, because I had seen her three or four times. I am not sure now. The average fee for an analytical hour was then 100 francs, and I was ready to pay accordingly. As I handed her the bills, she showed them to Laura, saying, "Here, sausages for you." I had suspected from the beginning that Laura had her paw in it. I then said very sincere words of thanks and heard the following: "Mr. Gambini, when you first came here, I realized that you were thin, pale, and depressed. Your creativity was just waiting to come out. I gave you a backing, so you could trust yourself and do what the unconscious wanted you to do. You don't owe me anything. The work you have done is yours." And so we bade farewell.

Years later, I wrote her again. My work would be published under the title *Indian Mirror—The Making of the Brazilian Soul.* Now in its second edition, both in Portuguese and English, it is a very beautiful book, illustrated with old engravings portraying ancient maps, Brazilian nature, Indians, and Jesuits converting them. I imagined that if she would write a preface I would be legitimized by the highest authority in the Jungian world. But she refused. So the book had to rely only on its own merits, if it had any.

I have since then been lecturing on this topic, adding thoughts and reflections that keep coming to me after all these years. I have definitely become a sort of a freethinker, in the sense that I always obey the inspirations of an inner voice that whispers in my ear the words I say in my impromptu talks or the new topics of research that I am to pursue. At the 1995 Zürich congress, I presented some of those ideas, shifting the angle a little bit, under the title "The Soul of Underdevelopment."

Quite recently, I was invited by the colleagues who work in the foundation that carries Jung's and Marie-Louise von Franz's names to lecture on my topic at the monastery in St. Niklausen, Switzerland,where training is given according to their teachings. Before I started my first lecture, I asked the audience for a moment of silence. In those thirty seconds or so, I saw again the two of us sitting together for the first time in her library. Then I clearly felt to its full extent the meaning, the scope, and the consequences of her way of being an advisor.

The Journey of Individuation

A Matter of Life or Death

GOTO KAZU

In 1975, I wrote a letter to Dr. Marie-Louise von Franz asking her if I could have a personal analysis with her in 1977, the year I was planning to leave Japan and come to Switzerland to undertake the training program at the C. G. Jung Institute in Küsnacht. By July 1975, I had already completed one hundred and fifty hours of personal analysis with two Japanese analysts, so that when I arrived in 1977, I was able to begin analytical work directly with Dr. von Franz.

In every session, I used to give her a written report of my dreams along with my interpretation of them. I also included my remarks about various things that were discussed in the previous session, things that I could not explain or understand well. When Dr. von Franz read my first written report on my dreams, she said to me: "You did serious work, good for you!" The next time, she said: "Excellent." And the time after that, she said: "Perfect!"

My dreams always betrayed and threatened me. In one such dream, a Mr. N appeared and said to me: "You don't need the [C. G. Jung Institute] diploma now." Dr. von Franz said, smiling: "If he is a nice person, let's listen to what he has to say." I explained to her that he was a male nurse at the ward for alcoholic patients at the mental hospital where I had worked as a clinical psychologist until December 1976. Mr. N had been an alcoholic himself when he was young, but he had stopped drinking and was now taking care of alcoholic patients. Once he had introduced me to an alcoholic patient in his early forties. I treated him by applying an "image-formation technique." He drew a total of fourteen images within the context of this treatment method, and soon after this he stopped drinking. The whole treatment lasted but two months.

Dr. von Franz said to me: "I will give you the diploma." And she wrote a letter immediately to the Curatorium of the Institute. I took the letter to Mrs. Heddah Baumann, the secretary of the Jung Institute. Mrs. Baumann said to me: "Even Dr. Barz, the president of this Institute, studied here for three years."

There are two interesting events I would like to mention in connection with Mrs. Baumann. When I wrote to the Jung Institute in 1970 requesting information about the training program, Mrs. Baumann sent the documentation to the wrong address:

Japan
Tenri University
Doctorantin
Miss Kazu Goto

The correct address, which I had sent to the Institute, was actually:

Miss Kazu Goto
Sekiya 886
Kashiba-cho, Nara-ken
Japan

The envelope with the information regarding the training program was delivered to Tenri University, then to Professor H. Kawai, who was a Jungian analyst trained in Zürich. I received the envelope from

Dr. Kawai later when he was giving lectures on Jungian psychology, not at Tenri but at Kyoto University.

The second occurrence was about the fact that I could not start studying at the Jung Institute until autumn 1977, even though I had applied for the spring term of that year. After my encounter with Mrs. Baumann, I saw Dr. von Franz again and related what Mrs. Baumann had said regarding the diploma, as well as the two things about the mistaken address and the delay in starting my training program at the Institute. Dr. von Franz commented that "Mrs. Baumann seems to have been hitting the head of von Franz's pupils instead of hitting the head of von Franz."

There is a dream I had in which Dr. von Franz appears that I would like to relate in this commemorative publication in her honor. It was a very vivid dream, and I woke up with a most intense impression. The dream took place in a dark forest.

> *Many animals had gathered in an open area surrounded by big trees. The animals made a blazing fire at the center of this open area. Dr. von Franz jumped into that blazing fire.*

The dream reminded me of an illustrated children's book with the title *A Hare in the Moon.* In this story, a hare jumps into a blazing fire. After I had related the dream to her, Dr. von Franz told me that she would not be jumping into the blazing fire (in the Chinese horoscope, Marie-Louise von Franz is a hare).

When I returned to Japan, I visited Hozokan, a publisher in Kyoto specializing in religious books. I found the picture book, *A Hare in the Moon.* The relevant passage reads as follows:

> A hare could not find any offering to Sakra Devānām who came down to the earth in the guise of a medicine man. The hare made up his mind to offer himself to Sakra Devānām and jumped into a blazing fire. Sakra Devānām Indra felt pity for the hare, took him into his arms and took the hare with him to the moon.

In another dream that occurred just before I left Switzerland to return to Japan, I dreamed that:

I am walking through a side gate of a white mud wall that surrounds a large private house which I am approaching.

The only thing I could recall about this dream was that my great grandmother had to leave from the Hanbei Yashiki in 1850 with her baby and a small child. "Hanbei Yashiki" means the house of Hanbei Goto, the *shoya,* the village's chief. This house was half public, half private. The size of the house was 3,305 square meters, and it was surrounded by a white wall called "Itsucho Dobei" which is 109 meters long. Dr. von Franz said: "You will do something in this house." At the time, I could not understand what that meant.

Of special interest to me was, and is, the work on fairy tales. The first fairy tale Dr. von Franz gave me to interpret was a Japanese fairy tale called "Hanasaka Jijii," about an old man who makes withered trees blossom again. I enjoyed very much interpreting this fairy tale. In the Institute of Japanology in Zürich, I found a nice old version of this fairy tale. When I returned to Japan, I looked for various versions of "Hanasaka Jijii" at the Kokkai Library in Tokyo. It was out of my interest in fairy tales that I translated Barbara Hannah's book *C. G. Jung: His Life and Work* and then Dr. von Franz's *Individuation in Fairy Tales.* This was in 1985. I feel very strongly that the journey of individuation is a matter of life and death and that at the end this process raises people from death.

After finishing the translation of *Individuation in Fairy Tales,* I felt a strong urge to investigate my heritage, the story of my ancestors and their graves. This research work, which is now finished and will soon be published, confronts me with mysteries and synchronicities. It also begins to reveal to me the hidden meaning of the connection between my life and my encounter with analytical psychology.

Marlus—The Mischievous One

E. J. HANNAH

I met Marlus (as we were asked to call Dr. von Franz) on only one occasion other than in Zürich, where she lived with my uncle's aunt, Barbara Hannah. This was in Scotland where my family were on holiday in Ullapool—a small fishing town on the upper west coast. Barbara and Marlus joined us for a few days. They were touring the country, and they both had fallen in love with the splendor of the mountains, the beauty of the lochs, and the waterfalls as they tumbled down the hillsides (it had rained a lot that summer). In turn, we became very fond of Marlus and enjoyed her quick wit and lively conversation.

In particular, Marlus was entranced by the color and variety of the Scottish stones. She carefully collected them—some big, some small—and put them in the boot of the car, and more, and more. When Barbara opened the car again, the boot was filled with stones of all shapes and sizes. "What nonsense is this!" said Barbara, "Far too heavy." And she threw them all out. Marlus tried again the following day with the same result.

When it was time for them to leave, I commiserated with Marlus on the loss of her stones. Her mischievous smile broke out. "I've hidden them in our gumboots," she whispered, "I hope it won't rain today."

This incident for me shows the determination and underlying good humor of two formidable ladies.

Four Swans Gliding Out to Sea

SUSAN HARRIS

I received your letter concerning the commemorative publication honoring Dr. Marie-Louise von Franz, and I feel very ashamed that it has taken me so long to get in touch with you.

You wrote to the Isle of Man, to my mother Ruth Markus, and the letter was forwarded to me. Sadly, my mother died in August 1999, peacefully in her own home after a long fight with cancer. My mother worked principally with Miss Barbara Hannah, but I know she knew, respected, and was somewhat in awe of Dr. von Franz. I know that Dr. von Franz gave my mother great encouragement to complete her book, *Mermaid on a Dolphin's Back,* which she completed about two years before she died. It has not been published because she did not want it to be. However, she did get it printed. My mother worked very hard on her individuation and was inordinately grateful for the insight she received from Jungians, which helped her to live with her huge and difficult responsibilities. I received wonderful and sustaining confirmation of how far she had come down the road to individuation when I looked out of her bedroom window a few minutes after she had died. Her window faced the Irish Sea. A small amount of grass, some rocks, and the sea only twenty-five yards away. It was a beautiful summer's day, the sun was shining, the water was blue and motionless, and it was high tide. There in front of the window were four swans, and they were gliding out to sea in a perfect square, two by two.

Contacting the Otherworldly Image

GEORGES HUDE

Please excuse my writing to you [Dr. Kennedy] in French; my German and my English are unfortunately very poor. I would like to respond to your letter of February 2002 concerning a future publication for Marie-Louise von Franz.

Marie-Louise von Franz and I were friends, and I went to see her frequently in Küsnacht. Our exchanges were very rich and profound. As my wife had unfortunately died in July 1994, Marie-Louise von Franz and I naturally spoke extensively about illness and death. Our conversations were very precious to me. She also spoke to me about her own illness, about her dreams, and particularly those dreams that dealt with death.

One day, I received a letter from Dr. von Franz dated February 12, 1996, which seemed to me of utmost importance and which would perhaps suit a commemorative publication, for it shows very well the profundity of her thought. It is written in French. Enclosed you will find a copy (which had been dictated, because at that time she could no longer write letters herself).

At your disposal and with cordial regards,
Georges Hude

Marie-Louise von Franz
Lindenbergstr. 15
8700 Küsnacht
February 12, 1996

Dear Georges,

I believe I have found the solution: One must struggle very hard in order to avoid attaching oneself to the image-memory of the deceased. The image-memory has become an empty mask. One must search for an image of the deceased person as he or she is in the beyond, and then try to establish contact with this otherworldly image.

With all my best thoughts,
(signed) Marie-Louise von Franz

Walking with Kings Without Losing the Common Touch

ROBIN LEA HUTTON

I've been sitting here at my writing desk for the longest time, thinking . . . and remembering. I was thinking back to the last time I saw Marie-Louise von Franz at Bollingen and remembering fondly the great fortune I had for all the time I got to spend with her for the almost twenty years we worked together and, more importantly, the friendship we developed that carved a deep groove in my heart.

Where do I start? How can I possibly put into words this little woman (little only in size, that is) who was packed so full of life and wisdom and love for her friends and analysands . . . how can I possibly do justice to what she has done for me, and what she has given to my life? There aren't enough words . . . and the words I find seem so inadequate . . . but I have solace in the fact that I'm sure everyone who is writing for her Festschrift is finding out for themselves this very truth, so I am not alone.

Marie-Louise von Franz gave my life more meaning in one hour of analysis than I have gotten from all the other analysts before and after her. And she put me in touch with my own inner analyst, which was one of the most important gifts of all.

As I sat at my desk trying to write this piece, a little bird tried for twenty minutes to break into the window right in front of me. He'd fly from the tree limb into the window and then back to the birdbath, only to do this again and again and again. The noise was making me a little crazy, not to mention my concern for this little bird. No matter what I did, nothing stopped him. I stood in the window and tried to scare him. It was like I wasn't there. I went outside and tried to shoo him away. Didn't work. My German shepherd, Henry, went crazy and attacked the window when the little fellow would fly just inches above his head. Didn't deter the bird at all. Instinct had gotten hold of this creature, and that was all there was to it. A friend finally suggested putting a towel up on the window so that the bird couldn't see whatever reflection it was that so fascinated him and drove him to this behavior, a behavior that could ultimately hurt him if he didn't stop it.

I did so, and the behavior stopped, just like that, and I thought to myself, "This is a metaphor for life. I know there's some profound psychological insight for me in here that I'm just not seeing (especially since this is the second time this has happened in the past month—and, a few months ago I caught a hummingbird at my dining room window that got trapped inside the house and was trying to get out; I gently wrapped my hands around him and safely carried him outside and released him back to nature). The Self is obviously trying to get my attention and tell me something. *What would von Franz say about this one?* She'd give me some profound insight, something I could go to work on for weeks, maybe months . . . something solid I could do to find out what it was the Self was trying to say to me through this little bird.

(As I write this, I remember a story von Franz told of either an analysand or a famous person she knew who had a bird try for the longest time to get into this person's home by flying into a closed window. No matter where the person went, the bird followed, always flying into the closed window. The person totally ignored the bird, even tried to shoo it away if I remember correctly. Von Franz said that the bird was the man's soul trying to get in, because like all of us, he had gotten so caught up in the existential world of ego goals and pursuit of power and success that he was totally ignoring his whole inner life, his soul. The bird was desperately trying to come in and call attention to the fact that he has to divert some attention back and take care of his soul. Unfortunately the man just saw the bird as a pest, so he ignored it and went off and had some sort of catastrophe. (Oh, dear.))

With that in mind, I put on "The Trout" by Schubert, lit my "sacred" vanilla candle, which I started burning when I heard of her passing and light only on those occasions when I write to her in my journal, and started to write this, because I obviously needed to connect with her.

I first met Dr. von Franz at the Panarion Conference in Los Angeles in 1979, where she gave a paper on numbers and the archetypal energy that surrounded them, or something to that effect. To be perfectly honest, it was so over my head that I'm still spinning from it and still don't understand what she was talking about, but that didn't stop us from becoming friends. That was what was so great about her. She was one of those rare people who "walked with Kings but never lost the common touch," and she accepted and loved you for who you were—shadow and all—and not for the persona you felt you had to live up to.

I was the friend who kept her supplied with tyrosine, the natural supplement that she needed to help treat her Parkinson's (she couldn't get tyrosine in Switzerland). She learned about the medical benefits of tyrosine from a dream that she had Tom Laughlin interpret for her, which told her clearly that the L-dopa she was taking for her Parkinson's was damaging her heart and that tyrosine, because it was a natural supplement and a precursor for dopamine production, would help her body create her own dopamine and help her manage this horrible disease naturally. After the interpretation of this dream, she stopped taking the L-dopa and started the tyrosine, which she took daily up until her passing. Thank goodness she did, because honoring that dream gave us about fourteen more years with her.

I must admit that every time I take tyrosine, I think of her. Every time I do a lot of things I think of her fondly and wish I could pick up the phone and talk to her. But I guess that's why God invented journals because I still have my chats with her there (only I lose the effect of her great accent and miss terribly the twinkle in her eye when she nailed me with some shadow quality I was having a hard time seeing (read: refused to see), though she could see it so plainly like it was on the end of my nose!).

In the last years of her life, the letters that I would get from her were addressed in Barbara Davies's hand, and since her passing, the correspondence I have had with Barbara over the years comes in very similar envelopes, and so whenever I get a letter in that same airmail envelope, I still get a rush for just a fleeting moment and think "Oh, great! I got a letter from von Franz!"

Getting a letter from her was always such a delight, for they always seemed to come just at the time when I needed them most—if for no other reason than to know that she had been thinking of me—but more often than not, she gave me some insight that I really needed to hear.

One of the many insights and gifts that Mar-Lou had given me was the confidence and strength to feel that I could do whatever I set my heart to, to follow my passion (and therefore the self), and as long as I followed what the self wanted me to do, that's all that mattered. She never judged me, she liked me for who I was because she truly understood and appreciated the uniqueness in all of us, and that gave me the strength and confidence to want to do more, to want to face more of my shadow and transform it. She never expected anything from me other than to become the person God wanted me to become from the moment He conceived me. She helped me understand the power and wisdom of my soul through my dreams and active imagination.

Through active imagination I learned how much I loved to write—which was a real shock to me! And because of Mar-Lou, I ventured off and wrote my first novel (which, if you asked friends and family who knew me growing up, they would say it was the farthest thing from their minds that I would ever do that with my life), but she encouraged me to follow my soul and do it. She made me see that my novel was actually one long active imagination, for I learned so much about myself in the process because she told me that each of the characters I wrote about actually stood for that part of my own unconscious personality that was being expressed. I have been able to write about things I never knew were in me, and it has taken me places I never thought I would go. And most important of all, Mar-Lou helped me see that writing is my greatest passion, and that is what my life's work is to be—no matter what topic I choose to write about.

I don't need to write the Great American Novel or the movie script that becomes the box-office champion of all time (though, of course, both of these are obviously in my fantasy or I wouldn't have just written it—oh, my!), but she made me see that the *act* of writing is what the Self/God needs me to do, and if I follow what the self needs me to do—if I follow what it is that God needs me to do to complete His creation of me—then she said the self/God will guide me and protect me and all will be right in my world.

Only when I do that can Merton's saying—"My work is my prayer. The results do not concern me, they are God's problem"—become a reality. (Unfortunately I haven't evolved enough yet to where the results do not concern me—but individuation is a journey, not a destiny, and God isn't finished with me yet so there's still time!)

Her teachings and insights made me see that it's the deviation from this path that will bring me pain, depression, illness, and worst of all, despair. And it's those times of despair that I miss Mar-Lou the most, for those were the times she always seemed to be there to help pick up the pieces and make sense of this crazy, crazy world—and she made me believe that no matter what, God had a plan for me and was looking out for me, and He would take care and protect me.

That's the greatest security to have—and the greatest gift she gave me—to truly believe that I am a unique creation of God, and by doing His will and developing all of the hidden talents, behaviors, potentials, and gifts He has given me along my path to individuation, no matter what crosses my path, I know that too is God . . . and He will see me through the darkness of night and the brightness of day and help me become all I was meant to become (come hell or high water!).

And even though at times I may forget it . . . (sorry Mar-Lou—you know more than anyone how that negative animus can get a hold of me) . . . to be given the knowledge of that incredible gift, all I can say is . . .

Thank you, Mar-Lou, for helping me find my path and setting me on it. I am eternally grateful and can never repay you for the map you have given me.

God bless you for all the love and support you gave to me along my journey. Your thoughts and insights I carry every step I take.

I love you, my friend. I miss you terribly.

I will see you in my dreams!

—Robin L. Hutton

(P.S. After some work, I found out what the little bird wanted from me. As I have said before, von Franz taught me to take everything that happens around me—even a little bird at the window—and look at what it is trying to say to me. Only then can I live a conscious life and not be stuck in an unconscious one, for once the self is activated, you can't simply turn it off, for if you try, it's to your own detriment.

(The little bird came to the window right in front of my writing desk where I write my novels and screenplays. I've been so caught up in the business/producing side of my work, the extroverted ego goals, that I haven't written creatively in a very long time, and the bird was telling me that I needed to get back to my writing. That's what my soul needs for me to do. So as I write my resolutions for 2003, I can't help but think that von Franz had a hand in guiding that little bird my way to help me start the new year off right and get back on the right path. Thank you, Mar-Lou!)

Living in Her Own World

RENATE INHELDER-BUECHEL

November 22, 2002
Rosenweg
9466 Sennwald

Dear Mr. Kennedy,

Your request for information regarding Marie-Louise von Franz came as a surprise. I first became acquainted with Dr. von Franz during her visits to the medical practice of Dr. H. Koch, who was serving then as the physician at the baths of Bad Ragaz where I worked from 1976 to 1984. Marie-Louise von Franz is for me invariably connected to Miss Barbara Hannah. The encounter with these two women at that time was for me—a twenty-year-old very young woman—quite an experience. Every year during their stay at the baths and later when they came back for checkups, I had the pleasure of talking to these two ladies.

Initially both of these women seemed quite foreign to me. But slowly I was able to get to know them and began to very much admire their knowledge and their way of life, at times being very much captivated by "their world." Naturally my curiosity to get to know Dr. von Franz was great. I cherished the visits of these two ladies and admired the loving manner in which Dr. von Franz cared for Miss Hannah. Little by little, I used the very short time of their visits to learn more about their work and the manner in which they lived.

In 1984, I gave birth to my son, Thomas, and dedicated my life fully to my family. I now regret that I lost contact with them. I was, however, immersed in another very instructive and fulfilling time of my life. It amazes me that I apparently left such an impression on Dr. von Franz.

I hope I have been able to help you a bit with these few details, send you kind greetings, and would like someday to see your work regarding Dr. von Franz.

With kind regards,
Renate Inhelder

The Teumessian Chase

WILHELM JUST

Ottensheim, May 2003

The course of the journey to Jungian psychology and the unconscious was set for me in summer 1964—without realizing it at that time of course—when I met William H. Kennedy in Bailey Island in Maine. I had traveled to the United States in the company of Manfred Michlmayr, a friend from university, to work with Professor C. G. Shull in his neutron diffraction group at the Massachusetts Institute of Technology in Cambridge, Massachusetts, during my vacations. Manfred had met Bill the previous summer when he was hitchhiking in Carinthia and Bill had picked him up on the road somewhere. On returning home to Austria from my stay at MIT, Bill asked me to take responsibility for receiving American students who came to Europe on a program of his and organizing meetings with Austrian students. We met each year in Vienna to prepare these visits. After finishing my studies of physics at Vienna University, I returned to the U.S. and took up a postdoctoral position in Professor Shull's research group for three years. At the beginning of my stay, I saw Bill several times in New York, then our contact vanished completely.

In 1972, I visited Paris—at that time I was working at the Institut Max von Laue-Paul Langevin (ILL) in Grenoble already—and was strolling through the avenues when I saw Bill sitting in a cafe together with Emmanuel, his adopted Greek son. Bill's hooked nose was not to be overlooked. The joy and surprise of this unexpected meeting was great. It turned out that Bill was just preparing to move from New York to Switzerland for good since he had reached retirement. From then on, we did not lose contact again until he died in 1983. I came to visit him and Vernon Brooks and Emmanuel Kennedy regularly in Gommiswald, where they had taken residence. Bill was fascinating when he was talking about arts, literature, theater, opera, history, politics, and the world—the outer and the inner one. He never tried to persuade or convert. So I heard a lot of interesting things about analytical psychology and C. G. Jung, whom he had known personally—but this was for me only of academic interest then.

What I myself was really devoted to at that time was ecology. I had become thoroughly disappointed by physics; especially at MIT, I had been shocked by the discrepancy, at the academic level, of the scientists I had the opportunity to meet and their differentiation as human beings. For many of them, outside their world of science there seemed to be a giant void. In my youthful naïveté, I had taken it for granted that the deep understanding of nature offered by modern physics must go along automatically with depth as a human being. So, in my disappointment, I had looked further to find an all-encompassing understanding of the world. And I thought I had found it now in ecology. Outside my work as a scientist, I was engaged with ecological issues—especially concerning nuclear power. Some friends and I formed a group which met regularly and tried to inform the public about the consequences of using nuclear energy. There I was surprised to notice that my French colleagues in Grenoble seemed to work on the basic assumption that ecological damage could be prevented if only research, technology, and economy were pursued honestly and freed of greed for profit. I was not quite comfortable with this approach; it seemed to me unrealistic, one-sided. So I prepared a seminar in which I wanted to show that the concept of nature as a completely calculable machine that could be subdued to man's will on his own terms had become obsolete with the discovery of quantum physics in the beginning of the twentieth century. By the same token, it had become evident that the object of physical observation can never be separated from the observer. A related development had taken place in mathematics and had culminated in the incompleteness theorem of Kurt Gödel in 1931.[1] As a consequence, the expectation that mathematics could be founded on absolute and final grounds had to be dropped. Reality, even the reality of exact sciences, always appears with a veil that cannot be lifted on principle—thus were the implications of their findings. The program of the sciences of enlightenment—the reduction of nature to a completely calculable machine or clockwork—had toppled.[2]

In both realms of science—physics and mathematics—man could no longer sneak out of the picture of reality which he draws up; rather, he is included in it inseparably forever. The picture man assumes as reality will always eventually turn out to be a projection.[3] The struggle to grasp reality consists of projections and their withdrawal when they no longer fit and begin to hamper the flow of life. Sciences seem to advance following the same pattern as the evolution of consciousness in man—in the individual as well as in mankind as a whole. The more light is spread by human reason, the darker will be the shadow as its Siamese twin and consequence. This shadow is irreducible. The parallel to psychology imposes itself, as was already noticed by the fathers of quantum mechanics.[4] Thus the discovery of the atomic and subatomic world wrought an essential revolution in the concept of reality which is still not sufficiently realized in the public and collective consciousness even nowadays. In psychology, it was C. A. Meier who first drew attention to the analogy of quantum physics and modern psychology in a paper in 1933; for C. G. Jung and W. Pauli, it was the central issue of their collaboration.[5] M.-L. von Franz also dealt with it extensively throughout her life.[6]

In the seminar I was preparing for my colleagues in ecology I wanted to show how modern sciences forced quite new and strange views on how man confronts his reality. In the context of ecology this means that man's understanding of the physical world and its control will always be a limited one. Since modern psychology had come to analogous findings, I wanted first to discuss the issue with an expert. Knowing that Bill Kennedy was familiar with the world of psychology, I asked him to arrange a meeting with a psychologist for me. He suggested Marie-Louise von Franz, whom I did not know up until then, and arranged an hour with her. I met with her in early spring of 1977 in her study in Lindenbergstrasse. Bill had encouraged me to tell her a dream on this occasion. I did not think much of dreams at that time, but nevertheless I was curious. So, after having discussed my scientific questions, I told her the dream I had the night before our encounter. Her interpretation and remarks struck and touched me deeply. In talking about the dream, she quite accurately addressed the essential issue of my life at that time as though she had known me quite intimately for a long time. Apparently something inside myself knew me better than I could have ever known myself, and Marie-Louise translated for me the strange language of the dream and showed me how I was seen from this other in myself. I asked her to recommend somebody near Grenoble I could work with. Thus I started Jungian analysis with Florence Bacchetta in Geneva, a pupil of hers. Becoming familiar with analytical psychology in the course of my analysis, I realized that Jung's approach to comprehending reality was exactly what I had been searching for. After some time in analysis, I wanted to penetrate still deeper into Jung's work on the collective unconscious. Encouraged by dreams, I dared to apply to the C. G. Jung Institute in Zürich for training in analytical psychology. While keeping my position as physicist, I began to attend the Institute in summer 1981. All my vacations and a lot of unpaid leaves were used to follow the training program in Küsnacht. Countless times I traveled the track from Grenoble to Zürich to Grenoble. Now I could take up my analysis with Marie-Louise again, later also with Gotthilf Isler. Luckily, I was able to spend two entire years in Zürich, the first one on a sabbatical leave and the other when the research reactor of the ILL in Grenoble had a serious breakdown—an absolute stroke of luck for me! Marie-Louise also supervised my diploma thesis at the Jung Institute. Her encouragement for my work, "Images of Creation in Physics and Mathematics" (*"Bilder der Schöpfung in Physik und Mathematik"*) and her deep and thorough understanding of the revolutionary implications of modern physics were a decisive help in tackling all hurdles. I still owe to her the publication of the subject as a book. In 1987, I finished the training and earned my diploma. Two years later, I gave up my career as a physicist in Grenoble and returned to Austria and my home village, together with my family. Since then I have worked as a psychoanalyst in Linz in private practice.

The encounter with Marie-Louise von Franz changed my life decisively; the religious dimension of my life was as much affected as was my understanding of physics. Her open-minded, deeply honest, unpretentious approach to comprehending things and penetrating them did not shrink away from any subject. She never halted at purely formal aspects or discursive approaches as is the temptation for scientists; always she went directly at the heart of the matter—where logos and eros are not yet separated, or rather, no longer separated. Once she told me very proudly and laughing that a French journalist had noted: "Vous avez échappé la culture, Madame." She never used sciences as apotropaically, but took and respectfully investigated them as an expression of the collective unconscious. What C. G. Jung said about his life—"The daimon of creativity has ruthlessly had its way with me"—holds also for her.[7]

The double aspect of this daimon is at the center of a relatively unknown story told by Ovid in his *Metamorphoses*—the story of the Teumessian chase.

> Boeotia was savaged [the story goes] by a fox which lived in a cave in the mountain Teumessos.[8] The fox was sent by Dionysus to punish the Thebans for excluding the descendants of Cadmus from their inherited right of the throne. Teumessos, the mountain, had been created by Zeus once upon a time to hide the princess Europa after he had abducted her at the shore of Sidon, where she was playing innocently with her playmates. This fox could take its victims at will and remain unpunished since it could run so fast that no other living being could catch up with it. The beast ravaged the land and demanded a youth as a sacrifice each month. Like the

> sphinx of Thebes, it was a terrible plague on the population; they were helpless in the face of its plundering raids. In this plight the Thebans asked Amphitryon for help; he brought the dog of Cephalus, which Europa had received from Zeus as a wedding present. This dog [the myth tells us] was faster than any other living being. Amphitryon let it go to catch the fox. A wild chase started. The dog from which nothing could escape was after the fox no other being could catch. When Zeus saw this from his Olympian abode, he threw a lightning bolt down on both animals and transformed them into a marble statue. Thus, by divine intervention, the outcome of the chase remains unsettled—in the stone image the chase is still going on today.[9]

First of all, the story of the Teumessian chase hints at the limits of logic of language in a vivid way. There are other antique stories which anticipated problems modern formal logic was faced with in the nineteenth and twentieth centuries. The most famous is the statement attributed to the Cretan Epimenides that all Cretans are liars—an antinomy. The statement would be false in the case where Epimenides spoke the truth. It only would be true if he was lying. It is a so-called *self-referential statement.* The statement makes sense only if expressed by somebody outside the system of Crete. Inside the Cretan world, it is an *undecidable statement.*[10] Bertrand Russell has put it in a funny tale—the story of the barber of Sevilla. A barber there extolled himself, announcing that he shaved all the men of the town who did not shave themselves. But then he was faced with the question of whether he should shave himself or not and got into a terrible quandary. The language of formal logic entangles us in paradoxes that make us wonder what we really can grasp of reality. From the psychological point of view, C. G. Jung states:

> Whatever we strive to fathom with our intellect will end in paradox and relativity, if it be honest work and not *petitio principii* in the interests of convenience. That an intellectual understanding of the psychic process must end in paradox and relativity is simply unavoidable, if only for the reason that the intellect is but one of many psychic functions which is

> intended by nature to serve man in constructing of his images of the objective world. We should not pretend to understand the world only by the intellect; we apprehend it just as much by feeling.[11]

As Marie-Louise von Franz shows in many of her books on fairy tales, the fox was considered malicious, insidious, cunning, shrewd, and also a demonic animal and a witch animal.[12] Greed, that is, never to have had enough, is generally attributed to the fox. In fairy tales, however, the fox also may appear as helpful and lead the hero on the path to the enchanted and magic realm. It knows about the treasure to be found there and also how one can get ahold of it. In Greek mythology, the fox is connected with Saturn (Chronos).[13] As we know, Chronos greedily devoured all his children because he was not ready to cede power to a son. In *Cabala, Speculum Artis et Naturae, in Alchymia,* there is a picture of a man chasing after a fox which has just disappeared into its cave in a mountain.[14] In the center of the mountain, in the dark of nature, the central mystery of alchemy—transformation—takes place. The fox is an animal side of human nature, the instinct in man, which may lead him to the essential whereas the man in the picture only trusts in his reason and blindly patters.

The fox symbolism has to do with instinct in man himself. The exceedingly vigilant, shrewd animal hints at such an aspect of the human instinct. The excellent sense of smell provides orientation—fox and dog still are able to follow a track where man is absolutely lost. Wherever the eye of reason has left us in the lurch, we have to rely on our instincts. Together with its proverbial greed, the Teumessian fox represents an instinctual, insatiable desire in man to look further, to hasten faster, to strike another prey and still another, a deeply rooted restless yearning in man which is always faster so that it cannot be caught and tamed, tied down and comprehended. It stirs up and gets us on our way; but what it tracked down needs to be brought to consciousness, otherwise it will fall prey to the unconscious again.

The effect of fox nature in man is beautifully described in the fairy tale "The Golden Bird."[15] Here the fox knows about the path the hero has to pursue and also the dangers. The hero ignores the fox's advice to remain

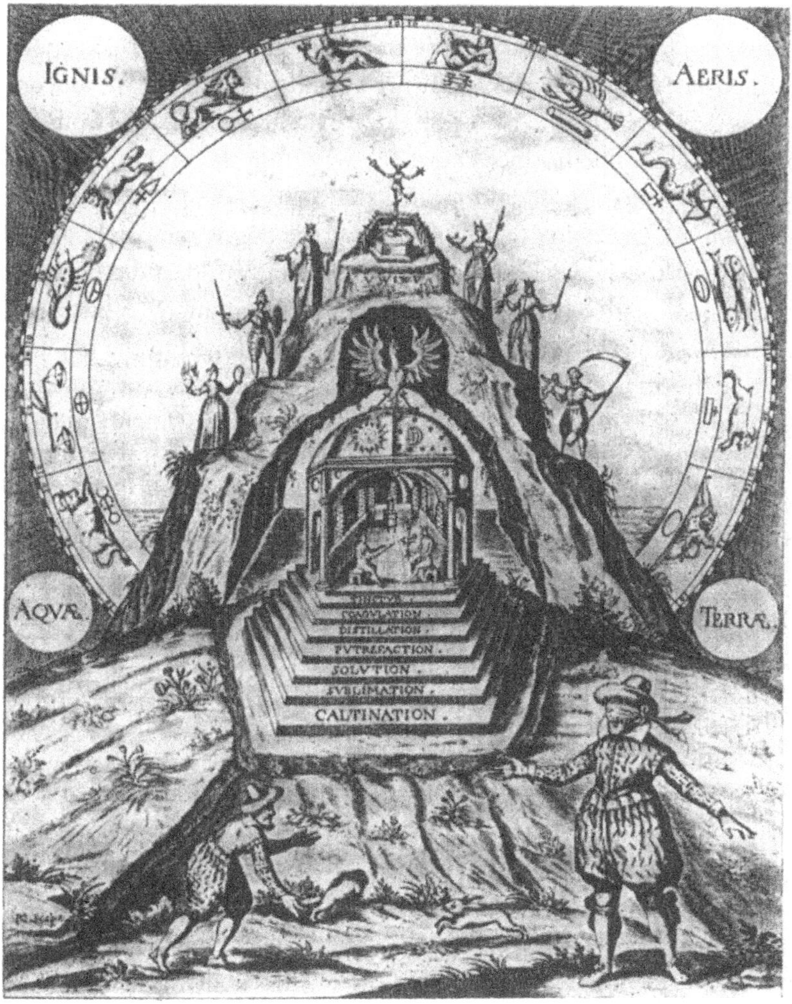

From C. G. Jung, *Psychology and Alchemy, CW* 12, picture 93.

humble in his feats—to take the wooden cage, not the golden one; to leave it with the wooden saddle, and so on. As though carried away by insatiable greed, each time he seizes more than he should against the advice of the fox and gets entangled in dangers, deeper and deeper but also closer to the essential treasure. The fox, however, rescues him again and again and leads him further. At the end of the tale, when all is solved and saved, the fox asks to be killed by the hero. Thus the animal is transformed back into a human being. The animal—that is, the unconscious—is sacrificed and thereby its human kernel is redeemed from unconsciousness. The instinct knows the way from the beginning, but it needs the ego to be brought to consciousness.

From the psychological point of view, the dog is the psychopomp. Cerberus is the guide of souls in the Greek underworld, and there is the black poodle which is Faust's guide and transforms into Mephisto, and so on. The dog is the animal of Hekate and attributed to the moon—that is, the light that shines in the darkness of the night. Like the fox, the dog represents an instinctual presentiment and knowing that guides consciousness and shows the way, where it would be lost if it depended only on itself. As dog, this aspect of the instinct is closer to man and consciousness than the fox. Its wild nature is domesticated and subdued to consciousness. The greedy and wild nature is transformed and may now work together with consciousness. The dog is a true companion of man and the extended arm and eye of the shepherd or hunter—fast and attentive. In alchemy, Mercurius—the great guide of the soul—is called *filius canis coelici coloris,* the son of the dog of azure color.[16]

The Teumessian fox represents an instinctual search in man that devours what it is after. It does not bring what it gets ahold of to consciousness and assimilate it. It mirrors us when we only appropriate contents greedily and obsessively without really integrating them, without holding them together in a meaningful whole (the herd!). Then the fox breaks into the human, that is, conscious realm and robs its contents by making them unconscious. The dog, on the other hand, would be an instinct that gathers the contents of consciousness, puts them together into a whole, protects and guards them. It saves consciousness from disintegration in the face of perils, like sheep held together by the dog in presence of danger. Finally, as Cerberus, it leads the soul on its transition to the otherworld where it is all-important not to become dissolved. The fox would be an excellent image for the accumulation and communication of knowledge as it rages nowadays. Greedily, knowledge is devoured, but the soul remains hungry and unnoticed since the devoured contents remain untransformed and are not really integrated, not brought into contact with each other and the whole.

It is meaningful that the myth of the Teumessian chase hints at Zeus and Europa, since it is this mountain Teumessos where Zeus hid Europa after having abducted her. He had broken into the idyll of the family of Agenor and Telephassa, her parents, as he and other gods have done on many other occasions—driven by desire and ruthless as the Teumessian fox. Zeus had abducted their daughter Europa when she was playing innocently and dancing with other maidens at the shore of Sidon. After carrying her away over the ocean, he celebrated the divine *coniunctio* with her. However, Zeus did not merely break into the idyllic family life and rape the innocent Europa, he also gave Europa—among other precious things—that dog as a present for the wedding. With that gesture, his wild, rapacious fox aspect was domesticated and a psychic potential working toward consciousness came in. That this double aspect is characteristic of the divine we know also from our Christian tradition. Jacob is attacked by God at the ford; Hiob is exposed to Yahweh's devouring side, and it has to be sustained and recognized before it can transform; Isaac should be sacrificed by his father on divine order; Jesus Christ becomes victim.[17] And it is all-important now that the suffering and sacrifice does not remain unconscious but brings forth meaning. The fox is, so to speak, the guide of the psyche which tracks down the new in the unconscious and tries to devour it; the appearance of the dog may bring about a more differentiated, higher level of consciousness by protecting against disintegration.

The mythological Amphitryon played a role similar to that of Joseph as the foster father of Jesus, the godson, in the Christian tradition. Each stood by his bride although she was made pregnant by outer—divine—intervention. Both had to cope with the breaking in and incomprehensible action of a god. Amphitryon had been the bridegroom of Alcmene; but before the wedding could be celebrated, he had to take revenge on the murderers of Alcmene's brothers. Amphitryon returns as victor, but Zeus had visited the waiting bride, taking the shape of the victorious hero the night before his return. In a long night of love—Zeus arranged the night to last three times as long—he engenders the splendid Heracles. It was the last time Zeus came over an earthly maiden. The hero Heracles remains unsurpassed. In Amphitryon, man not only stands up to the raving side of god, he also assumes responsibility for it. Heracles himself unites both sides in himself to an extreme extent; he is the raging hero and the suffering hero. At the end, he is deified.

By striking the two animals with lightning and transforming them into stone Zeus makes sure that the Teumessian fox and Europa's dog can never be separated. Both of them are needed. It is an aspect of the paradoxical nature of the unconscious which cannot be dissolved. On the one hand, it shatters and devours; on the other, it brings about the new, nourishes, gathers the dispersed. The lightning of Zeus transforms both animals into a marble statue, thus perpetuating the conflict forever and appointing the couple as antinomy. Whenever consciousness is to take a decisive step forward, it has to face the antinomical nature of the divine and come to terms with it. Perhaps it needs the inspiration of divine lightning to be able to accept both of them as belonging together and recognize the one meaning of the antinomy. In any case, the divine lightning does not burn fox and dog to ashes; rather they are transformed into stone. We are not told whether the insolvable contradiction is petrified in the statue or the "stone" is the fulfilment wherein the antinomy has found its solution. It remains the task of the individual as to which of the possibilities will be realized in his life—petrifaction or *lapis.*

NOTES

1. E. Nagel, J. R. Newman, *Gödel's Proof* (London: Routledge and Kegan Ltd., 1959); D. R. Hofstadter, *Gödel, Escher, Bach: An Eternal Golden Braid* (New York: Basic Books, 1979).
2. C. G. Jung, *Nietzsche's Zarathustra. Notes of the Seminar Given in 1934–1939,* edited by J. L. Jarrett. Bollingen Series XCIX (Princeton, N.J.: Princeton University Press, 1988), p. 1335.
3. C. G. Jung, *Psychological Types, CW,* vol. 6 (Princeton, N.J.: Princeton University Press, 1971), par. 793; M.-L.von Franz, *Projection and Recollection in Jungian Psychology: Reflections of the Soul* (LaSalle, Ill.: Open Court, 1980).

4. N. Bohr, *Atomphysik und menschliche Erkenntnis* (Braunschweig: Vieweg Verlag); E. Schrödinger, *Geist und Materie* (Wien: Verlag P. Zolnay, 1959); W. Pauli, *Physik und Erkenntnistheorie* (Braunschweig: Vieweg Verlag, 1984).
5. C. A. Meier, "Moderne Physik—Modern Psychologie," in *Die kulturelle Bedeutung der komplexen Psychologie* (Berlin: Springer Verlag, 1935), p. 349.
6. M.-L. von Franz, *Number and Time* (Evanston, Ill.: Northwestern University Press, 1974); see also M.-L. von Franz, *Psyche and Matter* (Boston: Shambhala, 1923) and *Time, Rhythm, and Repose* (London: Thames and Hudson, 1978).
7. C. G. Jung, *Memories, Dreams, Reflections,* edited by Aniela Jaffé (New York: Pantheon Books, 1963), p. 358.
8. Gr.: *Τευμησια αλωπηξ*.
9. Ovid, *Metamorphoses* 7.755.
10. See note 1.
11. C. G. Jung, *Psychological Types,* par. 856.
12. M.-L. von Franz, *Individuation in Fairy Tales* (Boston: Shambhala, 1990); *Shadow and Evil in Fairy Tales* (Boston: Shambhala, 1995); *Animus and Anima in Fairy Tales* (Toronto: Inner City Books, 2002).
13. Auguste Bouché-Leclercq, *L'Astrologie greque* (Paris, 1899).
14. Alchemical work of St. Michelspacher, Augsburg, 1654. See C. G. Jung, *Psychology and Alchemy* (1944), *CW,* vol. 12 (Princeton, N.J.: Princeton University Press, 1953), p. 195.
15. *Grimm's Fairy Tales.*
16. C. G. Jung, *Psychology and Alchemy,* par. 278, footnote 216.
17. Moses 1:32, 23; C. G. Jung, *Answer to Job* (1952), in *CW,* vol. 11 (Princeton, N.J.: Princeton University Press, 1958); M.-L. von Franz, "In the Black Woman's Castle: Interpretation of a Fairy Tale" in *Archetypal Dimensions of the Psyche* (Boston: Shambhala, 1997), pp. 174.

Oblomov and the Russian Mother Complex

MARIA KARDAUN

In Goncharov's much acclaimed novel *Oblomov,* the now proverbially lethargic "hero" suffers from a lack of ambition so complete that he spends his days in bed. To the extreme laziness of his protagonist the author dryly remarks that he created the character of Oblomov as a result of both personal observation and self-analysis.[1] At the same time, Goncharov allows for a more romantic source of his art: "I wrote, as if by dictation. And, truly, a lot came unconsciously; someone sat invisibly beside me and told me what to write."[2] In accordance with Jungian literary theory and in the wake of the illustrious Jungian scholar Marie-Louise von Franz, I will interpret Goncharov's novel not in the light of its author's personal psychic constitution or development but as a more or less autonomous piece of literature, showing an archetypal pattern of machinations of the Russian mother complex. Special attention will be paid to the function of the famous "Dream of Oblomov" within the novel as a whole.

In 1859, after ten years of artistic silence, the Russian author Ivan Alexandrovich Goncharov finally published his long-awaited novel, *Oblomov.* The novel is celebrated for its psychological and social insight but notorious for its lack of action. In the first one hundred and fifty pages, the main character, Ilya Ilyich Oblomov, a landowning nobleman who lives in his flat in St. Petersburg, does little more than lie on his bed, sleeping, dreaming, pondering life, sighing to himself, sometimes yelling at his servant Zakhar and then dozing off again. The most common expression on his face, when he is awake at all, is one of serene unconcern. He appears to be a totally insignificant hero to begin with, and our impression of him hardly improves as the story unfolds.

Nonetheless, as soon as it was published, the novel was recognized as a masterpiece of literature, in Russia as well as abroad. The "Dream of Oblomov" in particular, with its elaborate descriptions of the immobility and inefficiency of Russian country life, was well received.

The question is, Why? What makes a book about such a seemingly unattractive protagonist interesting? In what way does the description of such a sleepy and dull kind of human existence appeal to the reader? Surely it is not in itself exciting, or encouraging for that matter, to read about human beings who suffer from pathological laziness to such an extent that they quite literally do not bother to lift a finger.

And another question: What about the function of the dream in the novel? Is it merely an aesthetically satisfying, additional description of stagnation? (Apparently this is a central theme.) Could it have been omitted without diminishing our understanding of the rest of the book? Or does it perhaps, like a real dream, provide us with unexpected, interesting, essentially intuitive information through which we can grasp something of the deeper meaning of the daily events described?

For the answers to these questions, I suggest that we invoke the help of Jungian theory. More specifically we will investigate the symbolic content of the dream. We may thus gain some insight not only into how the dream of Oblomov fits in the context of the novel as a whole, but also into a collective dimension of Oblomov's lack of vitality.

Jungian Psychology and Art

Of special interest for our purposes is what Jung says about the correspondence between works of art and dreams.[3] As is well known, Marie-Louise von Franz has worked out this aspect of Jung's oeuvre in a variety of unparalleled interpretations of works of literature.[4] She also summarized and reformulated Jungian art theory in a short, but very clear and convincing theoretic article on the subject.[5] According to Jungian theory, works of art and dreams have a lot in common. Both are manifestations of the unconscious and both have a compensatory function in that they offer a symbolic representation of a state of affairs that is essentially compensating for existing conscious views on the same subject. As in a dream, in a work of art an autonomous unconscious reality takes over and essentially shapes the book, the painting, the symphony. Therefore the result may sometimes be surprising to the artist him- or herself, being something other than what he or she consciously intended to create.

Dreams and works of art differ in that art is seen as essentially a product of the collective unconscious, whereas dreams *can* but do not necessarily reflect something of collective importance; unlike (most) dreams, works of art are compensatory not only of the conscious views of the artist as a person, but also of the conscious views that dominate a culture. It is for this reason that undemocratic rulers often feel the need to suppress free artistic expression: depending on how tyrannical they are, they cannot allow alternate views on life, least of all views that, intentionally or otherwise, reveal a hidden, collective inclination to disapprove of the official perspective.[6]

The Contents of the Novel

In order to see our dream in its context, it may be helpful to sum up in a few words what happens in the novel.

The book consists of four parts, in the first of which the landowner Oblomov spends his days lying in bed, sleeping, eating, and developing some vague plans for his estate, which he himself takes seriously. He is wearing his soft Persian dressing gown. He has been living like this for about eight years.

When we enter the story, Oblomov's peace of mind is most cruelly disturbed by two terrible, more or less unexpected problems. He has received a letter with bad financial news about his estate: his income will be 2,000 rubles less than the year before. And second, he has to move to another apartment because the owner has plans to convert the building.

His strategy for coping with these problems is twofold. First of all, he forbids his servant Zakhar to bring him any more bad news, and second, he remains in bed. When he isn't asleep or quarreling with Zakhar, he sighs things like, "O dear, you can't run away from life. It gets at you everywhere." Or he suddenly cries out, "Mother of God, I'm in such a hurry." And then he quietly resumes his nap. This goes on for about a hundred and fifty pages.

In the second part, a certain Andrey Karlovich Stolz, a half-German friend of Oblomov who grew up with him, now a very successful businessman with a good nature and a lot of well-directed energy, forces Oblomov to get dressed and undertake some action. Among other things, he introduces him to a girl, named Olga. Stolz also manages to find Oblomov a temporary place to stay.

Oblomov and Olga start seeing each other. They fall in love. Olga is obsessed with the idea of redeeming her beloved. Stolz had asked her to make sure that Oblomov goes out, reads books, and develops himself, and Olga wants to make this project a success. As soon as she discovers the Persian dressing gown, it is given away to an acquaintance.

Oblomov has come very much alive now that he is involved with Olga. They want to marry as soon as he has settled his affairs so that they can live on his estate. Oblomov is full of plans, sometimes even deliriously happy.

However, there is also a somewhat less appealing side to his relationship with Olga. It cannot be denied that he often feels exhausted by her demands. He is, for example, always afraid that she will question him about the books he is supposed to be reading or ask him his opinion about the current political situation. In fact, she "does not permit the faintest shadow of somnolence on his face," and it is all rather fatiguing.

The beginning of the third part forms the turning point of the book. By some more or less criminal trick, of which Oblomov is of course an easy victim, he is forced to move into a house in the country. This house belongs to Agafya Matveyevna, a simpleminded widow of about thirty years of age who happens to be a very good cook.

The widow is very different from Olga. She takes care of Oblomov's every physical need, even before he realizes himself what he would like. First of all, she manages to get ahold of his old Persian dressing gown, mends it, and returns it to him. She cooks exquisite meals for him while he lies on the sofa again. In view of all this, it is not surprising that Olga waits in vain for her fiancé to settle his affairs and marry her.

In the fourth part, Olga marries Stolz instead of Oblomov. Oblomov marries the widow, and they have a child, a little boy, called Andrey after Andrey Karlovich Stolz. A few years later, Oblomov dies of a stroke caused by a combination of overnutrition and lack of exercise. Little Andrey is adopted and raised by Olga and Stolz.

The Dream of Oblomov

The dream of Oblomov was first published in 1849 as a separate work of literature. Later it was integrated into the larger context of a complete novel. It occupies about one third of the first part of the book, the part in which Oblomov spends all of his time in bed.[7] As Oblomov wonders, in a brief moment of lucidity between two naps, why he isn't like other people, he is unable to find the "hostile source that prevents him from living as he should." The unconscious then sends him a dream with the answer (in symbolic language, of course).

The dream describes how Oblomov used to live as a little child in his native village Oblomovka, how he is attentively looked after by his parents, his nurse, and all the serfs. The role of his mother is especially emphasized: "Seeing his mother, who had been dead for years, Oblomov even in his sleep thrilled with joy and his ardent love for her; two warm tears slowly appeared from under his eyelashes and remained motionless. His mother covered him with passionate kisses, then looked at him anxiously to see if his eyes were clear, if anything hurt him, asked the nurse if he had slept well, if he had woken in the night, if he had tossed in his sleep, if he had a temperature." His mother is overprotective and does not allow Oblomov to live. With all kinds of tricks she keeps him inactive, infantile, and helpless. Of course, she does not want him to study either and looks for every excuse to keep him at home. He once tried to escape her influence in a naughty attempt to participate in a quite innocent snowball fight. His mother immediately sent the serfs after him, who finally "got hold of the young master, wrapped him in the sheepskin they had brought, then in his father's fur coat and two blankets, and carried him home in triumph. At home they had despaired of seeing him again, giving him up for lost; but the joy of his parents at seeing him alive and unhurt was indescribable. They offered up thanks to the Lord, then gave him mint and elderberry tea to drink, followed by raspberry tea in the evening, and kept him three days in bed."

So we see that Oblomov's mother, at least his mother as she appears in the dream, is very caring indeed. She has nothing less than absolute love for him, but at the same time she kills any disposition or inclination for development the boy might have had spontaneously. Oblomov is "cherished like an exotic flower in a hothouse, and withers as soon as he enters real life."

Apparently Oblomov suffers from a devouring mother complex, represented symbolically in the dream by the image of his mother. Still, Oblomov's problem is not just a personal one. All of the three little villages, which together form Oblomovka, in which the dream is set, are dominated by the same complex. Each day in Oblomovka has two highlights: the first highlight is dinner and the second, the absolute climax of the day, is the after-dinner nap. The Oblomovka of the dream symbolically forms the realm of the mother complex. In this Oblomovka, there is no ambition in life other than having a good time. Stagnation and immobility are the rule, from time to time unexpectedly and unpleasantly interrupted by work. The dream of Oblomov depicts an idyllic mother-complex world—idyllic, but stifling.

I suggest we now return to our original questions. What makes a book about a figure like Oblomov interesting? In what way does the description of this sleepy kind of human existence appeal to the reader? And what about the function of the dream in the novel? Is the dream merely an additional description of stagnation? Or does it provide us, perhaps, with unexpected and interesting information? You will not be surprised by now that I wish to claim the latter.

As we saw, the dream clearly shows the reader what is the matter with Oblomov. Although Oblomov is an adult in years, from the unconscious point of view he is still a seven-year-old boy, living in total emotional and physical dependancy in the world of his mother, or better, of *the* Mother; the reader recognizes from the evident symbolism in the dream that Oblomov is in the sweet paws not of his own mother, who has been long dead, but of a very powerful mother complex, and that all his fake arguments in the rest of the novel against starting an independent life of his own are really the cunning tricks of this dominant mother complex. It is "she" who prevents him from marrying Olga, too. In most cases, like here, the mother complex is against individuation. Oblomov lacks the courage and determination that the Russian hero Ivan gives proof of in his confrontation with the Baba Yaga, and he is completely helpless against the Mother.[8] Oblomov himself badly wants to marry Olga, but he cannot. Whenever he seriously thinks about marriage, he starts to worry and comes up with the same kind of arguments his mother used to keep him home when he should have gone to school. What if Olga will be disappointed in him? Isn't she too young? What if she falls in love with someone else some day? And anyway, if they get too involved, it will be difficult to part. In short, the project is full of dangers.

The dream also helps us understand the symbolic meaning of many other elements in the novel, for example, why the mother complex, in the form of the widow, gets hold of Oblomov once more and finally kills him. One might say that she hugs him to death.

Apart from what the dream shows the reader, within the logic of the novel the content of the dream is compensating for the conscious insight of Oblomov, since the dream—in a very dreamlike way—represents a truth Oblomov himself is not aware of, namely that he is still this seven-year-old boy. He himself is under the illusion, at least at this stage of the book, that he is a grownup, efficiently devising valuable ideas about ameliorating the position of his serfs and inventing ways of enlarging the income he has from his estate.

It cannot be maintained, however, that the figure of Oblomov is of a totally negative nature, that he can be described only *ex negativo.* Oblomov may be a negative figure when looked at from the rational father-complex point of view, and indeed it cannot be denied that he lacks many good qualities, but there is also a hidden beauty in his character, a beauty which Olga, Stolz, and the widow do not fail to notice. There is something kind and genuine about him that is valuable. Also, he is always sincerely interested in the well-being of his fellow humans, be they masters or serfs. It may be true that Oblomov is not at all fit for the struggle of life, yet it is a loss when he dies. Even long after his death, he is still generally mourned, because they had all loved his "crystal-clear soul." There is no feeling whatsoever of "good riddance," neither in the characters of the novel nor in the reader.

The Novel in Its Historical Context

According to what we said at the beginning, art is supposed to provide some knowledge or insight compensatory of what is generally believed. In what way can we consider Goncharov's novel as compensatory of the contemporary conscious views held in Russian society?

As mentioned before, the novel was originally published in 1859. In Russia, the transition from a traditional feudal form of society to a pre-capitalistic one was rapidly taking place. Two years later, in 1861, serfdom was actually abolished by Tsar Alexander II.

Now Goncharov's novel is often considered a powerful condemnation of serfdom, albeit in an indirect and implicit way. But in 1859, this condemnation of serfdom comes somewhat late to be original. All educated people at the time of Goncharov, including the conservative tsar, knew that serfdom had served its time and that the feudal system was no longer working, so they did not need Goncharov to lift this insight into the realm of general awareness.

It is my opinion that the real message—or, if you wish, the real value or the real meaning—of the novel is to be found elsewhere, namely in the minute description of what is irrevocably lost. The novel, most of all in the dream of Oblomov, presents a warm, even lyrical description of the much-despised feudal mother-complex form of society. Maybe the contemporary common opinion was somewhat too enthusiastic about the miracles of modern life and too contemptuous of the old-fashioned, superstitious feudal society still existing in the country.

One final remark in this respect: Stolz has all the positive qualities one can think of—he is not just practical, intelligent, and successful but also sensitive, compassionate, and very benevolent; his name, Andrey Karlovich Stolz, has several positive masculine connotations, such as "brave," "man," "proud"—but he isn't convincing as a literary figure and one does not really identify or sympathize with him. Goncharov himself calls the character of Stolz "weak and pale, the idea peeping through him too nakedly."[9] Goncharov admits, in so many words, both that it was his intention to create in Stolz a convincing embodiment of modernity and that he failed. It is generally agreed upon that Goncharov wanted to write a novel to depict the negative qualities of traditional, feudal Russia and the "superfluous men" it created. If so, he didn't succeed. Against his own convictions, the novel became not a condemnation but a celebration of a lost world. As happens often in art, the objective psyche took over and overruled the conscious plan the artist had in mind.

The novel ends on an optimistic note: the son of Oblomov, who was already named after Stolz, is now adopted by Stolz and Olga. Little Andrey is the result of the old and the new couple and represents a kind of union between traditional life and modernity. The end of the book expresses the hope that in the unfolding pre-capitalistic, no-nonsense father-complex way of life there may still be room for the Oblomov offspring, the noncalculating, inefficient, but at the same time sincerely poetical, kind, quiet, and friendly Oblomov mentality.[10]

NOTES

1. Ivan Goncharov, *Oblomov,* translation and introduction by David Magarshack (London: Penguin, 1954, 1988), p. vii.
2. Letter to Lkhovsky, translated and cited in Nathalie Baratoff, *Oblomov, A Jungian Approach: A Literary Image of the Mother Complex* (Bern: Peter Lang, 1990), pp. 18, 26ff. See also Joachim Klein, "Zur Interpretation von Goncarovs *Oblomov:* Der Traum und das Unbewusste," in *Res Slavica: Festschrift für Hans Rothe zum 65 Geburtstag,* edited by Peter Thiergen and Ludger Udolph (Zürich: Ferdinand Schöningh, 1994), pp. 139ff.
3. C. G. Jung, "On the Relation of Analytical Psychology to Poetry" (1931, pp. 65–83) and "Psychology and Literature" (1950, pp. 84–105), in *Collected Works,* vol. 15 (Princeton, N.J.: Princeton University Press, 1966).
4. Examples include her interpretations of Apuleius in *The Golden Ass of Apuleius: The Liberation of the Feminine in Man* (Boston: Shambhala, 1992); Saint-Exupéry's *Le petit prince* (in *Puer Aeternus*), and in Bruno Goetz's *Das Reich ohne Raum: Eine Vision der Archetypen* (Bern: Origo Verlag, 1995, with a commentary by M.-L. von Franz).
5. Von Franz, "Analytical Psychology and Literary Criticism," in *New Literary History* 12.1 (1980), pp. 119–126.
6. A notorious example is Plato's attitude toward art. See Maria Kardaun, "Why Plato Banished the Artist: Some Jungian Observations," in Frederico Pereira, ed., *Literature and Psychoanalysis: Proceedings of the Thirteenth International Conference on Literature and Psychoanalysis* (Lisbon: ISPA, 1997), pp. 197–204; and "Platonic Art Theory: A Reconsideration," in M. Kardaun and J. Spruyt, eds., *The Winged Chariot: Collected Essays on Plato and Platonism in Honour of L. M. de Rijk* (Leiden: Brill, 2000), pp. 135–164.
7. Many interpreters have pointed out that, stylistically speaking, Oblomov's "dream" is not very dreamlike. Dreams, at least literary dreams, tend to be bizarre, wild, and very much at variance with everyday experience, whereas the imagery that Oblomov's dream displays could have easily belonged to a quiet conscious contemplation. The point is, however, that Oblomov's dream *isn't* a conscious contemplation: the text informs us that Oblomov is "peacefully asleep," and there is no doubt that in this condition he experiences a spontaneous flow of images arising from the unconscious, images that make sense in light of the novel as a whole. For an elaborate and persuasive argument against reducing Oblomov's dream to an uninteresting digression that

is only loosely connected with the rest of the novel, see Klein, "Zur Interpretation von Goncarovs *Oblomov.*"

8. Marie-Louise von Franz, *Shadow and Evil in Fairy Tales* (Boston: Shambhala, 1995), 157–178.
9. Goncharov, *Oblomov,* translation and introduction by David Magarshack, p. x.
10. I thank my friend and collegue Joke Spruyt for her generously bestowed advice about the English.

Care for This House

ROBERT C. KLINE

Knowing Marie-Louise von Franz for quite a number of years, I might disclose what first brought our relationship into being. It was one line from one of her books: "As for those who believe, we may only envy them their faith." I quickly responded in terms of believing and faith are, at base, matters of intelligence, that is, how could one not have faith? I next attached myself to one of her dreams, in which she and her father went back in time (which she did not wish to do), and they looked at the house of her childhood, and her father said, "It doesn't matter now." I was quite impressed with an unconscious which had such a good sense of time, and it reminded me a bit of the old prophets who seemed also to have knowledge of time in their dreams.

Not too long after thinking about her dream of the childhood house, the local public broadcasting station had a program featuring Bernstein presenting one of his songs from a show that never became popular (*1600 Pennsylvania Avenue*), and the lovely song sung by June Anderson was titled "Take Care of This House," the words going thus:

Take care of this house
Keep it from harm.
If bandits break in, sound the alarm.
Care for this house,
Shine it by hand
and keep it so clean the glow can be seen
All over the land
Be careful at night
Check all the doors.
If someone makes off with the dream,
The dream will be yours.
Take care of this house, be always on guard
For this house is the home of us all.

I dubbed a copy of the program and sent it to her.

The years passed, and at the time of Marie-Louise's funeral services, not being able to go to Switzerland, candles and Durufle's *Requiem* honored the event in a quiet, personal remembrance.

It was a few years later that I heard of a family member whose daughter had died of cancer. They had nursed her at home until her death. I sent a card expressing my sympathy and included a quote from Jung which said: "Life, so-called, is a short episode between two great mysteries—which yet are one."

About six months after sending that card, I unexpectedly had the most numinous dream of my life (and I'm pretty old). I walked toward two heavy wooden doors which were in semidarkness, and the doors opened as I approached, displaying an indescribably pleasant room full of light and with an air of peace—happiness—wholly lacking any cloud of worry whatsoever. I was told that this was my Swiss chateau. I was free to browse around at my leisure, the dream lasting (it seemed) about a minute or so.

Now one wonders if Marie-Louise was thanking me (from heaven) for the video. Or, perhaps, a message from God? The story is not yet finished, as a dream has again thrust into the future with a message that has yet to be fulfilled, and time will tell if it materializes into actuality or not . . . or if so, just how.

What I liked most of all was Marie-Louise's loyalty to Jung and his ideas and how she would leap to his defense whenever—and wherever—needed.

Bless her, indeed.

Relying on the Wisdom of the Self

WALTRAUT KÖRNER

Actually, I did know Marie-Louise von Franz for a long time, although I cannot claim that I got really close to her personally. I experienced her as a student at the Jung Institute in Zürich-Küsnacht, where she gave lectures and seminars; always I met her with great shyness and almost awe, which seems to be a quite natural feeling toward outstanding personalities. When I recall that time—the mid to late 1970s—I must admit that I was in a state of puberty then, barely grown out of my mental and psychological infancy, just at the beginning of analysis with the late Paul Walder, who himself still had supervision with Marie-Louise von Franz. He conveyed to me the impression of a very strict "Fräulein Dr. von Franz"—that kind of address for an unmarried woman that was still common then in spite of the feminist efforts to make all adult women "Ms."! Paul Walder, who adored von Franz greatly, taught me to respect her as almost holy; so I did not dare to come nearer to her personally. I regret this very much now. But very often she appeared in my dreams as an ideal image of a woman who has great knowledge; I knew she had worked her way through to the very depths of Jungian psychology. At her side, I felt myself very small. Therefore I took great pains to strive more or less unsuccessfully to achieve this ideal. How proud I was when, at the end of my training, she wrote to me that she found my written fairy-tale examination about "The Three Brothers" very good! And when she gave a lecture in the main hall at E.T.H. (Eidgenösische Technische Hochschule) in Zürich many years ago, to a packed house, I found her extremely admirable in her modest, quiet, and natural authority. She talked about fairy tales, and everybody listened so intensely that you could have heard a pin drop! She radiated deeply experienced knowledge, which others obviously also felt.

Probably Marie-Louise von Franz did not know what to do with me when we had short encounters at the institute because I did not dare to talk to her. Yet she was very human—enthusiastically loving the folk music that was played by a small rural band at her sixtieth birthday to which we were all invited. Gosh, how long ago this is! It was a very big party, everybody happily dancing and laughing, not knowing that there were dark times to come when her illness began and grew worse over the years. But her suffering was also filled with light, as I know from the persons who nursed her, and during that time my admiration for her lost this admixture of naïveté and puberty and gave room to the qualities of compassion and gratitude.

This new quality had already gradually developed when I began to translate her essays and books from English into German. Doing this, I became acquainted with her as an author who had a deep instinct to guide her in understanding and developing Jung's archetypal concepts; her thinking was grounded and always very much to the point.

Translating for me meant an ongoing process of learning and it still is, in the sense of approaching Jungian psychology which basically is not satisfied with superficial knowledge but tries to really grasp an inner truth and live for it. Dr. von Franz was never at loss for examples from her practice or her personal life, and I would say that she was the first and remains one of not many analysts who are able to connect Jungian thinking with our everyday "soul life"; she did that with an admirable, loving veracity. So, in the course of time, I learned to know her as a person whom one could face honestly and authentically. Finally, I dared to write a short note of condolence to her when her close friend Barbara Hannah died, overcoming the barriers which I myself had built up between the two of us. And she gave me an answer, in a very short letter, that I comforted her! Later, we had further contacts, sending notes to each other concerning questions of translation or sometimes even personal greetings. Everybody knew how difficult it was to satisfy her stylistic and linguistic demands in translating her books and lectures.

Our last personal meeting was at the fiftieth birthday of my analyst, Nora Mindell, who at that time was a close friend and pupil of von Franz; for a little while she attended in her wheelchair and obviously enjoyed the party and made us deeply happy. I kept this memory in my heart, grateful for her short visit which was also an encounter "woman to woman" and not anymore "Fräulein to Fräulein" in that distant way it had been. Her photo hangs on the wall facing my desk; it shows her in a blue dress in her garden. There she radiates a quiet but serene spiritual strength that reminds me of giving up any egotistic attitude in dealing with Jungian psychology and instead searching for deeper meaning in the manifestations of the unconscious psyche. This "unselfish" attitude which von Franz always demanded became also fundamental for my work as translator, trying to interweave her individual language with the underlying objective statements and thus creating a text that is authentic and understandable at the same time. Very often, I got frustrated, because in translating I did not have relaxing times to dive deeper into her thoughts, although I discovered always new dimensions and perspectives in her work; instead, I had to be very disciplined to formulate properly in German what her message was. But some content always stuck in my soul, and if I were to define very briefly what I learned, I would say that von Franz taught me deep confidence in the supporting archetypal structure of the unconscious. Without this experience, it would be impossible for me to do my work as an analyst. She herself was an outstanding model of confidence in the ways of the soul and encouraged me to risk ongoing encounters with my own complexes as well as relying on the wisdom of the Self. So I always keep in mind one statement she made: that all therapy should be in the service of the Self, and that each client has the right of being served by us in helping them to encounter the Self.

Memories of Dr. Marie-Louise von Franz

FRITZ LANDTWING

Foreword

In order to more clearly understand my contribution to the commemorative work in honor of Marie-Louise von Franz, I would like to write a short introduction. My memories of Marie-Louise von Franz, which go back to the mid 1970s, were suddenly called up again in February 2002 by a letter from the Psychological Club of Zürich. The letter was sent to "Members and Friends" of the club and served to orient the addressees of the forthcoming Festschrift. Attached to this letter was a short, personal note addressed to me by Dr. Emmanuel Kennedy, who wrote that "he had been a good friend of Marie-Louise von Franz for many years and knew that Dr. von Franz had held me in esteem, and that he found it desirable and meaningful if people who were not necessarily scholars would also share their memories of her."

Rather than "uncanny," I would prefer to say "unique" are the circumstances and serpentine the paths that the unconscious oftentimes uses to reach its goal. I visited the Psychological Club of Zürich only a few times; I was never a member. The name Dr. Emmanuel Kennedy was unknown to me, although during the many years of my own analysis I had had some contact with Jungian analysts. I asked myself how in the world did a Mr. Kennedy get my address, as my contact with Marie-Louise von Franz consisted of two one-hour sessions prior to the beginning of my own "official" psychoanalysis in 1976. And then I met her one other time for an hour in the mid 1990s. In the period in between, I occasionally corresponded with her and received a few brief answers. I thus had little reason to believe that she held me in any form of esteem. And dreams about her in particular I think would be far better coming from others. I asked Mr. Kennedy how he came upon my name and he answered that he had found reference to my name and business in an address book of Dr. von Franz's from the 1980s and then, after a few detours, had been able to track down my present residence. I am very grateful to you, Mr. Kennedy.

Memories

I hope that my foreword will help contribute to the understanding of the memories which now follow. I would like to say in advance that none of my direct encounters with Marie-Louise von Franz—not even the final one, her death—occurred in a "normal" manner.

It all began in 1975. As a young coiffeur-master, I had managed to survive the first difficult years building up my business. The fruits of my labor were beginning to mature. My energy then began to flow again toward my family. And then it happened: my wife "instigated" a marriage crisis—or, more fairly said, the crisis had to happen—and I was thrown abruptly out into open sea. After a while (I had by now learned to swim), my wife gave me a book that she had borrowed from a friend with an article titled "Woman in Europe," written by a Dr. C. G. Jung. The name C. G. Jung and the word *psychology* were foreign for me. I had somehow vaguely heard of them both, but nothing more. In any case, I at first casually leafed through "Woman in Europe," but then began to be seriously drawn into the text. It took little time to notice that I was quite personally addressed and that I actually understood what this man C. G. Jung was writing about. It was a form, one could say, of deliverance.

A good bit later, my wife's friend made it clear to me that I would hardly make it through my situation on my own. When she offered to help me find an analyst, I grabbed the lifeline. I had little idea of what analysis was but a lot of trust. And I had little money, but then found an analyst-in-training who was willing to work for a modest fee. Everything went very well right from the beginning. The best memory of this man, Ken Neumann, was that he did not feel that he had to know and explain everything. In all of the difficulties that I was having at that time, this was the balsam that healed. In particular, I soon noticed that Ken Neumann was not just some fledgling analyst but that he had considerable talent.

In the analytical hours, the name Marie-Louise von Franz kept coming up. "Frau von Franz said . . . ," "Frau von Franz thinks . . . ," "Frau von Franz writes. . . ." These allusions from Ken were always accompanied with a deep respect. After several months, I could contain myself no longer and asked Ken who this Frau von Franz was. He answered that she was one of the last close collaborators of C. G. Jung. By that time, I had at least some basic knowledge of Jung, what his psychology was about, and where it leads to. I could only answer with: "Ahh, so!"

The work between Ken and me developed fruitfully, the crisis with my wife receded a bit into the background . . . and I stepped forward a bit into the light. But then new clouds arose: Ken was beginning his final exams and knew that he would soon move to Jerusalem with his family. We thus had to find a new analyst for me. And good analysis was expensive. In my naïveté, the most obvious thing to do was to ask Ken to recommend me to Frau von Franz. He felt, however, that this would be practically pointless as he himself had been turned down. Without listening to his advice, I picked up the phone and called Frau von Franz directly to ask her for an hour. On the other end, a woman's voice (with a foreign accent) stated tersely that Frau von Franz was not reachable at the time and that I should phone back tomorrow at 2:00 p.m. That was it. I was relieved . . . yet irritated. How could domestic help allow itself such definitive airs. Nevertheless, I decided to try again the next day as requested. (I had no idea at that time of the presence of a Ms. Barbara Hannah.) The following day, I received an appointed time for a session and a week later I was courteously received at the front door by the "domestic help" and accompanied to the foot of the staircase. I noticed instantly that this woman [Barbara Hannah] was exceptional. Once upstairs, Frau von Franz then received me with straightforward warmth and ease.

Ken, who at first did not want to believe I had received an appointment at all, had recommended that I should do my best to keep both feet on the floor. This was, however, easier said than done. Frau von Franz opened our conversation with a monologue about some irritating situation she had recently had at the C. G. Jung Institute and how "some imbecile there simply did not want to grasp that it could not go on this way. . . ." I quietly listened but also felt more and more at home. It was human, very simply human.

Then suddenly things took a turn which pulled the floor right out from under my feet. Looking directly at me, she asked: "Who in the world has given you such a dressing down?" She had seen right through me. And I had so hoped to make the best possible impression. In any case, the hour flew by, and Frau von Franz offered me a second one in a week, which I felt was quite an honor. That hour occurred as scheduled. I no longer remember what we spoke about. But the end of the hour impressed me deeply: Frau von Franz said, short and to the point, "Mr. Landtwing, I would gladly work with you, but I would need about six months before I have an analytical hour free." My reaction was both elation and to be deeply aggrieved. Unfortunately, something in me took the upper hand, and I can only say today that I was a total idiot: I thanked her courteously but said that in due respect to the urgency of my situation, waiting for half a year would be too long, thus I could not take her up on her offer. Frau von Franz understood me fully and was in no way upset: she simply could not change her situation. She also would not accept any money from me, and in no time I was outside enjoying the refreshing air of a spring morning.

That night I had the following dream:

> *I descend the steps leading down from Frau von Franz's house after my hour. As I step onto the street, I am overcome by an imperative urge to urinate. It is quiet there, and there is no one in sight, so I urinate through the bars of the fence into von Franz's garden. It is a warm discharge with the force of a fire hydrant, and it is as if I urinate hundreds of liters. My feelings of shame are gone. I awake greatly relieved.*

Years later I read a quote from Frau von Franz regarding urine in her book, *The Golden Ass of Apuleius: The Liberation of the Feminine in Man.* She wrote: "In alchemical texts, urine is a particularly productive and positive substance. . . . Urinating is a symbol of the expression of one's own innermost nature, thus indeed something of the highest value."[1]

Another memory that lies close to my heart are the ten lectures of a lecture series from Frau von Franz that was organized by the Vereinigung der Zürcherischen Volkshochschule (the Association of Adult Education in Zürich). These lectures occurred around the beginning of the 1980s in an auditorium of the University of Zürich. The theme was the legends and myths regarding the creation of the planet Earth from various ethnic peoples and cultures. Each of the weekly lectures was brimming with people; there was not even any room left on the staircases and in the aisles. Looking back, one sees how much this woman was already loved and respected. I retain little memory of the Pueblo Indians, the Eskimo cultures, and other ethnic groups that she discussed, but the atmosphere in the auditorium I will never forget. Although my memories are quite subjective, I believe that I can say that many of those who attended would agree with my impressions. Frau von Franz spoke of these cultures, "of peoples, to people," with an unerring respect for their integrity, their natural dignity, and their knowledge. The whole auditorium sat on edge, hearkening to the "Great Mother" who was telling her "grandchildren" myths and legends of the peoples of the world. Now, what can parents tell their children today, in the year 2003? They can speak of little more than superpowers who have the capacity to set loose a nuclear arsenal that in a matter of days could reduce the cultures of the world to dust and ashes and lay the entire planet to waste. Everything would have to begin anew. And this all had come to pass in just a few short years.

It would have only needed a little glowing fire near the speaker's lectern with an exotic fragrance of incense wafting in the air and the entire auditorium would have been transformed into an oriental palace for one hour, week after week.

Arousing, if not to say outright alarming, was the tenacious repetition of her sentence: "As you surely know. . . ." Frau von Franz said this phrase two to three times a lecture and each time it was followed by a general hesitation and—as I experienced it—a quiet glancing about from left to right to see if one neighbor or the other had actually known the point. I do not know whether or not Frau von Franz intentionally said this, but in any case it was always fitting.

During the third to the last lecture, something quite special occurred which was also typical of the eloquence of Frau von Franz. In the middle of the hour, a young man stood up in the center of the audience, leaned forward, vigorously interrupted Frau von Franz point blank, and posed a question that had nothing whatsoever to do with the context of what she was presenting. The entire room reeled back in trepidation. Marie-Louise von Franz raised her head from her lectern, turned slowly toward the man, and courteously requested that he please give her a minute to answer his question. By that time, it was clear to most members of the audience that she was dealing with a man who was psychologically unstable. Frau von Franz then answered his question as best she could—it was in regards to some psychological issue—and then asked the man if he was satisfied with her answer. He thanked her, returned to his seat, and the hour continued as if nothing had happened.

Like a beautiful celebration, or a festive theater production, or a harmonious concert, a journey through ten lectures for the "grandchildren" with the "Great Mother" also comes to a close. The lectures were completed, the fire extinguished. The last spark of that fire, the closing words of Marie-Louise von Franz, I will share with you in my conclusion. They will be repeated in honor of this grand woman for they say everything . . . and even more than pages of text could portray.

But first: my last personal encounter with Frau von Franz occurred on Friday, April 24, 1992, at five p.m. at her house on Lindenbergstrasse in Küsnacht. I had had a visionary dream that I wanted to share with her. I knew that her health was not the best, but something within me forced me at least to try. I had the help of Dr. Dieter Baumann, with whom I had been in analysis for a long time. He assisted me by writing her a letter of recommendation. The "unusual" once again played its hand: Frau von Franz gave me an appointment in the middle of our spring vacation. My partner and I were at that time in Cinque Terre (northern Italy). Our decision was clear. We drove back to Zürich for those two days in April. Frau von Franz never knew. The hour of analysis was everything other than speaking about the dream. Rather, it was mostly a mutual, very respectful conversation between two *Menschen.* I had immediately noticed that she had just been to the hairdresser and was wearing a lovely dress. I had put on a suit and tie. At the end, I asked her what I owed her and the terse, yet humorous answer was: "Mediums are always broke, so let's leave it be." Marie-Louise von Franz had apparently heard of my mediumistic abilities from some other source. I answered: "Please. You see can that I do not have a full beard and do not wear tattered sandals. I have put on one of my best suits for you and have brought my wallet along." "Okay," she said, "then you can give me one hundred francs for the hour." The world was again in order. It was a mutually dignified farewell.

This farewell brings me to my last memory, which I will share. It is in regards to how the news of her death reached me. It was February 19, 1998. My partner Lyss Oeschger and I were spending our winter ski holidays in the village of Pontresina, that is, in the glistening powder and blinding sunshine of the Engadin (not far from San Moritz). I was sitting in the reading room of the Hotel Steinbock after breakfast and was leafing through the Zürich newspapers. There I came upon the obituary of Marie-Louise von Franz. It had finally occurred. That which we had long awaited had come to a close. Now, the word *Steinbock* means both "mountain goat" (more precisely, the *Capra ibex*) as well as the astrological sign of Capricorn, in which Marie-Louise von Franz was born.[2] (I am also strongly influenced in my astrological sign by Capricorn.) It was as if the Steinbock had called for its *Capra ibex* in the Hotel Steinbock at the very heart of its natural habitat in the alps and glaciers of the Engadin. I knew one thing for certain; I had to see this woman one last time before we bid her farewell in the church. The next morning, I drove over the Julier Pass totally covered in snow to Küsnacht, joined the memorial service, and returned the same day, deeply moved.

In her honor, and as a gesture of thanks to Marie-Louise von Franz, I would like to offer the last spark of that modest and imaginary fire here in the conclusion: as the lecture drew to a close, Frau von Franz picked up her notes, shook and shuffled them first vertically, turned them on their side, reshook and reshuffled them horizontally, and then tapped them into place. The tension in the auditorium had unmistakably increased. Then she quietly repeated the full procedure with a reflective yet astounding self-assuredness. All the pages then appeared to have found their place. Frau von Franz looked up, her glance passed across the room into the eyes of the people, and she then spoke with her so poignant and sonorous voice:

"So . . . now I am finished."

NOTES

1. M.-L. von Franz, *The Golden Ass of Apuleius* (Boston: Shambhala, 1992). In the German edition, p. 169ff.
2. The *Capra ibex* is the very pride of the Swiss Canton of Grisons, the central valley of which is the Engadin. It appears as an emblem in the flag of this canton. Also, see Theresa Loetscher's contribution on M.-L. von Franz's astrological chart in this Festschrift.—*Ed.*

Two Remarkable Moments

TOM LAUGHLIN

The First Remarkable Moment—Jung's Religion

There are so many remarkable things to say about von Franz, so many remarkable moments to remember, life-changing moments that to do them justice would require a book, not just an essay for a Festschrift.

You see von Franz, Mar Lou, had achieved that status that belongs to the rare few who have spent their lives developing what Jung discovered as the "living thing" "down there" in the unconscious. Mar Lou no longer belonged to this world; she belonged to that other world that belongs to those who have so developed within themselves the transpersonal psyche that they no longer see the world and everything in it the way the rest of us see it, but instead they see everything from the "world view."

Having begun working for Jung as a researcher at only eighteen years of age, and ending up literally cowriting Jung's last four major works, Mar Lou knew as much about Jung's work and life, his psychology, philosophy, spirituality, and religion as anyone. I did not use the word *religion* loosely, for one of the two most remarkable moments in my life occurred when I realized for the first time, through a private conversation between von Franz and Edward Edinger during lunch at a Panarion Conference after Edinger's lecture on the new dispensation, that Jung had in fact established a new religion, and although that sounds exaggerated, even disturbing, you will see in a moment, as I did during that conversation, how non-exaggerated, realistic, and accurate that statement is.

(I would be remiss if I did not acknowledge the tremendous gift I received by being blessed to work for more than twenty years with both von Franz and Edinger simultaneously, two of Jung's most towering intellects, both living out of the transpersonal psyche. My Jungian blessing began with my first introduction to Jungian therapy being with the equally gifted Joseph Henderson, an incredible launch, and then going on to work with many of Jung's other personal colleagues such as Schärf-Kluger, Hilde Kirsch, and James Kirsch.)

Edinger had just given a lecture that could, without exaggeration, be accurately described as astonishing. He had laid out very carefully how Jung had indeed created a new dispensation. In simple terms, a new religion. Ed, Mar Lou, my wife Delores, and I were seated at lunch when Mar Lou became very pensive, as she often did when she was about to say something important and meaningful. "We all know it's true," she said to Ed, "but you are the first to have the courage to say it publicly."

The word *religion* derives from *religio, religiare,* "to bind back to," "to reconnect the smaller to the greater, the piece to the whole." All religions have at their nuclear core the purpose of reconnecting man, the lesser, to God, the Greater, the Whole, which is exactly what Jung's new psychology does. It provides the way for the ego, the lesser, to reconnect to the Greater Living Thing in the unconscious, reconnects man to God.

Later, in a private conversation, Mar Lou described the importance of Edinger's essay by showing how the incarnation of the divine into human form was a universal religious theme. She showed how in the Greek religion Zoë was the goddess of life itself, eternal life, and when Zoë entered into an individual unit, a tree, a dog, a human being, it became bios (from which we get our words *biology, biography,* and so on). Zoë, the principle of life, was eternal. You could never kill Zoë. Though you could kill a million trees, or a million people that Zoë had incarnated in, you could never kill Zoë, life itself . . . a theme present in all religions, the theme of relating the lesser to the greater, man to God.

In Christianity, the theme is the same. God, the greater, enters into an individual man, the lesser, and thereby God becomes man, and through this incarnation in man, man is reconnected to God. From this nuclear core reality, endless series of symbols, rituals, and dogmas flow, all designed to enrich and deepen the reconnection of God to man by each individual developing the newly incarnated life within.

What Jung had given us, and as Edinger had laid out so clearly, von Franz emphasized, was an entirely new way to understand how God incarnated in man, and how man could develop this veiled deity within.

Von Franz pointed out a seminal moment in Jung's discovery of this new reality. It occurred, she said, when Jung—struggling with his very different theories from Freud's of how the psyche is formed, developed, and functions—suddenly realized that "there was something alive down there," meaning in his unconscious or his soul. Von Franz shared that Jung then and there committed his life to trying to discover what this "living thing" was, and how he could best develop it within himself, and should he succeed at that, how he could help others to do the same. All of Jung's work, all Jungian therapy, has that purpose, that goal, to reconnect the lesser conscious personality—the ego, the intellect, and the will—with the greater "living thing down there," that far greater personality, far greater intelligence lying dormant in the unconscious waiting to be developed. Everything Jung wrote and did was to that end—to help everyone develop the far greater living personality begging to be developed in each of us.

Jung said God and man were two sides of the same coin. To the side pointing inward and creating the entire person Jung gave the word *Self*, the side facing into eternity was God. Mar Lou then explained that the reason Jung used the word *Self* instead of God was because he was already, at that beginning stage, being crucified for being too mystical and his psychological theories and treatment were being dismissed as not being practical. Jung wanted his discovery to be judged on its merits, not prejudged out of fear and Freudian bias.

From the psychological standpoint, Jung's discovery of the "living thing" down there to be developed is self-evident and indisputable. From the very beginning of working with Mar Lou, she helped me to understand this reality. A newborn baby has no capacity to function as a human being, no ability to sit up, talk, walk, or take care of itself, and certainly no capacity to do all of the tens of thousands of things every adult human being is able to do. But lying dormant in that baby, in that unconscious, is the potential capacity to do all of these things, to become a far greater person than one is at birth. Just as the DNA has in it a greater intelligence containing a blueprint for the physical adult each person will become, so Jung discovered there was a psychological DNA that has in it a greater intelligence with a blueprint of what that human being should become, containing thousands of capacities, abilities, skills, talents, and behavior patterns that are to be developed if only the environment does not hinder, damage, or even destroy them. In fact, the newborn baby does not even have an ego, intellect, or will, but this "living thing," this greater intelligence is what creates the ego and the conscious personality from seemingly nothing, intending those as vital tools to continue to develop the greater personality and greater intelligence lying dormant in the unconscious, in the soul, bringing them up one by one from the unconscious and adding them to the conscious personality.

All of the great religious figures and teachers the world has known are examples of the greater personality being developed to its highest form, a level of development, von Franz pointed out, that we all can reach if only we know how to reconnect back to the living thing, the God within, and find out what we are to develop next. Truly, Jung has given us an entirely new way to reconnect the lesser to the greater, the piece to the whole, man to God; truly, a new religion for those who have been lucky enough to discover the reality of the unconscious and the objective psyche that lives in each of us.

On one occasion, Mar Lou pointed out, Jung summed up his belief that "life is nothing but the story of the self-realization of the unconscious. Everything in the unconscious seeks outward manifestation." Jung went so far as to say that virtually all neurosis and many physical illnesses are because some aspect of the personality is being prevented from being developed. The secret of healing lies in creating an environment that allows each of us to consciously develop this hidden aspect of the personality, an environment that frees us to live up to our full potential instead of someone else's expectations. Above all else, von Franz made this crystal clear in the environment she created to work in, and in her constantly insisting that my expectations come from the living thing within and not from her.

> Hidden in the neurosis is a bit of still undeveloped personality, a precious fragment of the psyche lacking which a man is condemned to resignation, bitterness, and everything else that is hostile to life. (Jung, *CW* 10, par. 355)

The word *God* is tricky and difficult to use because it has so many different meanings for different people. Jung said he didn't care what image or concept you had of God as long as you recognize that God was the superior power. Man's ability to conceive of God is severely limited by man's limited intellect, so the most we can ever say about the infinite God falls hopelessly short because of our limited intellect's ability to conceive of God. The ballbearing upon which all of Jung's life revolved was that superior power.

"My *raison d'etre* consists of coming to terms
with that indefinable being we call God."—Jung

Once, sitting with Franz Jung in Jung's study, I asked him if it was true that Jung was preoccupied in the last half of his life with the reality of God. Franz assured us that indeed, from the age of thirty-five on, the central thrust of Jung's work was God and religion, although he was reluctant to use those words openly because he was already being ridiculed as a mystic and did not want the extremely important realities of his psychology and therapy to be further dismissed.

(Later, Franz took my wife, Delores, on a joyful tour of Jung's tower at Bollingen, Jung's "sacred place," and through Franz's endless stories, she learned things about Jung that are priceless. Although I have been a guest in Mar Lou's and Barbara Hannah's home in Bollingen, I never had the pleasure of seeing Jung's tower.)

The next day, von Franz reiterated Franz's words and shared with me two decisive quotes regarding Jung's belief and work in his journey to discover this new religion, this new way of reconnecting man back to God. The first was from a letter of August 8, 1945, in which Jung replies, "You are quite right, the main interest of my work is not concern with the treatment of neurosis but rather with the approach to the numinous." Von Franz explained that Jung used the word *numinous* to describe the overpowering experience one has when one meets this indefinable God. "But the fact is," Jung went on, "that the approach to the numinous is the real therapy, and inasmuch as you would attain to the numinous experiences, you are released from the curse of pathology. Even the very disease takes on a numinous character."

To drive home the point of how intensely Jung felt that all healing depended upon reconnecting man back to God, that is, the numinous, the living thing down there, von Franz shared with us another deeply held conviction of Jung's that he felt so strongly about he stated it publicly. "Among all my patients in the second half of life—that is to say, over thirty-five—there has not been one whose problem in the last resort was not that of finding a religious outlook on life. None of them has been really healed who did not regain his religious outlook. This of course has nothing whatever to do with the particular creed or membership of a church" (*CW* 11, par. 509).

The discussion that began that day between Edinger and von Franz, and continued with each of them individually for the rest of my life with them, was a life-transforming experience for me, and to be graced with the opportunity to work with both of them through the years, enriching my understanding of this precious information delivered that day, is truly one of the most remarkable moments of my life. To become aware that Jung had indeed established a new religion, a new way for man to find God, both within and without, was, to be honest, numbing. The implications of this discovery were so enormous. One of the greatest, most important books in all of Jungian literature is Edward Edinger's masterpiece, *The Creation of Consciousness*, in which he discusses magnificently what Ed and Mar Lou discussed that day, Jung's new dispensation, the new way that God becomes incarnate in man, and the way all of us can participate in this new divine drama by incarnating this "living thing" within ourselves.

(Of course, *the* epic work of this millennium is Jung's *Answer to Job,* a book so profound and with such far-reaching implications that it will take mankind at least a hundred years or more to begin to understand the completely new approach to religion Jung has posited there. "Christianity hangs by a thin thread . . . the problem of evil," von Franz said to me once as she introduced me to *Answer to Job.* "The Christian must believe that only good comes from God and all evil comes from Satan or man himself, never daring to face the harsh reality that God, if not the author of evil, at least clearly allows it—but for what purpose?" Jung is the first to answer that question thoroughly and completely, but unfortunately, it is difficult reading and even more difficult to comprehend these fundamentally new ideas about the nature of God. "God needs us to become conscious," von Franz explained, echoing Jung, "but who can understand that?" With her help, many of us were able to embark on the process of learning that almost unspeakable truth.)

For the first time, the full impact of the inscription Jung has over the door to his home hit me with a force it never had before: "*Vocatus atque non vocatus, deus aderit*" ("Summoned or not, the god will be there"). As Jung himself explained, "Here another not less important road begins, not the approach to 'Christianity' but to God himself, and this seems to be the ultimate question."

This is exactly what it became for me from this luncheon onward, and the center of all the rest of my life with von Franz.

The Second Remarkable Moment von Franz Gave Me

The second of the hundreds of remarkable insights and moments Mar Lou gave me and that I wish to share in this Festschrift had to do with "how Jung interpreted my (von Franz's) dreams."

The most important gift I got from von Franz and all the other great Jungians I was privileged to work with and know throughout my life, was the secret to life itself, the secret that if you learned how to reconnect with the living thing within, with the Zoë incarnate in you, this greater intelligence would always be available to you and the greater personality waiting to be developed would always be available for your growth and enlightenment. Von Franz had a special genius for showing one how to reconnect to the living psyche, how to take the most abstruse esoteric concepts of Jung's and make them into simple, practical, easy-to-understand tools that one could use in everyday life. Often, I had people who found Jung too difficult, and I would turn them on to von Franz where they immediately grasped Jung's most arcane and difficult theories. Still the very best introduction I know of to Jung is von Franz's chapter, "The Process of Individuation," in *Man and His Symbols,* and the best, most impressive introduction of Jung's psychology of dreams is von Franz's, *The Way of the Dream.* Her written words were always as juicy with life as were her personal sessions. Above all, the one word that sums them up better than any other is they were *real.* Mar Lou put me, and everyone I know, in touch with the inner and outer reality as no one else was able to do.

Once I had learned from Mar Lou that my real authority, my real teacher, lay within, and once I learned how to develop this dialogue and relationship to the greater intelligence alive within me, I began to discover a wisdom even beyond Jung, von Franz, Edinger, and the rest, the same wisdom that is available to us all if only we are given the gift to have the courage to face our shadow and transform it.

An example of how this works in our day-to-day life might be helpful.

Early on I was not just honored, but thrilled, when von Franz asked me to interpret one of her dreams, which I was privileged to do from then on whenever I was in Zürich. My knowledge of interpreting dreams came, of course, from how von Franz interpreted my dreams, how Edinger interpreted my dreams, as well as all the other Jungians mentioned above that I had the good fortune of doing dream work with for many years. All were basically the same, although each had his or her own way of finessing the approach.

After a while, I became dissatisfied with this method of interpreting dreams, which all of these great Jungians were using. My dreams, my own inner work, and my own method of interpreting my own dreams told me there was a better way. Now imagine the egregiousness of this assumption of mine—that I had found a better way to interpret dreams than von Franz, Edinger, Henderson, and so on. I was terrified at what I feared was a serious inflation and wanted to abandon my approach, except it produced such beautiful results, far better than I got doing it the "gold standard" way.

In the summer of 1984, I was in Zürich for my semiannual trip, and von Franz invited myself, my writing partner, Robin Hutton, and Barbara Hannah to lunch at the restaurant in Bollingen where they had celebrated so warmly and joyfully Jung's eightieth birthday. Toward the end of the meal, von Franz told me about a dream she had that was still puzzling her even though she had worked on it intensely, as had one or two others she trusted to try to help her with it. She asked if I would work with her on it. I was always delighted to help von Franz interpret one of her dreams.

I say "help" interpret because I believe it is essential that a good therapist knows he or she is not interpreting the patient's dream; the same creative intelligence that created the dream will also provide the richest interpretive material if only it is allowed to do so by the therapist, who is merely a skilled helper.

I then, with great trepidation, dared to say to Mar Lou—who could always see right through me as though she had x-ray vision—"I would like to do it a little differently. I've discovered a new way to interpret dreams and with your permission I'd like to try it on this dream"—the meaning of which was still alluding her. With the tremendous confidence and security the great ones have, instead of being threatened by this seemingly outlandish claim, von Franz said, "Of course, go right ahead."

My "new" way takes a lot more time than what is typically done in an analytical hour, and two hours later, with poor Barbara sound asleep, I finished. For a long time, Mar Lou just looked down at the table and said nothing. Finally she spoke, "But that is exactly the way Jung interpreted my dreams."

She went on to say that after doing sixty thousand dreams you get lazy and you start to skip the associations. She confirmed my belief that the key to interpreting dreams lies in providing the same superior intelligence that created the dream the opportunity to comment thoroughly on all of the images it created in the dream; it will basically interpret the dream for you, for it alone knows why it created the dream . . . to "tell you" what the dream means. If the associations are done correctly, the same intelligence will basically interpret the dream for you and why it used these symbols as the language it wanted to use to tell the patient what the patient needs to know.

Obviously, von Franz's approval of my "new" method and learning that it was exactly how Jung interpreted her dreams (though, of course, Jung adapted to every individual patient because every patient was unique and every dream was unique) was not only a remarkable moment for me, it was a transforming one, and not just because of the approval of von Franz and the comparison to Jung, which of course was heady stuff indeed, but because it verified Jung's basic premise, that everyone of us has "down there"—this transpersonal intelligence that if only we learn how to listen to it will transform our lives. The same supernatural intelligence that gave Jung all of his discoveries is real and exists in all of us if only we understand what Jung has given us—though, because each of us is unique, it gives each of us what we uniquely need to have to develop the greater personality within us to its fullest. I say "supernatural" because this intelligence is superior to our conscious intelligence, and "natural" because it is beyond the nature of our human intellect and book learning, which is exactly what the word *supernatural* means—beyond our human experience and existence.

Two Footnotes

The information that came out of this dream had to do with von Franz's medical condition and the medications she was taking as required by her excellent doctors. Although von Franz gave me permission to share this dream in detail, space limitations require that I simply share with you the fact that the medicine von Franz was taking, while beneficial in some ways, unbeknownst to any of us, contained within it an ingredient that was extremely dangerous for her heart condition, especially in this high altitude. It is extraordinary, to say the least, that this information should come from a dream when neither von Franz nor I, nor her doctors, had any knowledge of the side effects of this medicine or the ingredients it contained and would have never even thought of a medicine prescribed by top medical doctors to be dangerous for her.

Von Franz was also taking the standard drug for Parkinson's called Levodopa, which is a precursor to the creation of dopamine, essential to Parkinson's patients because the cells in their brain that produce dopamine, a brain chemical essential to having energy and a feeling of well being, are being destroyed. Instead, the dream advised von Franz to take an amino acid, which is a fancy word for a protein found in nature, called Tyrosine, which was also a precursor to developing dopamine in the brain. Tyrosine had no side effects whatsoever and was far more useful in developing a better chemical balance in Mar Lou's brain. She stopped taking the Levodopa and continued to take Tyrosine up until her passing. (Subsequently science has learned that while Levodopa has a temporary salutary effect, within a year or two it wears off and the more debilitating symptoms of Parkinson's develop more rapidly. What science subsequently learned, Mar Lou's dream knew years earlier.)

Obviously this was a remarkable moment and a life-transforming experience that showed unmistakably the supernatural power and supernatural intelligence hidden in the transpersonal intelligence of the dream maker and dream interpreter in the unconscious, first by giving to me a "new," more effective method of interpreting dreams than I had thought available, and second, by giving von Franz information about her medicine that none of us, including her medical specialists, even knew existed. Never again would anyone be able to deprecate the power and supernatural wisdom of the dream. The only time a dream fails to deliver this kind of intelligence and advice is when the interpreter, Jungian or otherwise, fails to interpret the dream correctly, which sadly is all too often the case today.

The second little footnote occurred when I later shared with Joe Henderson this experience, with Mar Lou's permission of course. "The skipping! The skipping! That's the biggest mistake they do in interpreting dreams," he said, confirming that that was how Jung also interpreted his dreams. Joe went on to lament with a broken heart that at the Jung Institute in San Francisco they no longer teach not to skip while interpreting a dream, they don't even bother to teach the interpretation of dreams—which is the alpha and omega of learning what the unconscious wants us to do next to solve our problems and improve our lives.

So indispensable is the correct interpretation of dreams to Jungian psychology that during the last several years of our work together von Franz didn't even want to know what the problems I was bringing to her to help solve were, nor what I felt about them. "Let's see what the unconscious has to say the problem is, and what you should do about it," she would say. And we would always begin with whatever dream I had brought, for in working carefully on the dream, everything would be revealed to both of us.

How tragic it is today that so few Jungians know how to interpret dreams correctly.

There are so many hundreds of other moments I could share, so many wonderful stories I could tell about von Franz, as could my wife Delores, who also worked with her for all those years, my daughter Teresa, and our partner Robin Hutton. I don't think there was a time that we came back from Zürich and didn't have a dozen laughs to share along with all the magnificent insights each of us had gotten. Delores especially had experiences there in Küsnacht, and at the Hotel Sonne, some magnificent and some horrific, that would also fill a small book.

I'll never forget the time, early on, when Delores came back and shared the story that they sat there and watched von Franz's dog, Laura, chew through the handles of her beautiful purse and was too in awe of von Franz to stop her. When Delores later told Mar Lou about it, she was embarrassed, but then chuckled, "Laura was just trying to teach you to be more assertive."

A last note: the tremendous empathy, feeling, and sympathy of Mar Lou was experienced by us all countless times in countless ways, but one small thing touched me very deeply: after Laura died, we urged von Franz to get another dog, but she refused. The reason was as kind and thoughtful as Mar Lou was herself. She knew she would die before the dog, and she did not want the dog to suffer the loneliness that loss was certain to bring.

Genius in the true sense of that word: von Franz was a genius. She had to be in order to become such an essential and indispensable part of Jung's genius and work, for no one lesser would do. Although von Franz, for the most part, was in the background, her work with Jung's and separate from Jung's is for the ages. She will live with me forever . . . as she will with everyone of us whom God chose to be blessed by her presence in our lives, to show us how to develop the "living thing" within us as she had within herself.

As she pointed out at that memorable lunch, and as Edinger has written so beautifully in *The Creation of Consciousness,* it is the responsibility of those who are called to put their life in the service of transforming the primordial psyche, the raw living thing, by offering himself as a vessel for the incarnation of the Deity and "thereby promote the ongoing transformation of God by giving Him human manifestation," which is why God became man in the first place.

Marie-Louise von Franz offered herself as a vessel for the incarnation of God, and she achieved it superbly.

Thank you, God, for Mar Lou. Thank you, Mar Lou, for allowing me to see and experience God in a way I never would have without you.

Horoscope of Marie-Louise von Franz

THERES LOETSCHER

The interpretation of a horoscope shows the possibilities of how a particular constellation could be lived. It always depends on the stage of development of the individual and the inherited and acquired tools he or she brings (or fails to bring) to the task of working on—and fulfilling—his or her life pattern. It is essential for the interpreter of a horoscope to discern the archetypal pattern represented in the quality of the planets and their relationship to one another and then to understand and analyze the person, who is a transforming being, within the fabric of this relationship.

Ascendant (AC) Scorpio

A person with a Scorpio ascendant radiates a powerful force. She or he is a very good observer, masters crisis situations, detects that which is hidden (repressed or, in Jungian terms, in the shadow), is interested in the nature of processes, and is oriented to that which is essential and substantial.

Scorpio is the sign where one is confronted with the deepest abyss, but where one can attain the highest forms of knowledge. In life, and in particular during puberty, this can lead to experiences of divine exultation or aggrieved sadness.

The ruler of the ascendant Scorpio is Pluto. Pluto is located in the 8th house, the house of "dying and becoming." It represents the descent into the unconscious, themes of life and death, the ability to detect secrets and taboos in others, and to help others in crisis. (Dreams are of considerable help here.)

With Pluto in Cancer in the 8th house, one has the gift to help lead others to their roots (Cancer equated with roots). (But one can only help others if one has descended oneself into the depths of the psyche, that is, into the abyss.)

The Conjunction of Saturn/Pluto

Saturn is the ruler of the 3rd house, Pluto is the ruler over the actual birth.[1]

Individuals with this constellation presumably experience considerable fear in their childhood, and in particular, in the context of ambiguous situations, connections, or contiguities. Thus an intense urge to do research was developed in order to get to the bottom of things (Pluto) and to fathom the secrets of life (8th house), an urge which was realized and expressed, for example, in Marie-Louise von Franz's books such as *Shadow and Evil in Fairy Tales, Psyche and Matter, On Divination and Synchronicity,* and *On Dreams and Death.*

Another characteristic of Saturn in conjunction with Pluto constitutes the necessary endurance coupled with a sense of duty to go level-for-level down into the depths, past that which is concealed (8th house) in order to reach the most basic archetypal pattern (Pluto).

This aspect enables one to draw another person's attention precisely to his or her blind spots, and often with remarkable clarity.[2] For some, this may seem merciless or hurtful, in particular when a person is not prepared to descend into the depths or when a person is particularly superficial. (The strongly occupied 3rd house points to frankness in speech.) But there are people who concern themselves with the essence of things, with the depths, and with the process of becoming conscious (Pluto in quincunx to Venus, the planet of eros relationship).[3] These types of people are reliable and faithful, their friendships are enduring, and they are separated from their friends only by strokes of fate.

Alchemy, physics, and psychology each provide a means of understanding the symbolic language not only of these depths but of the basic fundamental needs and values (Pluto, 8th house) of mankind.

Second House: Venus in Sagittarius

The 2nd house is the house of values, values of materials and of things, of nature, of personal values and self-esteem. There may be pleasures, but here they are in relationship to Neptune so that one may tend not to know when they are enough or what does one good. (In extreme cases, this constellation can be related to addictions.) With a 9th house—Neptune trine Venus—there could also be a yearning for higher knowledge.[4]

There is a preference for art (possibly symbolic objects connected with religiosity: Sagittarius). On other levels, the power of imagination in regards to values and religion is present while security and values are directed toward religiosity (Sagittarius).

Or we may also interpret this as nature quickened by means of querying into the background of natural objects and events (Venus trine Neptune) and their relationship to one another (physics).[5] This leads to the "quickening" of matter, that is, to the discovery of the "soul" of matter; in the concepts of the alchemists and of Jung, matter then becomes "gold."

Synastry Horoscope of C. G. Jung and Marie-Louise von Franz[6]

In a synastry horoscope, C. G. Jung's midheaven (*medium coeli*) and Lilith (black moon) constitute a conjunction with the Venus of Marie-Louise von Franz as if it were to say: closely examine the unredeemed (Lilith) problem of matter (Venus, 2nd house) and seek that which is missing, for example, the divine in nature (Venus trine Neptune).[7] The concordance of psyche and matter became of paramount value to both Jung and von Franz.

Naturally, Marie-Louise von Franz's Sagittarius in the 2nd house of Venus can be lived out in a very different form, for example, new impressions along with new styles and qualities of life can be won when traveling or collecting artwork from cultures throughout the world. Traveling can also mean journeys of an inner nature where, through the search for meaning, inner forms and qualities can be discovered. On this level of development, Marie-Louise von Franz was inspired to pursue questions regarding the hidden nature of matter and fathom its secrets (with the help of Pluto in the 8th house).

The planet ruling the 2nd house (Sagittarius) is Jupiter. Jupiter is found here in the 4th house in Aquarius, which implies the inner quest (4th house equated with home, roots), but in this case not only on a personal level but also on that of the collective (Aquarius). It concerns itself not only with the family and home on the personal level but also on the universal level. It appears that Marie-Louise von Franz not only pioneered these issues at the dawning of the age of Aquarius but showed us our own new home country, a home that can only be reached through a journey (Jupiter) to the inner world (descendant, 4th house) where we gain the greatest freedom (Aquarius).

In this synastry horoscope, C. G. Jung's Saturn stands in a precise 1° conjunction with Marie-Louise von Franz's Jupiter. Jung's authority and earnestness (coupled with criticism when necessary) constituted a stabilizing effect on her inner journey.

Third House: Sun/Mars/Mercury in Capricorn

Communication and writing are central themes. Thoroughness, concentration, and ambition are the main attributes of those born in Capricorn. Such persons must occasionally assume responsibility already in childhood, or their parents appeal to their reason (that is, more with words than with feelings). The person presumably has an authoritarian father.

Mars acts quickly. With Mars in the 3rd house, communication is frank and direct. The spirit is so fleet and agile that the person is often too fast, that is, the person may tend to overrun others. This can create tension, power struggles, and rivalry among siblings when, for example, the other does not catch on as quickly. When one feels threatened in one's authority, Mars is constellated as a warrior and stabs back with his sharp knives (rather, sharp tongue, because Mars is in the 3rd house, the house of communication). This situation escalates to intellectual conflicts.

On the other hand, this aspect (Sun/Mars/Mercury in the 3rd house) can also mean that one inspires others to develop their own ideas. (Now, next to such a powerful personality, who dares to differ in his or her opinion? And rightfully so, because who actually then has the strength needed to go into the depths and develop his own mature opinions?)

This constellation also indicates that a woman will probably be confronted with themes regarding the animus (both hers and that of others). Marie-Louise von Franz once said in a lecture that when she was uncertain whether or not she was in the animus, she would only have to speak to a man, and then she would know where she was.

Sun/Mars/Mercury in 3rd House, in Quincunx to the Moon in the 10th House/Midheaven

One has the need to express one's ideas outwardly in public (10th house) in either oral or written language (3rd house). (The Great Mother nourishes the society.) One receives emotional security in public (moon), thus one often chooses a profession where the "helping mother" can be integrated. But here there is also tension between reason and feeling, between the head and the heart; the moon stands in opposition to Uranus on the *immum coeli*, the lowest point of the chart. Stepping out into the public eye with one's own thoughts is problematical at first. One has perhaps many new and progressive thoughts and creative ideas but does not trust oneself to make these public. (In his exchange with Marie-Louise von Franz, Wolfgang Pauli strongly encouraged her to publish her own creative works under her own name and not that of Jung.)

It is interesting to note that in the synastry horoscope Jung's Uranus stands in conjunction with Marie-Louise von Franz's moon. One could thus say that she may have initially taken over many of Jung's ideas (Uranus) but, by means of the force of Jung's Uranus, her own Uranus was activated. She was thus profoundly inspired by Jung's Uranus and deeply connected to him on a mental level through his sun in conjunction with her Neptune (9th house equated with the expansion of consciousness and the search for meaning). Thus one can well understand her comment in later years when she said that she had remained set on Jung.

The moon in opposition to Uranus is also a constellation that can indicate lack of belief in oneself and uncertainty of feeling. Maybe here a dominant mother represses the creativity of her daughter. With this constellation, the child then seeks safety and security. With this aspect, safety and security has to be sought in the development of one's own individuality. Once secured, a genuine relationship to the outer world could be lived. Mental and spiritual nourishment could (and still can) flow outward to the public.

The moon in the 10th house/midheaven in Leo reminds one of the queen who gives herself fully to her people. With the moon's opposition to Uranus and to the North Node (4th house), the pressure to pursue one's own roots is great (it is, in essence, a karmic task).[8] Here, however, with Uranus and Jupiter in Aquarius, new knowledge could also be extended to the well-being of mankind. (It is similar to a revolution that leads down to the fundamental, primordial roots. These roots then connect one to a deeper understanding of the totality in oneself, the complete man/complete woman, thus providing, so to speak, a mental and spiritual home country.)

In the synastry horoscope, Jung's Saturn stands in conjunction to Marie-Louise von Franz's Jupiter. This could mean that Jung (here as critical teacher: Saturn) supports von Franz in approaching her roots through discipline and hard work (Saturn). The moon in opposition to Uranus can also mean a fear of feeling bonds. One may prefer to remain single, or at least one needs a great deal of tolerance, and this in one's own home (Aquarius). This home then is one where friends from all over the world (Jupiter) who are interested in spiritual and mental development can come in and out.

Lilith in Taurus in the 7th House

The I-thou axis (1st and 7th houses) is concerned with partnership. With Lilith in this house, one often meets levels of respect and esteem in a partnership or relationship that may be overvalued (for instance, inflated) or undervalued (for instance, depreciative). (Lilith does not want to be submissive, yet she also does not want to be dominant. She seeks equality.)

According to this archetypal pattern, one often sets high expectations on relationships that can often lead to a battle between the sexes. Here there are animus-anima themes that eventually point to a conjunction of the opposites.

Lilith in the earth sign of Taurus in the 7th house can also mean discrepancy between bodily and mental or spiritual relationships. One dedicates oneself perhaps more readily to spiritual relationships and love than to physical sensuousness. An ambivalent attitude toward closeness and distance may prevail, an ambivalence that may occur as well toward the pleasure principle. (Or, one may repeatedly end up with a partner who is so inclined.) Attraction-rejection is a frequent theme with this aspect.

I recall a lecture by Marie-Louise von Franz in Einsiedeln in which she spoke about the theme of the single woman (probably in the context of individuation). During a subsequent discussion, a single woman in the audience said that men always want "that same thing." And von Franz answered, somewhat emotionally, "Yes, yes, and the woman then runs away, yet looks back to see if he is not coming after all." (In this example, we see the quality of the above-mentioned constellation.)

This constellation forces one to work on the animus (or anima) and promotes the process of becoming conscious in particular in the context of projections (I-thou axis).

In the synastry horoscope, Jung's Lilith stands in conjunction to the Venus of Marie-Louise von Franz, and his moon stands in conjunction to her Lilith. One could say here that under his aegis, Jung's care and concern (moon) gave von Franz the necessary strength to pursue these painful themes.

The moon also leads us into the world of images and symbols. Von Franz learned the language of symbols through Jung and thus understood her own process, which naturally is a good prerequisite for helping people involved in intense conflict with their partners.

The ruler of the 7th house (and also the 12th house) is Venus. Venus is in aspect to Neptune (9th house) and to Pluto (8th house). Venus, the planet of (eros) relationships, is thus colored by Neptune (this also indicates a preference for spiritual relationships). With this aspect, one is capable of guessing the wishes of others. One can feel one's way into the other person (in extreme cases, to a point of total identification). With Venus trine Neptune, one is very effective in drawing to oneself people who are "seeking," that is, people in search of a deeper relationship to the inner world.

NOTES

1. Conjunction here means that Saturn and Pluto are at a 0° (zero degree) angle to each other, that is, they lie at the same point. [The translator wishes to thank Ms. Jody Schlatter, Jungian analyst, Zürich, who provided the extra notes and commented on and corrected the English translation of astrological terminology.]
2. "Aspect" is used to refer to an angular relationship, for example, a 0°, 90°, 120°, or 150° relationship.
3. "Quincunx" is a term specifying a 150° angle of relationship between two objects.
4. Venus and Neptune constitute a "trine," a triangular aspect of 120°, here a harmonious relationship.
5. "Quickened," literally "imparted with a soul."—*Ed.*
6. A synastry horoscope is the horoscope of two people calculated by placing one horo-

scope on top of the other. Such horoscopes are employed, for instance, to determine qualities of the "match" between two people.—*Ed.*

7. In regards to the elliptical orbit of the moon around the earth, there are two foci, one closer to the earth and the other farther away. Lilith is the focus that is closer to the earth.—*Ed.*
8. The North Node is one of two points of conjunction between the sun and moon.

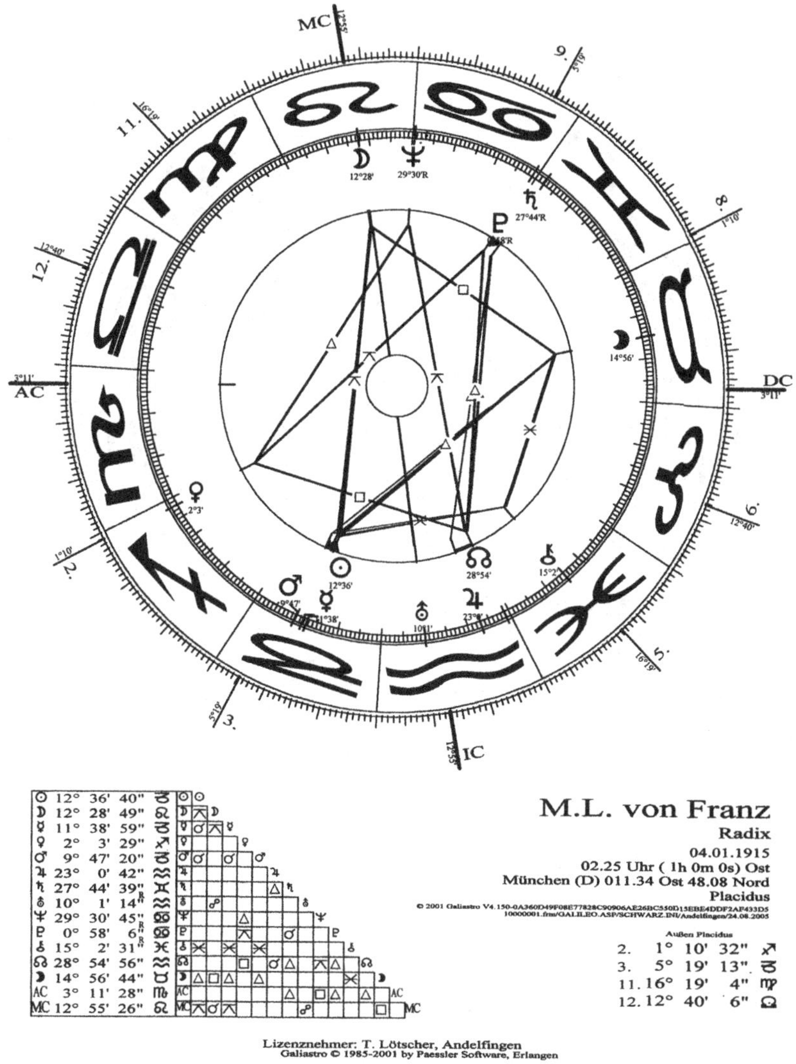

Figure 1: Horoscope from Marie-Louise von Franz

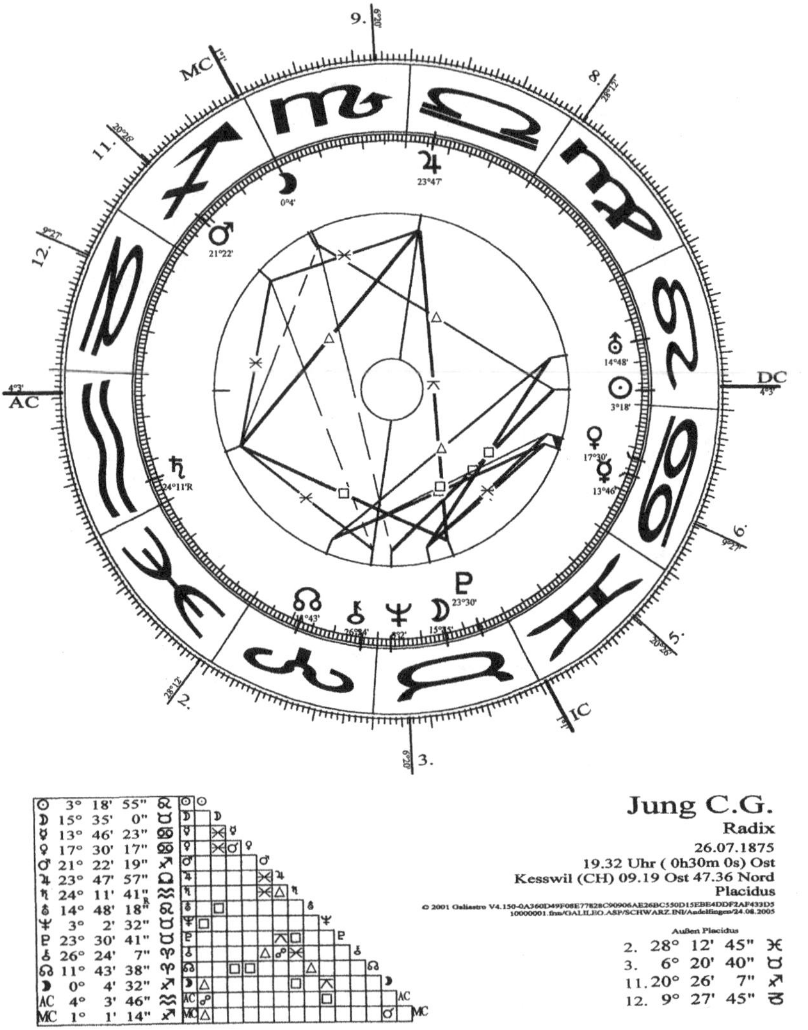

Figure 2: Horoscope from C. G. Jung

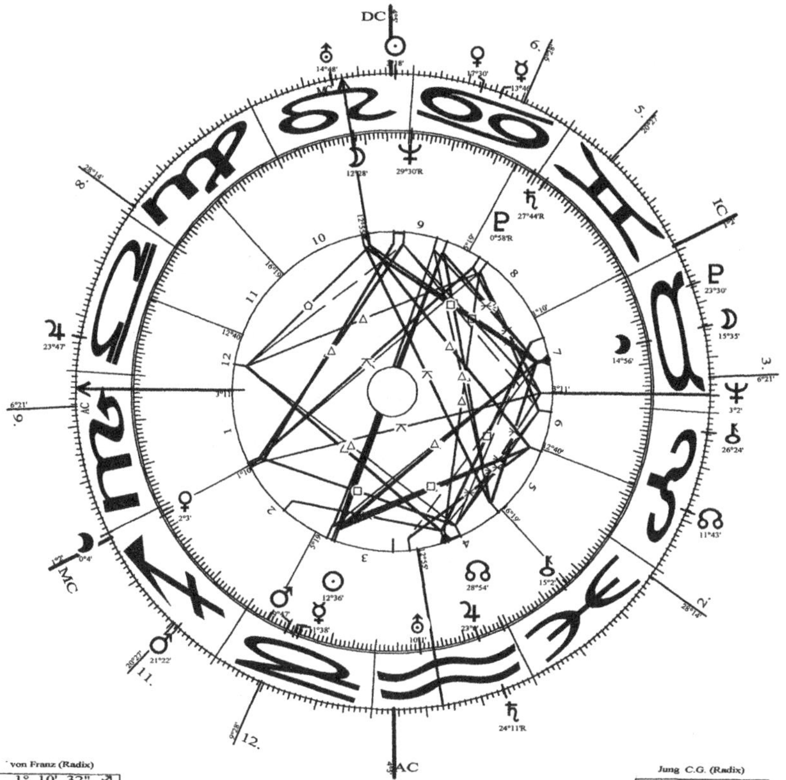

von Franz (Radix)

2.	1°	10'	32"	♐
3.	5°	19'	13"	♑
11.	16°	19'	4"	♍
12.	12°	40'	6"	♎
☉	12°	36'	40"	♑
☽	12°	28'	49"	♌
☿	11°	38'	59"	♑
♀	2°	3'	29"	♐
♂	9°	47'	20"	♑
♃	23°	0'	42"	♒
♄	27°	44'	39" R	♊
♅	10°	1'	14"	♒
♆	29°	30'	45" R	♋
♇	0°	58'	6" R	♋
⚷	15°	2'	31"	♓
☊	28°	54'	56"	♒
⚸	14°	56'	44"	♉
AC	3°	11'	28"	♏
MC	12°	55'	26"	♌

von Franz

Innen: Radix (Placidus)

04.01.1915, 02.25 Uhr, 1h 0m 0s Ost

München (D) 011.34 Ost 48.08 Nord

Jung C.G.

Außen: Radix (Placidus)

26. 7.1875, 19.32 Uhr, 0h30m 0s Ost

Kesswil -tg (CH) 009.20 Ost 47.36 Nord

Jung C.G. (Radix)

2.	28°	14'	20"	♓
3.	6°	21'	52"	♉
11.	20°	27'	1"	♐
12.	9°	28'	44"	♑
☉	3°	18'	55"	♌
☽	15°	35'	0"	♉
☿	13°	46'	23"	♋
♀	17°	30'	17"	♋
♂	21°	22'	19"	♐
♃	23°	47'	57"	♎
♄	24°	11'	41" R	♒
♅	14°	48'	18"	♌
♆	3°	2'	32"	♉
♇	23°	30'	41"	♉
⚷	26°	24'	7"	♈
☊	11°	43'	38"	♈
⚸	0°	4'	32"	♐
AC	4°	5'	10"	♒
MC	1°	2'	11"	♐

Lizenznehmer: T. Lötscher, Andelfingen
Galiastro © 1985-2001 by Paessler Software, Erlangen

Figure 3: Synastry Horoscope from Marie-Louise von Franz and C. G. Jung

Dream Analysis with Marie-Louise von Franz

ROGER LYONS

Before I went to Zürich as a student of Professor Jung in the spring of 1946, he had written to me that he wouldn't be able to take me on full-time, but that I would have an opportunity to become more fully acquainted with his psychology through some of his pupils. Fortunately, I had the chance to work with Marie-Louise von Franz as my principal analyst and teacher. Although we were both relatively young, having been born in the same month of January in 1915, she turned out to be an excellent choice.

Jung said in one of our sessions, "Switzerland is the place where you dream." How right he was is borne out by the fact that, despite years of analysis before and after, I have never had the rich confrontation with my unconscious that I did in Zürich. In particular, during my analysis with von Franz, I had two dreams about Jung on the same night which I never had the opportunity to discuss with him, but which were as important to me as my actual meetings. When I told von Franz these dreams, she immediately said, "These are big dreams, dreams you could spend your life on." And in fact, to me these dreams relate to certain historic events that have occurred since then right up to the present time. There is a mystery about some dreams that constantly beckons and challenges. Even today, I am sure I have not exhausted their meaning.

But at that time, more than half a century ago, it was only after we discussed them at length that I realized how important these dreams were. For the next six weeks, my homework and analysis was spent mainly elucidating, amplifying, and reflecting on these dreams and reading materials relating to them. Jung would describe this process with the alchemical term *circumambulatio.*

Some time after these dreams, von Franz made a classic remark I will never forget. She said, with something of a twinkle in her eye, "Your unconscious is a nice fellow!" It was kind of a left-handed compliment since my conscious will had nothing to do with it. Nevertheless, I felt encouraged.

First Dream

Jung and I were examining the reason why sensation is my weakest function. He showed me a series of drawings illustrating the development of the human embryo. He told me these drawings were made by a sensation type. In making these drawings, Jung said, this man was aided by a professor with good intuition who, by means of his hunches, filled in where the greater genius was not fully developed. Jung asked me, "In which of these drawings do you first find the blastopore?" I chose twice, but both times I was wrong. He said I should have pointed to a drawing of a later stage of development. The drawings were painted yellow on white which made it difficult for me to discriminate them. I wondered why a more contrasting color had not been used. I asked Jung if he had read a book that fascinated me, a book by a biologist, H. S. Jennings, entitled The Biological Basis of Human Behavior.[1]

In college, I had majored in biology, and the course that most fascinated me was the one that covered the then budding sciences of genetics and embryology. In fact, the Jennings book interested me so much that it was one of the few books I brought along with me to Switzerland. Since my interest was more philosophical than scientific, I had long since forgotten, if I ever knew, what the term *blastopore* meant. It was only some time after the dream that, to my astonishment, I ran across the actual word in the text. But when I did, I found that the blastopore referred to a very early stage in the embryo's development. "In the hollow spherical mass of small cells that constitute the gastrula," writes Jennings, "there begins at a certain spot, just in front of the depression known as the blastopore, some organizing or differentiating influence, of unknown nature, which passes from cell to cell causing each cell to alter internally . . . . so that all together they constitute the organized structural pattern of the embryo. Experiments show," Jennings continues, "that this center sends out messages to the cells which determine from then on how the various tissues and organs of the body will be constituted."[2]

From a Jungian point of view, of course, the dream does not refer to the external physical world, but to the inner world of the psyche. In fact, the unconscious uses the stage when the blastopore appears to symbolize dramatically the incarnation of that wholeness Jung calls the Self. In the dream, Jung tests me to see if my dream ego can detect where the Self first appears. I try twice, but both times I make the wrong choice. Obviously, my development has not reached the stage where I can differentiate the Self properly.

But how do the dream figures fit into Jungian typology? Why was the sensation type who drew the series on the development of the embryo called a "genius"? The fact is that sensation in waking life is truly my weakest function and one of its manifestations was a strong disinclination to draw or paint. Nevertheless, because of the gentle urging of von Franz, and my determination to try to understand Jungian psychology, I forced myself to spend many hours on these activities.

To get over my distaste, the first thing I often did was to slash colors haphazardly on the blank paper. The resulting product was often quite crude, but, like a Rorschach test, the unconscious images that I discriminated from what at first often looked like chaotic abstractions were extremely valuable in my analysis. Von Franz called these pictorial efforts thoughts. She said it was even an advantage not to be artistic because then my unconscious could come through without being hindered by consciously learned techniques. I still look at these drawings, paintings, and mandalas from time to time and find them both mysterious and enlightening.

In her lectures on "The Inferior Function" von Franz writes,

> The inferior function is the door through which all the figures of the unconscious come into consciousness . . . it is the ever-bleeding wound of the conscious personality, but through it the unconscious can always come in and so enlarge consciousness and bring forth a new attitude.[3]

It is a Jungian principle, derived from alchemy, that the treasure (in this case, the "genius") lies in the dirt of the unconscious, in the *prima materia,* the *nigredo*—in my case, the sensation function. By being forced to differentiate this function, I learned by means of my pictures a new way to dialogue with the unconscious. In the dream, the personalized sensation type draws the series on the development of the embryo. But he needs the help of his opposite type, "a professor with good intuition, who by means of his hunches fills in where the greater genius was not fully developed."

The yellow color on white symbolizes the embryonic egg yoke enveloped in the translucent placenta (egg white). Even though I could not find the blastopore stage, Jung's question shows where I am in my spiritual development (individuation process) and at the same time indicates the direction I need to go for greater maturity.

Despite the revolutionary developments in embryology and genetics since 1930 when Jennings's book was published, his description of the physiology of the blastopore stage is still valid. Today, the cells at this stage are called multipotent stem cells, and they are believed to be the most effective for therapeutic cloning. This involves generating different kinds of tissues and substances for transplantation into the patient.

The promise of this procedure for improving the quality of life and the treatment of some of the world's most devastating diseases has created a whole new field of medical research. But the religious and ethical problems raised by the use of stem cells and their potential for misuse have stirred passionate debate between those who want to slow down or ban such research altogether and those who want to allow the process to continue under careful supervision. Still others would like to go full speed ahead. An advisory panel appointed by President Bush to study the question failed to reach a consensus.[4]

But what is the inner psychic significance of these developments relative to the dream? In mythological terms, it is as though the Self (the blastopore)—or, if you will, God—is enabling scientists, through His inspiration, to wrest from nature yet another creative power—this time the power to evolve into a being with a higher consciousness or, alternatively, the power to destroy the human race spiritually as well as physically.

Second Dream

Jung showed me a man who was another kind of expert. He was interested in hockey. Jung said, "Even here, the local moral problem comes up." He opened a folio and showed me a very complicated diagram of a play in field hockey. I couldn't for the life of me see how that had anything to do with the moral problem, but Jung explained to me that although the good side was one goal ahead, the problem was how to prevent the devil from scoring the next goal. That, it seems, was the thing occupying this man and kept coming up in all his work.

As I watched, the figures in the diagram began to move, and suddenly, from the sidelines, the devil ran onto the field, got ahold of the ball, and began to make his way toward the "good" side's goal. When the devil was about to make his shot, he put on a welder's mask. To prevent the devil from scoring, the goalkeeper rushed out of his cage, leaving the goal unguarded. The goalkeeper then tried to grab the ball from the devil's arms. But it was no good. The ball disappeared. I knew the devil would score, although I did not see this in the dream. I remember that in the diagram demonstrating this, the goalkeeper left behind him a thick black spiral track. This was all presented by Jung as a demonstration of how even this man, though just a very ordinary man with a hobby, is so obsessed by the moral problem that it comes out in his work.

When I left college, I became obsessed with the idea that devoting one's life to reducing unhappiness and/or increasing happiness on a universal scale was the best thing a human being could do. After much reading in utilitarian ethics, I came to the conclusion that none of the utilitarian philosophers had expressed this idea adequately, and I thought I could develop a semantically precise ethics that might lead to motivating others to adopt this goal. This was for my conscious self the "moral problem."

Although she didn't mention it directly, I have reason to believe my first analyst, Beatrice Hinkle, thought I was a bit messianic about it.[5] She was right. I have long since given up trying to convince others that this standard is the highest good. For myself, I still believe it is, and it continues to give meaning to my life and has helped me to survive a strong tendency toward nihilism and the disaffirmation of life.

Since I didn't have the necessary philosophical background to write this ethics, I decided in 1942 to become a doctoral candidate at Columbia University. In that same year, because of my lifelong bouts with depression and floating anxiety, I started Jungian analysis. As I continued my graduate studies, I became disillusioned with the purely rational analytical approach of philosophy at that time. It seemed to me that only one man was coming to grips with the crucial problems of mankind, and that man was Carl Jung. I wrote him in December 1944, but it was not until September 1945 that he finally accepted me as a student.[6]

When I discussed my philosophy with Jung, he told me that the fact that I never dreamt about it indicated that it was probably not my destined path. I strongly disagreed with him, but the fact is that I did not pass my oral exam and so did not get my degree. Also, no journal wanted to publish my philosophy, and when I put it on the Web, I got very little response. This certainly seems to bear out Jung's conclusion. At the time, however, I was comforted by the fact that at least my unconscious shared my interest in the "moral problem," albeit from a completely different angle.

In the dream, the Self is symbolized by the ball and also by the Wise Old Man archetype (Jung). Von Franz said that the hockey game represents the play aspect of human nature. She maintains that "play is the beginning of all spiritual and civilizing conscious occupations."[7]

For homework, von Franz assigned me a book, *Homo Ludens: A Study of the Play Element in Culture* by the Dutch author Johan Huizinga, which is based on the same argument.[8] Huizinga defines play for humans as "a voluntary activity or occupation executed within certain fixed limits of time and space, according to rules freely accepted but absolutely binding, having its aim in itself and accompanied by a feeling of tension, joy, and the consciousness that it is different from ordinary life." When human beings are not totally occupied with the practical necessities for survival and ethical duties, they naturally turn to play.

Jung tells of how, after much resistance, he followed the impulses of his unconscious and reverted to his childhood by playing games. He played almost every day on the shore of the lake in Zürich, building a whole village from the materials he found there. He says it was a turning point in his fate. This activity continued on and off for the rest of his life.[9] Von Franz, in a filmed interview, tells how she used to watch him quietly for hours.

"The great archetypal activities of human society," writes Huizinga, "are all permeated with play from the start." Case in point—the archetypal stonecuttings in Jung's second home in Bollingen are a product of his play activity. The play element is an irrational function anterior to culture, says Huizinga. It is culture's origin and roots. Language, myth and ritual, the arts, science, philosophy, law and order, commerce—all arose out of play.

Huizinga, however, is careful to point out that not everything is play. "Play . . . lies outside morals. It is neither good nor bad."[10] Acts motivated by the necessity for survival, moral considerations, compassion or forgiveness—acts driven by the striving for truth, peace, and justice—

are ultimately outside its province. In fact, in much of what we call play, there is a nonplay aspect.

From Huizinga, I learned that in *The Laws,* Plato says, "God alone is worthy of supreme seriousness, but man is God's plaything, and that is the best part of him."[11] The gods in the *Iliad* and the *Odyssey* taking sides in the Trojan War illustrate this. The tragedies and comedies of ancient Greece were more than just plays as we consider them today. They were deeply spiritual experiences; in fact, they were a religious outlet for their audiences. Although sports today are considered to be secular activities, for millions of people, spectators as well as participants, the emotional intensity they generate sometimes surpasses the numinosity of many religious experiences.

One of the fascinating things von Franz told me was how play enters into the religious rites in the jai alai–type ball games played in pre-Columbian meso-America. She told me that, incredible as it may seem, in some of these games it was the winning side, not the losing side, who had the honor of being the human sacrifice!

In the dream, Jung says the game fascinates the "expert" because of its bearing on "the local moral problem," which in the dream is how to prevent the devil from scoring the next goal. Since good and evil enter the picture, this aspect of the dream goes beyond play. As the figures begin to move and the drama unfolds, we know he does not succeed. By coming in from the sidelines, the devil breaks the rules, and in so doing, he lures the "good" goalkeeper to leave the cage he is supposed to protect in order to grab the ball from the devil. Thus, like the devil, he too breaks the rules and, what is worse, deserts his function of guarding the goal. He thus succumbs to the devil's temptation.

In my drawing (see plate 7), as the goalkeeper rushes out of his cage to confront the devil, he leaves behind him an angry black spiral of evil which looks like a threatening serpent. The series of black dashes that extend outside the playing field indicates that the devil has come in from the sidelines to invade the protected mandala which is the playing field. As a result of the clash between the goalkeeper and the devil, the ball (Self) disappears, and it is inferred in the dream that the devil will score the next goal. This emphasizes what we already know, namely, that we cannot always prevent the devil from leading us into temptation any more than we, as human beings, can avoid sinning. Von Franz said the devil in the dream represents the archetype of the spoilsport or trickster. As for the devil putting on a welder's mask, this could mean that the devil himself needs protection from the light of consciousness.

The dream illustrates that we should not resist evil in a manner that leaves our goal unprotected. Despite Jesus' injunction in Matthew 5:38–49 not to resist evil and to love our enemies as well as our neighbors, the vast majority of mankind does not interpret this to mean that we should not defend ourselves, our families, or our countries, as we did in World War II, from actions taken by evil, psychotic, or misguided people. But if we do, we need to try as much as possible to resist being totally controlled by shadow projections that elicit emotions like arrogance, vengeance, hate, or anger which endanger the soul.

However much the national interest may have played a role, the United States, in offering the Marshall Plan which benefitted our axis enemies as much as our allies, was definitely in line with Jesus' teaching. On the collective level, by far the most admirable example of this was the position on amnesty taken by the Truth and Reconciliation Committee in South Africa toward those who committed racial crimes during the era of apartheid. On the individual level, Jesus would certainly approve of the principle of nonviolence as adopted by Gandhi, Martin Luther King, Nelson Mandela, Archbishop Tutu, and the Dalai Lama.

Jung uses Jesus himself as his model when he writes:

> It was the power-intoxicated devil of the prevailing Caesarian psychology that led him (Jesus) into dire temptation in the wilderness . . . Obeying the inner call of his vocation, Jesus voluntarily exposed himself to the assaults of the imperialistic madness that filled everyone . . . Far from suppressing or allowing himself to be suppressed by this onslaught, he let it act upon him consciously and assimilated it . . . Jesus (thus) fulfilled his Messianic mission by pointing out to humanity the old truth that where force rules there is no love and where love reigns force does not count. The religion of love was the exact psychological counterpart to the Roman devil-worship of power.[12]

The I Ching also has this to say about the problem:

> The struggle must not be carried on directly by force. If evil is branded, it thinks of weapons, and if we do it the favor of fighting against it blow for blow, we lose in the end because we ourselves get entangled in hatred and passion.[13]

In my diagram of the hockey play, the good side is represented by the red circles. The yellow circles surrounded by blue represent blond Nazi Aryans with blue eyes. Remember, the Nazis had surrendered only one year before this drawing was made. The goalkeeper has the shape of a red man whose arms resemble a grappling iron or the pincers of a lobster. He thus represents the influence of primitive instinct.

I wrote pages and pages of material circumambulating around these two dreams during the month and a half I was occupied with them. But that wasn't the end of it. Three years after I left Zürich, I began again to apply Jung's thesis that archetypal manifestations of the unconscious in dreams often not only relate to the problems of the individual psyche but can also have implications for the collective. What I had in mind was a series of historical events that were beginning to unfold that I saw as vividly illustrating the moral problem of this dream as it applied to the United States involvement in the Vietnam war. The first hint of this came to me in a premonition stated in a dream I had in 1949. In that dream, a shadow figure said to me, "Beware of Saigon!" I was so impressed by this dream that I specifically mentioned it to my wife and said she should never forget this phrase.

It was not until fifteen years later, in 1964, that the United States began a full-scale war against North Vietnam, a war that did not serve the interests of the United States in the least. And, of course, it was Saigon that was both the launching point of that war and the evacuation point of the defeated U.S. troops in 1975.

In its moral self-righteousness and communist paranoia, the United States did not perceive that in its decision to fight that tragic conflict, it succumbed to the devil's temptation with the result that the cream of its youth left their homeland (the goal cage in the dream) to fight the U.S.

"devil," communism, on the other side of the world. In the name of what its leaders promoted as a "good" cause, the United States ended up perpetrating the same evils it was fighting against with the result that not only fifty-eight thousand Americans lost their lives, but so did more than a million Vietnamese, on both sides, leaving a whole country in ruins and ours in a state of low morale and suffering from which it has not yet recovered.

Can we further interpret the dream, this time as a warning to the United States not to execute a preemptive, unilateral strike against Iraq with or without the support of the United Nations, however "good" the cause? Are we again coming out of our homeland to grab the ball from the devil, now in the form of Saddam Hussein? Even though we have an arsenal of weapons a thousand times more powerful than his, this familiar scenario should at least lead us to ponder the frightening consequences of what could be another tragic error of much greater magnitude.

Obviously, to derive such an implication from a dream goes far beyond ordinary rational human thinking, although many have arrived at the same conclusion by normal rational means. On the other hand, many others, including the executive branch of government under President Bush, have apparently reached the opposite conclusion using a different set of premises.

When I went to Zürich, I had the idea I might become an analyst, but by the time I left, I had decided I wasn't suited for that profession. Then I thought I might teach philosophy, but when I didn't get my degree, I returned to my former occupation with the United States Information Agency. I had no idea that my Jungian studies and analysis would lead to any consequences other than a better opportunity to continue my own individuation process.

But von Franz had a premonition she expressed in a letter she wrote me in 1952. She said, "It does not matter that you shifted out of philosophy and Jungian psychology—you will return to it under better conditions in the second half of life!" I had no inkling of how right she was until 1975, the year of my retirement. At that time, I gave a talk to a group of Jungians in Washington, D.C., about my experience in Zürich, and to my complete surprise, after the talk, one of my listeners, a professor who taught at Georgetown University, asked me if I would like to teach a course in Jungian psychology in the adult education department of that institution. I was delighted with the idea and, to make a long story short, I started teaching an introductory course, "Jungian Psychology as a Means to Self-realization," in the spring semester of that very same year. I continued to teach that course every semester for the next twenty-two years. I also added a more advanced course on "Jung and the Problem of Evil" and later one on "Jung's Challenge to Religion." In the course on evil, I used von Franz's *Shadow and Evil in Fairy Tales* as well as Jung's *Answer to Job* as texts.

In addition to giving lectures on various Jungian topics, I also had the privelege of being the discussant in a two-day seminar on a series of twenty documentary films featuring dream interpretations by von Franz of thirty men and women. The film series, titled "The Way of the Dream," was sponsored by the Smithsonian Museum's Resident Associates.

There is little doubt that von Franz will be remembered as the most creative of Jung's disciples. What I will remember most, however, is a wonderful and modest human being who was utterly devoted to the cause of the redemption of the human soul through the increased consciousness of the individual human being. At the end of von Franz's book, *C. G. Jung: His Myth in Our Time,* these sentences express what for her is the challenge humanity faces in the present millennium:

> When the Tao, the meaning of the world and eternal life are attained, the Chinese say, "Long life flowers with the essence of the stone and the brightness of gold."
>
> How many heroes will meet at the stone, now, to set out upon the great adventure of individuation, the journey to the interior? The fate of our Western culture depends, if I am right, on the answer to this question.

NOTES

1. Published by W. W. Norton, 1930.
2. Ibid., p. 94.
3. Von Franz and Hillman, *Jung's Typology* (New York: Spring Publications, 1971), p. 54.
4. "Bush panel has two views on embryonic cloning," *Washington Post*, July 11, 2002.
5. Beatrice Hickle was one of Jung's earliest American disciples and English translator, in 1915, of "The Psychology of the Unconscious," originally *CW*, vol. 8, later revised and published as *Symbols of Transformation* (1952), *CW*, vol. 5 (Princeton, N.J.: Princeton University Press, 1956).
6. See R. Lyons, "My Experience with C. G. Jung," *Harvest*, vol. 44, no. 2 (1998), pp. 137–157.
7. Von Franz, *Archetypal Patterns in Fairy Tales* (Toronto: Inner City Books, 1971), p. 41.
8. Boston: Beacon Press, 1977; written 1938.
9. Jung, *Memories, Dreams, Reflections* (New York: Vintage Books, Random House, 1989), pp. 173–174.
10. Huizinga, p. 213.
11. *The Laws*, 7.803.
12. Jung, "The Development of Personality" (1934), *CW*, vol. 17 (Princeton, N.J.: Princeton University Press, 1954), par. 309.
13. Hexagram 43, translated into English by C. F. Baynes (New York: Pantheon, 1950), p. 178.

The Psychology of the Archetype of the Veiled Kabir

The Genius of C. G. Jung

ANNE MAGUIRE

I am deeply honored to be asked to contribute an offering for the Festschrift in celebration of the life of Marie-Louise von Franz.

I was privileged to be the friend of Marie-Louise during the last thirty years of her life, and I would like to express the thought that her death has left the world a vastly poorer place. Never has her knowledge of psyche, her thought processes and intuitive insight been so sadly missed as now in the history of humankind.

The article that follows is a transcript of a lecture I gave recently to the Guild of Pastoral Psychology in London. In that lecture, I explored the lifelong relationship between Dr. Jung and his genius Telesphoros.

Marie-Louise von Franz was also a genius and was the most creative human being, a creativity substantiated by her many published works,

Originally published by The Guild of Pastoral Psychology, Guild Lecture No. 280. Reprinted by permission.

her magnificent lectures, and her researches into the archetypal world of psyche. She was an intrepid explorer in that world and was able to describe and communicate her findings in a way that made it easy for students to comprehend, absorb, and integrate them into consciousness. She possessed great teaching gifts. I admired her intellect and profound depth of knowledge immensely.

She had a great sense of fun and a lively sense of humor. She was also a wonderful hostess, an extremely good cook, a connoisseur of wine and her hospitality never varied. She was a woman of great independence of mind and spirit and had a true and deep eros. She was a wonderful human being and a good friend to me.

We live our lives in times of a frenzied rate of change, probably never before experienced in quite this way by mankind. It is a pace of progress without time to reflect upon yesterday, because tomorrow has begun to overtake today. We are out of time, which means out of reality. It is a state of unwellness, a destabilization; a condition, be it said, which appears to have silenced the priests and the doctors, those who care for spiritual and physical welfare. The priests' duty is to recognize loss of soul, but do the doctors recognize the soul?

One thousand two hundred years ago, there lived a doctor in the land of Persia who worshipped Allah every day. He wrote an ode to the soul which is both beautiful and immensely moving; quite possibly it has never been bettered. Because he recognized and loved his own soul, he always treated the body and the soul of his patients. His name was Ibn Sina and, in my view and that of countless others, he was a physician by divine decree and thus a very great doctor indeed. What makes a physician so? It is, *au fond,* a mystery. However, here I thought we might explore those inherent qualities and necessary gifts bestowed by deity at the birth of a human being destined to practice medicine as a physician. The required attributes at birth are *in potentia,* and which may in the course of life be realized, *Deo concedente.*

We are indeed fortunate in that a doctor of great renown, in his mature years, wrote an excellent autobiography in which he describes his relationship with a divine, inner companion, the genius Telesphoros of

Asclepius, the veiled *kabir,* who was the constant companion of the Greek god of physicians, Asclepius.

Since it is now more than forty years since Dr. Carl Gustav Jung died, perhaps it is the right time to think about and look at his great healing qualities, not simply as a psychologist but as a physician, a doctor of medicine.

Telesphoros

I would like to read these words by Dr. Jung written to describe a genius a long time ago: "The true genius nearly always intrudes and disturbs. He speaks to a temporal world out of a world eternal. . . . Yet, the genius is a healer of his time, because anything he reveals of eternal truth is healing."[1] The Romans believed each individual had a genius, a protective spirit, who was born with him and accompanied him through all the years of his life and died with him. The Roman genius is identified with the Greek daimon, and in the course of time the effects of Greek culture upon Roman civilization introduced the idea, and the development, of individuality, so it became natural to think of the genius continuing to exist after death. The idea of a personal immortality had its inception in Rome at that time and was later inculcated into the Christian religion. Mention of the genius has been found on archaic fragments of writings of the *Indigitamenta,* the ancient pontifical (Christian) books, relating to the duties of the ancient deities of those days. Later, every house and statue had its genius. The *genius domus* was the spirit of the home, the *genius locus* was the spirit of the place. Sacrifice and offerings of cakes, incense, and wine were made to one's genius on birthdays as thanksgiving for one's life, with prayers for the future.

In his autobiography, *Memories, Dreams, Reflections,* Dr. Carl Gustav Jung describes how the inner world permitted him to be conscious of the nature of an inner companion, the genius Telesphoros of Asclepius. This little god of the antique world visited Jung from time to time bringing extraordinary effects and priceless gifts—to name but two, creativity and healing. Telesphoros, a mysterious, little-known, archaic god, is the guide of Asclepius, the truly great Greek god of doctors. This antique god always appears as a child-god who wears a pointed hooded cloak. Only his face, fingers, and feet are visible. As he accompanies Asclepius, he is often found to be reading from a scroll which is unfurled. He usually carries a lantern to light the way, but when he is reading from the scroll the lantern is gripped between his knees. Sometimes he carries a cock in the front of his chest, as would a small human boy. The cock is the meaningful solar bird of Asclepius, the bird of the sunrise, the dawning of the light.

Telesphoros is a great mystery, for he is the pointer of the way, a guide of the souls of the dead or psychopomp, like Hermes. He is no less than the announcer of life and sometimes is named "the finisher." Death too is the finisher. He is described as a *kabir*. Now this little *kabir* played an immense role in the life of C. G. Jung, a man of Switzerland, the mountainous heart of Europe, who was himself to become a light-bringer of incalculable stature for mankind during the twentieth century. In his autobiography, written toward the end of his life, he describes those occasions when, unexpectedly and without preamble, the little veiled god, silently and secretly, entered his life.

C. G. Jung was born on July 26, 1875, it being St. Anne's Day. St. Anne, the mother of the Virgin, is the patron saint of France, where she is often represented as teaching the Virgin to read. Jung's birth took place at Kesswil, Canton Thurgau, where he lived for four years in the parsonage, a house situated on the Swiss side of the river Rhine near Basel. At an early age he felt oppressed by the somber atmosphere around him. Because his father was the pastor, he could not avoid the frequent burials and entombments of those persons who were alive and then who disappeared and were taken into the earth in the graveyard of the church. Not to mention, also, the sad-faced mourners in their dark clothes with shiny boots and black top hats, who were always present. These experiences, frightening for any child, had also a darkening effect for him on the Christ-image itself, that of the loving Jesus who, it seemed, came to take people away. It was an image accentuated also by the prevailing atmosphere of those days at the center of Europe. Religious faith, it appeared, had lost its original living quality, its lustrous nature, and become a collective way of life.

Marie-Louise von Franz (Jung's pupil and later the eminent analytical psychologist) writes: "Jung's father, Pastor Paul Johannes Jung, had in the depth of his being gradually lost his faith; he tried desperately and with great suffering to replace it with a consciously assumed viewpoint."[2] She continues: "Jung's mother had a dual attitude, as is so in persons where feeling is the first function. On the surface she concurred in the collective Christian way of life, but at bottom her 'religio' was different."[3] Her respect for a dominant or "supreme" value lay with nature, the animals, the forests, and the waters, although she never discussed such with her son.

The experiences which troubled Jung as a boy can be understood when seen reflected in the cry of Friedrich Nietzsche (German philosopher, 1844–1900), "God is dead." What does such a cry mean when people say this? The point of issue, in von Franz's view,[4] is rather that our image of God or our definition of him is dead, although the word is a name for something which was, for past generations, alive in the highest degree and which represented the supreme value. She continues: "That something which was so alive in their image of God, that psychologically effective power which evoked in them an impressive reverence for their 'God' is however not dead (as Jung learned and later sought to verify). God was never really 'captured' in that man-made image, still less in the definitions, so that he is free to leave them behind and 'reveal' himself anew." Instead of saying with Nietzsche, "God is dead," it would have been closer to the truth, in Jung's opinion, to say, "the highest value which gives life and meaning has got lost."[5] "He has put off our image, and where shall we find him again?"[6]

We know that cultural communities do lose their gods. Long ago there was the terrible cry which reverberated throughout the Greek world of the Mediterranean, "Pan is dead"; but nature was not dead. Such communities fall into severe psychological and social crises. It is a phenomenon repeated historically, time after time, during the passing of centuries. It is, of course, in our day the most pressing problem for deep deliberation by all conscious individuals!

In the Christian mystery Jung draws our attention to the death of Christ as being central to the image of the Crucifixion, the entombment, and his Resurrection. He said: "I am expressing what countless other people know—that the present is a time of God's death and disappearance. The myth says he was not to be found where his body was laid. 'Body' means the outward, visible form, the erstwhile but ephemeral setting for the highest value"[7] (like the rose of summer whose petals must fall). Writing just before the Second World War, he states: "The [Christian] myth further says that the value [the entombed body] rose again in a miraculous manner, transformed."[8]

I have said that, as a child, Jung had been aware of the disturbed and somber psychic atmosphere surrounding him. In his memories he tells us of his earliest remembered dream which was a profound experience and which occurred at that time. A childhood dream of such a nature sets out, symbolically, the innate essence of an entire life, or first part of a life. It reflects part of the inner fate to which the child will be subjected in maturity.

The Dream

The child, Jung, found himself in the big meadow near his home. There was a stone stairway leading down from a rectangular hole. At the bottom of the stairway was a doorway with a sumptuous green curtain which he pushed aside and saw, in the dim light, a chamber. The ceiling was of hewn stone and arched. The floor was laid with flagstones. In the center a red carpet ran to a low platform on which was a golden throne. Something was standing on it, about fifteen feet high and two feet thick, reaching to the ceiling. The child thought it was a tree. It was made of skin and naked flesh and had no hair. On the top of its head was a single eye gazing motionlessly upward. About the head was an aura of brightness. It was huge. Jung said he was paralyzed with terror. At that moment he heard his mother's voice. She called out: "Yes, just look at him, that is the man eater!"[9]

Imagine, he was four years old. But in the dream he had already the curiosity to go down the steps and into the chamber, and the courage to do it and to stand firm although terrified and, according to his view, paralyzed with fear. The courageous attitude evident then remained throughout his life.

The creative phallic god, the giant phallus enthroned in the dream, was the hidden (hermetic) or subterranean god, not to be named; the aforementioned "something," the thing of the greatest value. Jung said, later, he felt it was something underworldly which fed on human flesh. He added, it was "an initiation into the realm of darkness."[10] In later life, he realized that the phallus of the dream was a grave phallus. The hole in the meadow represented a grave, and the green curtain was symbolic of the green vegetation covering the earth.

In his tenth year, Jung again found himself at odds, as do so many children at that age. However, he was led to an action both baffling and utterly incomprehensible to him. One day, quite simply, he took his school pencil case, extracted the ruler, and carved a little manikin about two inches long at one end, sawed him off, and put him back in the box with a stone from the river Rhine, a little wool for a coat, and a bed to lie on. The pencil box was his *kista,* and it was taken to the attic and hidden in the rafters. It was Jung's secret, and inviolable. It was not to be touched or ravished in any way. It held a great value for him. From time to time, the child Jung used to visit the attic to see his manikin. Sometimes he added a little scroll of paper on which were words of a secret language of his own creation. The manikin was his invisible secret companion, to be visited when he felt at odds with himself. Each little scroll, added from time to time, had the character of a solemn ceremonial act. Jung said in later years that the story depicts the quality of eternity in his childhood. It was the first attempt to give shape to the secret which he did not know, but which was endeavoring to express itself in his life, in this way.

Twenty-five years later, when he was already a physician, a psychiatrist, and a psychologist, he read a paper about a cache of soul stones found at Arlesheim, comparing them to the Australian churinga, itself also a soul stone. The churinga is hidden by its owner in a rock cleft or a hollow tree, where it stays for a long time. If the owner feels low, or his libido leaves him, or he has a bad attitude, he goes to the secret place, takes out the churinga, puts it on his knee (like a child), and rubs it. By this rubbing, the bad humor, ill health, and ailing libido are all imparted to the stone, and the power of good medicine that has been breathed freely into the churinga whilst in its nature place, is transformed to the body of the owner. By the exchange of his libido with that of his churinga he is healed, in balance again with nature and himself. This is equivalent to what Jung did, quite unconsciously, with his little manikin. He gave it his libido and received its in return from the inner world. The point is, as Jung tells us, the dead stone is alive; it has spirit and is alive. His instinctual act, which had cured him of his malaise, is the first glimpse afforded to us of the inner healer-to-be in the mature Jung.

When he was at his more advanced age, he remembered his little manikin and then realized that the manikin was a little cloaked god from the ancient world, such as is seen so frequently on monuments dedicated to Asclepius. It came to Jung then that there are archaic components, age old, which have entered the individual psyche without any direct line of tradition. A child of nine, in the heart of Europe at the end of the nineteenth century, performs an act as a rite of ceremonial, which itself is akin to those acts performed by early man for thousands of years, since the "Dream Time," far away on the island continent of Australia in the heart of the Southern Seas! Neither was there any possible evidence of this information having been acquired from his father's library. Again, the little hooded and cloaked god entered Dr. Jung's consciousness in his seventy-fifth year, but more of that later.

In seeking to understand the inherent meaning of this genius, it is helpful to uncover the provenance of Telesphoros; not an easy task to lift the dust of thousands of years. He is described as a veiled *kabir.* "Veiled" because of his encompassing habit which makes him virtually invisible, thus proclaiming his mysterious being. He, as a *kabir,* was one of the *Kabeiroi,* the great gods, deities who were secret and had to be kept secret (Jung's manikin). Their mysteries were age old, and their principal site was Samothrace off the Thracian coast, far removed from the Hellenic sphere spatially, and dating from the eighth century B.C. in time.

In both Samothrace and Phrygia in Asia Minor, rock altar shrines dedicated to the Great Mother goddess, monuments of archaic cultic practices, had been found just at the beginning of the Second World War by the German archeologist, Max Lehmann. Long before the Celts, themselves pre-Greek settlers, there existed an indigenous people in these areas who had their own language of Sai, a name which was applied also to the priests of the *Kabeiroi,* the great gods of this region and children of the Great Mother. These gods were mystery gods, pure and simple, and so they have remained. Some were dwarfs, others children; all were small, often deformed in some way and not infrequently criminal.

Now the worship of Asclepius rose out of the millennium which preceded Christ's birth but may well be older. It is difficult for modern man to comprehend the magnitude of this religion and how reluctant were its participants to relinquish the tenacious adoration they afforded their god when Christianity began to intrude into their world. Asclepius was greatly loved. One of the great temples to him was at Pergamum, a town in Asia Minor famous for its parchment (*pergamon* means parchment) and close to the mountainous regions of Kabeiros in Phrygia—known to be sacred to Rhea, the Great Mother Goddess, and home of Telesphoros. In this region, Rhea was known as Berekyntia.[11]

At first, Asclepius himself went through a strange metamorphosis, from mortal physician to an oracular demon in the form of a snake, with the same snake eyes possessed by all heroes. Piercing, compelling, and hypnotic eyes, a snake is also symbolic of pure objectivity. Thus clarity, sharpness of vision, and objectivity are qualities befitting a physician. Later, Asclepius became an Apollonian deity. In the myth, his father was Apollo and his mother Coronis. She was actually pregnant with Asclepius, for Apollo's child was *in utero* when she was unfaithful to him. Upon learning of her infidelity, he killed her but took the child from her womb as her life's blood was stilled.

Imagine the unborn child entrapped in the silence of that maternal, quiet body before experiencing even the first breath of life. It is believed, today, that the child *in utero* suffers emotional reactions. Such terror engendered in that experience of Asclepius's birth is difficult to envisage.

His father saved him. So the legacy which the mighty, effulgent Apollo gave to his son would be a profound reverence for individual life, and a desire to protect and fight for life. From his mother? Passion certainly, eros possibly—she made a cuckold of Apollo for which she was doomed. One can only surmise that Apollo's attentions had caused her to be above herself, and she had forgotten that her good fortune was by the grace of a mighty god. Asclepius's legacy to those vocational doctors who carry in psyche the archetypal image of the physician is to retain reverence for life and give human assistance to enable the cure, as a divine event. One of the dicta of Apollo is, "Physician, know thyself." Never was this more true than in the life of C. G. Jung. Sometimes I ponder just what Apollo may think of the present-day medical practice which indulges an unconscious lack of reverence and even disregard for life, and, perhaps, also for those who carry it. The "Far Shooter," a name for Apollo and as he is sometimes described, is swift to punish those who do so at their peril.

In an illness, something of the life energy or vitality has died, and the individual stands before the possibility of death. But it is just there the opportunity exists for a cure. It is not a birth, rebirth, or a resurrection; it is an event acted out on the boundaries of the realm of the dead at the gateway to the beyond.

At Epidaurus, the temple was the place of divine healing, situated in the valley guarded by the dog, ruler of the adjacent mountain, and the snake, ruler of the valley below. The sick sought the cure away from their fellow men and the physician, in the innermost sanctuary of the temple. There the individual surrendered himself to a process within himself. Slowly, the dog, the snake, or the god himself came in a dream or vision, with the cure. *Au fond,* a cure is a mystery, the meaning of which lies in the world eternal. However, the dog's place was crucial. It stood for a transitional situation. As the animal of Hecate, it carried this darkness of the underworld, but as the animal of Asclepius, son of Apollo, it carried the gold of sunrise, the dawning of light. The cult brought a new intuitive aspect to the healing process. The dog symbolizes intuition. The cure appeared to lie directly in the capacity for intimate relationship with the god himself and in his animal aspects. The dog is a wonderfully related animal; it was a new, personal relationship to the Self or greater personality, and it had not happened before. It prefigured the individual relationship to come with Christ.

I have dealt at length with the attitude of the ancient world toward healing in order to compare it with modern thought. The role of psyche is generally not considered in the pathogenesis of disease today. The spontaneous cure and the miracle of healing are rarely envisaged as possibilities in medical prognostication, but they do exist. Prior to the birth of Christ, an upsurge of the Greek spirit brought a burgeoning of culture, and the developing rational caste of mind ousted the centuries-old adoration and devotion to divine powers in the realm of healing. A rational explanation rejected the inherent mystery. Scholarly men lost contact with the instinctive world and with it their gods.

As I have intimated, the archetypal image of the god of physicians included the god himself. Monuments show him to be at first, some 1,500 years before Christ, a handsome Apollonian god, whereas in the early centuries of the Piscean era he was aged, bearded, and seated. With him always were the serpent, the dog, the cock, and, later, the child-god. The exact time-moment when Telesphoros joined Asclepius eludes our consciousness. In Pergamum, where it is believed he first appeared, it was the second or third century B.C. He came from the mountainous region of Kabeiros in Phrygia, the land of the mighty Phrygian men, where he was greatly renowned as a divine healer.

The wisdom of the ancient physicians ascribed the mysterious process of healing to the night and sleep, rather than to the day and waking. One indication of this, as we have seen, was the "temple sleep." Another is the dwarflike nocturnal figure—a child in a hooded cloak. In the Asklepieion of Pergamum as Telesphoros, he was known as "The Finisher," for death too is a finisher, but elsewhere he was known as Akesis, "healing." He was nocturnal but concealed beneath the dark habit was his bright nature which was manifested in his epiphany, "when the opposite wall gleamed as though reflecting sunlight."[12] Here again he is a light-bringer. He was identical with the *genius Cucullatus*, a figure found in many parts of the Roman Empire. (A relic from those days is the *Munchener Kindl* of Munich.)

Thus, the veiled *kabir*, one of the great gods, came as a youthful double of Asclepius. He was his genius, to use the Roman term. His hooded cloak was pointed, like all the mysterious gods of the Great Mother, but his feet were bare. To my mind, this denotes his standpoint, which indicated a close and immediate attachment to the earth. He was grounded upon reality. He came with his lantern, giving light to the seekers who sought him and all those he chose to accompany. "He was the pointer of the way."[13]

Like all the dwarf gods of Rhea and also the Tom Thumbs of fairy tales, the *Kabeiroi* have a phallic aspect, because they are personifications of creative forces of which the phallus is a symbol. A symbol, you will recall, "is an indefinite expression with many meanings, pointing to something not easily defined and therefore not fully known. . . . It has a large number of analogous variants, and the more of these variants it has at its disposal, the more complete and clear-cut will be the image it projects of its object."[14]

When I said that Telesphoros is the phallic *kabir*, it means that he has the same creative libido or energy as the phallus. Thus, the creative dwarfs toiling away in secret for the Great Mother are analogues of the phallus as, when working in the darkness, it begets a human being. The name "Telesphoros" means "he who brings completeness."[15] He is none other than the god of inner transformation. When he enters a life, either in a dream or a vision, that life is to be transformed. The actuality of the transformation depends on the attitude of ego toward the inner daimon and the grace of the Self, as fate. In the first remembered dream of the enthroned phallus, Jung saw in it that the birth of his intellectual life started then. According to ancient Roman view, the phallus symbolizes man's secret genius, the source of his physical and mental creative power, the dispenser of all his inspired and brilliant ideas and of his buoyant joy in life. Every Roman, as I have mentioned, offered sacrifices to his genius on his birthday.

In speaking of Jung, von Franz said: "This genius often radiated from his personality in the jovial festive atmosphere he created around himself, in his cheerfulness, good humor, and also his truly enormous vitality, but above all his lifelong commitment to the inner creative spirit which drove him relentlessly to ever more and more research and creativity."[16] Barbara Hannah, the eminent analytical psychologist, his former pupil and longtime friend, told me that this spirit was also the source of an unusually large capacity for love, which both enlivened and burdened his existence. Von Franz also said that he had, to an extraordinary degree, the gift of empathy to the point of being mediumistic, and of participation, with sympathy and human warmth, for his family, his friends, his patients, and in the end, for all mankind. I concur with these words but, I might add, in reading his writings (his own works and not those which someone had interpreted), one cannot but sense through the clarity of his thinking an intensive eros, which grips one to the extent that one feels oneself to be there, with him, in his enveloping presence.

In antiquity, the ancient phallic god of Jung's first remembered dream embodied both the principle of eros and creativity, but he was also known as Telesphoros. In Epidauros, there were images of Eros, the god of love, and also Methe, the god of ecstasy. In ancient Greek, this word meant "to be entranced, rapturous, or transported with joy." It also meant "drunkenness," one can be drunk with joy also. Both these gods represent healing powers. When Jung was in Africa, he was enchanted by those wonderful sunrises. Each morning he got up to savor the moment. His exact words are: "I drank in this glory with the insatiable delight, or rather, in a timeless ecstasy."[17] That is a transport of joy, that is ecstasy, it is Methe, the god.

We have seen that Telesphoros entered Jung's life at various intervals. First, as the unmoving, huge phallus upon a golden throne. This was his primal form as the god "not to be named," the carrier of eros and the creative life force. However, there was something else. Jung, in later life, recognized it as a grave phallus, but also something invisible and transpersonal, that is, of a higher consciousness beyond the individual human. For in the dream, the question is posed and an answer given. The question concerns the problem of the death of God, the problem of the age in which Jung was born and our problem also. The dream contained an image of a grave phallus of the kind which the Etruscans, Romans, and Greeks used to erect on a man's grave. Von Franz has this to say: "It was a symbol of the afterlife of the spirit, and a guarantor of the dead man's resurrection."[18] The dead man, she continues, was obviously a king who, as a grave phallus, was awaiting resurrection. In ancient Egypt, honor was bestowed likewise to the sun god and king, in this way as Osiris, and was represented by the phallic *djed* (pillar). The erection of this pillar in the grave chamber signified the resurrection of the dead man who had become identical with the god Osiris, the god of the underworld who embodied the spirit of regeneration. In Greece, likewise, Hermes was represented as a phallus, but also as Kyllenios, the god of love and fertility as well as, like Osiris, the psychopompos and king of the dead. Again, Hermes as Hermes Mercurius was the god of alchemists. He was a peacemaker, a god of scholars, interpreters, and cooks—all aspects which Jung realized in his own life.

As I mentioned, Jung realized himself as an alchemist. He had retrieved alchemy from near oblivion. For the alchemist, inorganic matter was not dead but alive, and Mercurius was thought of as a god of the earth, the spirit of nature. The god hidden in the earth became Jung's life's work and led to the immense exploration of, and eventual understanding of, the profound "ocean depths" of psyche. It was this work which led to the scientific discovery and description of the collective unconscious. It seems to me this was prefigured in the waiting, patient attitude of the great phallus in the dream. At the end of childhood, the little *kabir* came as a visitation of the genius, permitting the creative urge to manifest itself through the medium of the child-Jung's hands.

Hands, symbolically, represent work or how one handles something. Again, a question was posed and answered in this manifestation. It seems to me that the tiny human form which evolved from the ruler of the pencil case revealed itself as "the pointer of the way," the psychopompos which led to the world of the unconscious and to Jung's future. The "scroll" in Jung's life was unfurled at that time and his future as a physician decided. It came to pass because it had been written and was being read. It was an edict of divine intention. The message came, indubitably, from the deepest layers of collective psyche. Jung was born to be a physician, and so he was.

Lastly, Telesphoros not only came as a visitation but revealed himself to the seventy-five-year-old Jung. A stone delivered during some building work at Jung's country house was of the wrong measurements, but Jung kept it and decided to do some carving with it. It stands in the garden by the lake. It is a striking cube of limestone. Limestones are organic and formed from the skeletons of animals. The pyramids are made of limestone, formed from the shells of Mediterranean molluscs. As Jung chiseled the stone with phrases in Latin and Greek, suddenly a small circle emerged which was an eye. Chiseling deeper in the center, he made a tiny homunculus which, he explained, corresponded to a *pupilla,* a little doll, which is yourself and which you can see in the pupil of another's eye, a kind of *kabir* or Telesphoros of Asclepius.

When I was about three or four years old, I was sitting on my mother's knee. She had the most exquisitely beautiful emerald green eyes, and I remember looking into them and seeing a little person. I said, "Mama, you have a little person in your eye." She said, "Why, my darling, it is you." I puzzled over that because I thought it was "her little person"!

There it was vis-à-vis the inner companion of the passage of his years, revealed to him at last! The following words came to him, he chiseled them in Greek and dedicated the stone as a thanksgiving offering for his seventy-fifth birthday.

> Time is a child—playing like a child—playing a board game—the kingdom of the child. This is Telesphoros, who roams through the dark regions of this cosmos and glows like a star out of the depths. He points the way to the gates of the sun and to the land of dreams.

Some months after this, Jung wrote his paper on synchronicity. The principle of synchronicity is a psychic factor which is independent of space and time. (Telesphoros's appearance in the stone was independent of space and time, as he came to Jung from the depths of psyche at that moment.) Jung's revolutionary concept of synchronicity forces us to a reconstruction of the meaning of chance, coincidence, and probability, together with the apparently unexplained events. Jung described a synchronistic event as the coincidence between an inner image, or hunch, breaking into one's mind, and the occurrence of an outer event conveying the same meaning at approximately the same time. Synchronistic events are acts of creation in time. I will explain. About a dozen years ago, I was giving a lecture at the C. G. Jung Institute, which I have done regularly for many years. It was a cold gray winter's morning and the snow was falling in flakes. The subject of my lecture was the Telesphoros of Asclepius. The lecture room, the Sala Terena on the ground floor, faced the gardens, not the lake. I became aware of peals of laughter floating up from the garden as a little boy of about five years old appeared chasing a dog. Both, somehow, had got into the garden, an unusual occurrence. They flashed past and were gone. The boy, whose laughter rang out, was dressed in a thick, gray overcoat with an attached pointed hood. His face was rosy but partially obscured by the hood. About one hundred and fifty students were with me, and we were stunned into silence as my descriptive words of the *kabir*'s dress hung in the air of the still room. We gazed at each other. I said, "Telesphoros and his dog!" And so it was!! That was synchronicity, and it had a powerful effect on us all.

Epilogue

As we have observed, Jung was an illuminator, a bringer of light for mankind. His influence cannot yet be judged adequately, it is too vast. Nor can its magnitude be fully comprehended. Jung was one of the very great physicians of all time, a fact not generally appreciated. He was, moreover, a physician by divine decree. He treated the ephemeral body with reverence and kindness. He turned to the soul, which itself often calls upon the body to manifest in illness its own plaintive cries of distress—a situation which is ubiquitous today and yearns for healing.

Jung was a rare doctor of the body and the soul. I have often been told, by many who knew him well, that he was always the physician, a physician utterly convinced of the awesome, mysterious, unknowable, hidden God who reaches the individual from the depths of his psyche, revealing himself in a form which He chooses.

Jung brought great gifts of understanding and healing to countless of his fellow men. Effected by his relatedness, his objectivity, the Apollonian clarity of mind, together with a truly Asclepian-reverence of eros for all life, both human and the world of nature. The greatest service he bestowed upon the human race, in my view, was the scientific discovery and description of the collective unconscious, that vast, underworldly, and uncanny realm which he entered in the dream of his childhood. The collective unconscious, the nighttime of ego's daytime world, uncharted until Jung, with the identical courage exhibited early in his childhood, explored it himself. He was at the time a psychiatrist and knew the inherent danger. His exploration accomplished, as a pathfinder he was able to guide others (who also had courage) to accompany him and examine this strange, but wonderful, world of psyche which he once described as the greatest of all cosmic wonders. From this discovery, he increased the value of his findings by opening up a psychological approach to religion, which this discovery of the collective unconscious made possible.

In his quiet house, by the lake, in the seclusion of his book-filled study, this modest, whole, human being translated into words the thoughts and ideas which came to him from the inner world of objective psyche. He spoke to a temporal world out of a world eternal. He spoke to the individual, not the collective man. His written words are the healing balm for all who come to read them. He is the healer of his time, because what he reveals of eternal truth is healing for those who care to heed his words.

I feel the greatest gratitude for the life of this truly individuated human being and very great healer. He was, and is, "a Basileus of Cos"—a prince of medicine.

NOTES

1. C. G. Jung, "What India Can Teach Us" (1939), in *CW,* vol. 10 (Princeton, N.J.: Princeton University Press, 1964), par. 1004.
2. M.-L. von Franz, *C. G. Jung: His Myth in Our Time,* p. 15.
3. Ibid., p. 16.
4. Ibid.

5. C. G. Jung, "Psychology and Religion" (1938), in *CW,* vol. 11 (Princeton, N.J.: Princeton University Press, 1958), par. 149.
6. Ibid., par. 144.
7. Ibid., par. 149.
8. Ibid.
9. C. G. Jung, *Memories, Dreams, Reflections* (London: Collins and Routledge and Kegan Paul, 1963), p. 26.
10. Ibid., p. 28.
11. C. Kerenyi, "The Mysteries of the Kabeiroi," *Eranos Yearbook,* Joseph Campbell, ed. (Princeton, N.J.: Princeton University Press), p. 48.
12. Aelius Aristides Roscher, Lex: V.col.310.
13. C. Kerenyi, *Archetypal Image of the Physicians Existence* (New York: Pantheon), pp. 56–58.
14. C. G. Jung, *Symbols of Transformation* (1952), *CW,* vol. 5 (Princeton, N.J.: Princeton University Press, 1956), par. 180.
15. M.-L. von Franz, *C. G. Jung: His Myth in Our Time,* p. 23.
16. Ibid., p. 19.
17. C. G. Jung, *Memories, Dreams, Reflections,* p. 252.
18. M.-L. von Franz, *C. G. Jung: His Myth in Our Time,* p. 24.

Memories of Marie-Louise von Franz

ROBERT MERCURIO

Over the years, the image of Marie-Louise von Franz has appeared in my dreams numerous times, as I know it has in the dreams of many, many other people. I have seen her, for example, as an ancient Chinese sage, as an animal trainer ("the only one not afraid of the great lioness," the dream informed me), as a traveler in a smart red outfit seated on a train, and as an invalid condemned to a strange four-wheel wheelchair. Her great honesty and her absolute dedication to the mysterious life of the psyche are no doubt the reasons why the unconscious so often chooses to use her image to represent its own deepest processes.

There is one dream which I had over twenty years ago that struck me particularly then and which has provided food for thought and reflection ever since. At the time, I had been in Zürich for only a relatively short period and had not as yet actually met Dr. von Franz, though I had read a number of her books. The dream is the following:

Von Franz and I are on a beach similar to one on the Italian island of Ponza. A terrible storm is raging with flashes of lightning, thunder, and an incredibly strong wind blowing in off the sea. Huge waves come

> *crashing onto the shore. Von Franz and I are huddled behind a big rock standing there in the middle of the beach, facing the sea. Suddenly, she raises a hand and worriedly exclaims, "I wonder what Yahweh has up his sleeve for us this time."*

Encouraged by my analyst, Dieter Baumann, I sent the text of the dream to von Franz, who immediately replied with a very brief but pointed note. The fact that the collective unconscious appears to be so agitated (the storm) makes our times particularly dangerous, she explained. In the event that some new content should arise from the unconscious ("what Yahweh has up his sleeve"), our individual and collective consciousness must not be caught unawares; hence the importance of being especially attentive to dreams and to all that happens both inside of us and around us.

For a long time, I was curious as to why the name "Yahweh" was used in the dream; a passage from Jung's *Answer to Job* and part of the interview with von Franz in the film, *A Matter of Heart,* cleared the question up for me. Jung recognizes that the god-image of the Old Testament, especially the one which Job encounters, is lacking in eros and corresponds to what he calls in a letter one of the "not-yet transformed aspects" of the divinity, something each one of us is likely to run up against as our own psychological work goes more and more deeply. Finding ourselves face-to-face with such content could very well be compared to facing the raging storm of the dream, and it is vital to somehow manage to set up any sort of relationship with it.

In the film interview, von Franz forcefully talks about the risk of mankind destroying itself and the world and says (almost in the manner of an Old Testament prophet) we must *stand up to God* and tell him not to allow it to happen; thus our consciousness and ethical stance affect the divinity itself. What she says here strikes me as a very important part of her relationship with the unconscious. Although she deeply believed that if we do our best to stay in contact with the unconscious and loyally follow its lead, it will show its benevolent helpful face and lead us toward completeness, she also felt that we should never be naive or overly romantic about the way this pure nature in us might manifest itself. Everything seems to depend on the sort of relationship we foster with it, for the parts of it that are not in relationship with consciousness remain "beyond good and evil" just as Yahweh was, in Jung's interpretation, unconscious of the moral value of his actions. The fact that in the dream von Franz uses the expression "I wonder what Yahweh has up his sleeve" seems to describe him, for the reasons mentioned above, as a kind of great unpredictable trickster, and the phrase "*this* time" seems to imply that this ambiguous side of the godhead has indeed made itself seen and felt many times before. These would be the moments when a person's own ethical position is of the utmost importance since it can effect a form of differentiation in an unconscious content, just as Job's way of dealing with his misfortunes created a form of moral differentiation in Yahweh. The times we live in bear this out only too well, as archetypal forces seem to be pushing many toward the acceptance of war.

There was, to my mind, something extremely poetic about the way M.-L. von Franz dealt with the unconscious and its manifestations, and yet she was deeply realistic about the risks any contact with the unconscious carried with it. It was probably for this reason that she was so insistent that each man and woman develop a degree of independence and autonomy in approaching dreams and other unconscious manifestations. She seemed to be intolerant of childishness in people who were perfectly capable of developing a more mature and differentiated approach to their own dreams and to their process of individuation and this comes over most pointedly in her essays on active imagination. I recall her telling me once, in her inimitable style, during a preexamination meeting, that what she had written and published on fairy tales was, in the context of the examination, to be considered "chewed-up, predigested baby food" and that we had all better be able to come up with our own individual interpretations. A few years ago, I and a small group of analysts in Rome were considering the possibility of launching an independent series of talks and discussions in the true spirit of Jung; before making any final decisions, we decided to wait and see what sort of dreams each of us had. Needless to say, the image of von Franz promptly appeared: she was standing outside a lecture hall where the audience was waiting for her to give a talk. All of a sudden, she tells me she's leaving, and I object, "but those people are expecting to hear you." Her response was, "You people take care of it!" and off she went. We tried to take this responsibility seriously and went ahead and acted on our idea, which is now in its third successful year of activity.

Hers is indeed a difficult legacy to carry forward—how could we ever hope to study and master all that she knew or to have her amazing powers of concentration and analysis? How could we ever hope to have the courage she showed in always making choices she felt were sustained and supported by the unconscious regardless of her own personal desires or ambitions? But none of these things can be used as excuses for not cultivating as dynamic a relationship as possible with the mystery of the psyche or for not accepting complete responsibility for the results of this. I'm sure there isn't one of us who has not over the last few years found himself or herself thinking, "I wish I could ask von Franz about that." But as I realized yet again recently while working on a dream, we can't go and ask her anymore, we've got to do the work ourselves. The dream that I was working on was one that I had had while writing a short article about the mandala of Niklaus von Flüe that a magazine had asked me to submit. Naturally I reread everything Jung himself wrote about Brother Klaus and carefully studied von Franz's book on the visions of Niklaus. The dream was the following:

> *A strong authoritative voice announces: Marie-Louise von Franz has died! Then I see something that I know is the result of this event: a gigantic "cosmic" mandala which has a square white frame and a round violet center that is swirling around as if it were taking shape. I also see, farther over to the right, what looks like an infinite series of small, light green mandalas, again each with a square white frame.*

I can't help feeling that the life and death of Marie-Louise von Franz has somehow constellated in the unconscious a form of order (the gigantic violet mandala) which affects us all and from which we all somehow benefit. I like to think of the small green mandalas as a series of "echoes" or "ripples" emanating from this event and touching each of us in the everyday events of our lives. This is no doubt, to a certain extent, the result of the life and death of each man and woman who tries to live honestly in contact and relationship with the unconscious. In the case of Dr. von Franz, her death and the way she participated in that event was a special occurrence indeed and bore out yet again her absolute dedication and devotion to the mystery of the psyche as well as her complete trust in it—a perfect example of the *pistis* Saint Paul speaks of and which Jung comments on in various places.

Once, during a control session years ago, I needed to "confess" something that I feared she would harshly disapprove of. After telling her what I needed to say, she remained silent and, without the slightest hint of judgment, simply asked, "What do the dreams say?" I told her that, even though I had tried to be particularly attentive, it didn't seem that I had had any dreams, something which frustrated me greatly. Her answer was simply, "Well, I think we can take that as a 'no comment' on the part of the unconscious. Keep trying to do your best." The fact that she abstained from any sort of ego-based judgment and immediately turned with absolute trust to the unconscious was the greatest lesson she could have given me, and the sense of responsibility she communicated to me was highly important.

And this takes me back to the dream mentioned above. "Marie-Louise von Franz has died" is the sad fact, but the mandalas seem to point to the personal responsibility I (and obviously each of us) need to accept in carrying on the work of individuation—a work that is without a doubt clearer for us thanks to the life and death of a truly great woman.

On the Tao of Uselessness

LARA MINDELL

Dear Marlus,

When I was a little girl, I stood in awe of you, my godmother. With time my feelings blossomed into a deep affection and a special kind of fascination. During my university studies more than ten years ago, I occasionally helped out in your household for a couple of weeks at a time, and you said things to me now and then in your loving, spontaneous manner that intuitively struck to the heart of the matter. These indelible insights will accompany me through the rest of my life.

Looking back, I would summarize the two most central features of my experience with you as, first, the natural matter-of-fact manner in which the reality of the unconscious pervaded the entirety of your being, your orientation, and your daily life. Your unique mixture of brilliant intuition, extensive knowledge, keen discernment, together with your profound capacity of eros rooted in nature and the unconscious was interwoven with a mercurial sense of humor that sparkled. I will gravely miss these precious qualities of yours.

Second, on a more personal level I was deeply affected not only by your humanity but by your ability to be open to doubt—despite the clarity of your own standpoint—as you genuinely wrestled with the opposites in the course of your life. Your extraordinary integrity and humility permeated this courageous attitude. In your incomparable manner, you also perceived deeper aspects of my and others' personalities, responding to each of us in kind although our capacities for self-perception were just beginning to emerge. That is why I once promised you that even if I was not capable of relating to your farsighted point of view, I would always remember your statements to me, for they struck such a deep resonant echo. I thank you for the invaluable gifts from that time. They have left a permanent impression on me.

An unforgettable expression of your outlook toward life is embodied in a humorous story (which I heard from you more than once, your face lighting up with pleasure each time).

> There was once an Indian novice who was terribly afraid of the elephants in the jungle. In order to overcome his fear, he went one day to his guru and asked him what he could do. The guru answered: "The next time an elephant crosses your path, you must say to him that you are Atman." In relief, the novice thanked him for the advice and set out with courage and conviction through the jungle. When finally he came upon an elephant, he repeated just what he had been told. The elephant trampled him mercilessly and went on its way. The man crawled back on all fours to his guru and told him that his advice had not impressed the elephant whatsoever. The guru answered: "Well, of course, because you did not realize that the elephant is Atman too."

With such playful humor you wove wisdom and laughter into daily life and often made us aware that the ego all too easily overvalues itself; the reality of the Self is not only efficacious in man but penetrates everything.

You knew of my interest in ancient Chinese culture and philosophy, in particular the school of Taoism, and once suggested that I delve into this material in connection with Jungian psychology later on in life. Now I have made a beginning by examining the writings of Zhuangzi.[1] After a big dream about the teachings of C. G. Jung, Richard Wilhelm, and the origins of Tao, I felt encouraged to undertake the following rather modest attempt to interpret one of Zhuangzi's short stories.

The Old Oak Tree: A Taoistic and Depth Psychological Approach to the Value of Uselessness

Zhuangzi's short story "The Old Oak Tree" particularly captivated me. On the occasion of this publication commemorating Dr. von Franz, I wanted to take a closer look at it. As my literature research began, I discovered that out of approximately one hundred and fifty-five parables and anecdotes from Zhuangzi, Dr. von Franz had analyzed precisely this tale and, as far as I know, practically no other one out of his collected works (other than "The Death of Chaos-Unconscious").[2] Furthermore, she treated this version of the story, and no other, out of the four very similar stories from the particular chapter of his work in which "The Old Oak Tree" is found.[3] After my initial surprise, the feeling slowly grew within me that this "coincidence" beckoned to me to amplify Dr. von Franz's insights on the meaningful spirit of this story.

Zhuangzi (originally named Zhuang Zhou) is known as the greatest historical figure of Taoistic philosophy. Based on observations of the famous historian Sima Qian (145–92 B.C.E.) in his *Shiji (Historical Chronicles),* Zhuangzi lived between about 370 and 300 B.C.E. He was born in Meng, in the state of Song within the Henan Province. Song existed at the time of the Eastern Zhou Dynasty (period of the Warring States, 476–221 B.C.E.). At that time, Meng was called "Nan Hua" (literally, "Southern Land of Blossoms"). Zhuangzi's writings survived the great book burning of Qin Shi Huangdi (the first emperor of China) in the year 213 B.C.E., despite the loss of certain portions and the addition of certain commentaries by later authors. During the Tang Dynasty in 742, when Taoism was widely honored, his works were canonized by order of the emperor, and the book received its present title: *The True Book of the Southern Land of Blossoms.* Zhuangzi was purportedly a comprehensive scholar who nevertheless was devoted to the life and teachings of Laozi. Although he was repeatedly offered ministerial posts by the royalty of that time, he preferred to be the custodian of a lacquer tree garden where, in calmness and tranquility, he went about his daily affairs with the same attitude he professed toward life in general. He was married and his family often lived in poverty. His lively spirit was, however, not affected by this condition. Quite the contrary! He enthusiastically sparred with other important philosophers of his time, and his criticism of society ranged from the gentle to the caustic.[4]

Zhuangzi's writings reveal an additional dimension rising out of the background of the epoch in which he wrote. During the period of the Warring States, marked by constant combat and hostilities, the state of Song suffered particularly bloody conflicts. The Zhou followers pursued the descendants of the conquered Shang Dynasty in Song with extraordinary brutality, evidenced by frequent invasions, massacres, mass repression, and internal intrigues. It is not surprising then that the state of Song, the very heart of political and social oppression and despair, was the initial breeding place for Zhuangzi's philosophical outlook. His central theme was a response to the widespread dilemma of his times, namely, how men and women can survive in a world dominated by war, suffering, and absurdity.

All of the great philosophical schools of China have grappled with this question and provided different answers. Confucius, for example, drafted political, social, and ethical proposals for reform, concretizing the ancient cultural tradition of exactly defined roles and duties within the family that is the embryo of society. Zhuangzi's school of Taoism was based on a diametrically opposed point of view. His mystical thinking, detached from convention and judgment, declared: free yourself from the world!

Zhuangzi gave no preference to poverty or to wealth, to death or to life. He did not hide himself from the world—for that would be a form of bias or judgment. Instead, he based his behavior within society not upon the motives of the common man who generally seeks wealth, fame, success, and security. Thereby he sought to achieve a state that is called *wu wei* (nonaction). This does not indicate a condition of indifference, laissez-faire, or passively letting life flow by. It also does not entail enforced tranquility, but rather a way of life, free of goal-oriented thought and striving. In this condition one acts as nature does: spontaneously without designs. Man becomes one with nature (or the heavens, as Zhuangzi says) and enters Tao (the way, the meaning) which embodies the underlying unity of man, nature, and the universe. The concept of Tao is a necessary bridge to the ineffable; in terms of experience, it means pure inwardness. Zhuangzi acknowledges no mental constructs.[5] His thought leaves much open and always allows a place for doubt. (In this sense, C. G. Jung shares much in common with him.)

The writings from Zhuangzi are handed down today in the form of a book divided into seven so-called "inner or esoteric chapters." It is confirmed that these chapters were written by Zhuangzi. They are followed by an "outer or exoteric" part that was probably composed by some of his followers. Richard Wilhelm divided the latter part of the book into twenty further chapters.[6] Each chapter contains a varying number of anecdotes, parables, and short stories. "The Old Oak Tree" comes from the inner section, chapter four (entitled "In the World of Man"), which encompasses eight short stories. The tale goes like this:

> On their travels, a carpenter and his apprentice passed a gigantic old oak tree in a field near an earth altar. It measured one hundred feet in diameter and was practically as tall as a mountain. Although the tree was regarded as a magnificent sight, the carpenter ignored it and went on his way. The apprentice marveled at the tree and did not understand his master. He spoke to him about it, and the master said: "It is a useless tree. If you were to make a ship out of it, it would sink. If you were to make a coffin out of it, it would quickly rot. If you were to make tools out of it, they would snap. If you were to make a door out of it, it would swell. If you were to make a column or a post out of it, it would quickly be infested with worms. Out of this tree nothing can be made; one can make no use of it." That very night, the oak tree appeared to the man in a dream and said, "With

> what kind of trees do you think you are comparing me? You wish to compare me to your fruit trees and whatever else bears fruit and berries? They can barely bring forth their fruit before they are violated and damaged. Their branches are broken, their twigs torn. Their gifts endanger their very lives, and rarely do they live out their full life span. This is the way it happens everywhere. That is why, my mortal friend, I have long since made every effort to become completely useless. In this way I have managed to make my uselessness become my greatest value. Moreover, you and I are both creatures of nature, so how is it that one creature sets itself so high above another to judge? You mortal, useless man, what do you know about useless trees?" The carpenter awoke and tried to interpret his dream. He realized that the tree grew intentionally at that earth altar because otherwise those who did not recognize the tree would have mistreated it. Furthermore, its use was different from all other trees, so to apply normal criteria to it would have been totally wrong.[7]

In order to avoid overlapping with Dr. von Franz's text, I would like to pursue two further trains of thought based on her considerations.

The theme of "usefulness versus uselessness" plays an important role throughout the above mentioned chapter and is for Zhuangzi an analogy to the issue of purposeful thinking. The four short stories—"The Gnarled Tree," "The Suffering of Usefulness," "The Cripple," and "The Fool's Song"—speak again and again of the unconventional usage of things that society deems worthless.[8] The carpenter who finds the old oak to be useless at first does not realize that it fulfills a particular function indeed, a religious one. Its unique qualities and its size have enabled its function to manifest and protect it from premature death in contrast to fruit-bearing trees. The cripple is judged by society and by old magician-priests as both a useless invalid and a harbinger of disaster. In contradistinction, Zhuangzi describes how despite (or just because of) the cripple's role as an outcast, he finds a niche where he can live out his life undisturbed as opposed to the soldier who dies a premature death in a bloody battle. The short story "The Cripple" goes so far as to end with the idea that crippled virtue is preferable to being simply virtuous.[9]

Zhuangzi's attitude in regard to uselessness culminates in the "The Fool's Song." According to the parable, Confucius passes the fool in the ruling state of Chu, where he hears the fool addressing the darkness of the times in the following lament:

> Fortune is as light as a feather: it will never be captured.
> Misfortune is as heavy as the earth: it will never be
> circumvented . . .
> Thorns, thorns! Do not obstruct the way!
> Madness! Confusion! Do not hold us up.
> The oil in the lamp consumes itself. The cinnamon tree is edible, that is why it will be cut down. The lacquer tree is useful, thus it will be split apart. *Everyone knows how useful it is to be useful, and nobody knows how useful it is to be useless.*[10]

As Dr. von Franz has explained elsewhere, when goal-oriented thinking is put into question, the one-sidedness and the relativity of the island of ego consciousness becomes more obvious—and in typically Chinese fashion—wholeness (or the unconscious) is given precedence.[11] Thus greatness and merit will not be measured by conventional, that is, psychologically speaking, *outer* criteria but rather by the degree of attaining *wu wei*—a state of outwardly aimless, internalized being following the course of nature, which Dr. von Franz compares with the development of the individuation process.

Aspiring to be useless, as the oak tree describes itself, is considered, like *wu wei* ("nonaction"), to be worthless by the standards of the collective. That is why it is compared to a cripple and a fool in other short stories in the same chapter by Zhuangzi.[12] Taoism, however, considers precisely this characteristic to be "true greatness." This is revealed in the *Daodejing* by Laozi:

> Conventional people hoard more than they need, but I possess
> nothing at all,
> know nothing at all,
> understand nothing at all.

They are bright; I am dark.
They are sharp; I am dull.
Like the sea, I am calm and indifferent.
Like the wind, I have no particular direction.
Everyone else takes his place and does his job;
I alone remain wild and natural and free.
I am different from others: my sustenance
comes directly from the Mother.[13]

It seems essential to me that, on the one hand, "The Old Oak Tree" (as well as other similar short stories of Zhuangzi's) emphasizes that the "carrier of individuation" (if we may say) is not only the inferior function, revealing stumbling blocks and sign posts that point the way toward the unconscious, but above all the "incapacity to live" in us—the greatest suffering in life, the greatest personal "abyss," the point of greatest inferiority and target of inner criticism, the greatest psychic and/or physical frailty, our Achilles heel—which holds the key to individuation.[14]

Now, to be honest: are we really capable of recognizing and bearing this inverted outlook in consciousness?

For the most part, we feel that everything in us that is not up to life's demands stands in our way; we experience it as annoying, depressing, and basically useless. In this context, "The Old Oak Tree" invokes the feminine, vegetative life which the hectic, rootless spirit of the times holds in such low esteem. I am referring here not only to the earth and its atmosphere, which we have defiled with our civilized ways, but above all to the feminine principle contained within the material and spiritual totality of each human being. For instance, when a life that is based on activity and (even positive) achievement is brought to a standstill, this is experienced as a hindrance that must be overcome as quickly as possible: one must "get the situation under control" and then "put it behind oneself."[15] Our modern interpretation of societal norms, scientific creeds, Western and often alternative medicine as well, numerous psychotherapeutic procedures, and the great world religions ultimately propagates this goal by focusing on conquering pain, stress management, resource-oriented coping, the rational as well as irrational disposal of blame and self-recrimination as means to avoid or repress suffering and painful episodes in life containing a deeper message. The delusion of being able to accomplish everything remains still deeply ingrained in our consciousness, despite C. G. Jung's discoveries of the collective unconscious, the Self, and the unitary background of psyche and soma.[16] Thus, even "becoming whole" has become an increasingly popular and desirable goal; it is, after all, worth striving for and ought to be achieved as quickly as possible, shouldn't it? A countertrend appears in the form of equally ineffectual and passive fatalism. We are most likely to encounter this attitude when a person is confronted with unexpected blows of fate or other adverse circumstances in his or her life. (See plate 8.)

As C. G. Jung and Marie-Louise von Franz have impressively demonstrated, one of the initial and major steps in the individuation process takes the form of a kind of wounding or suffering that the ego experiences as a humiliation. This condition provokes one to realize the existence of influential, transpersonal powers which demand our recognition and dedication.[17] The shamanistic initiation ceremonies of indigenous peoples throughout the world have always paid full tribute to this fact in ritualized forms.

It is precisely this quality of the neglected vegetative, feminine, and irrational that is so powerfully expressed in ancient Chinese thought. Needham's exposition of Taoism contains a beautiful passage on the symbol of the feminine (and on the water symbol):

> The observation of Nature . . . requires a receptive passivity in contrast to commanding activity, and a freedom from all preconceived theories . . . This is the sense . . . in which we may interpret the symbols of "water" and "the feminine" so dear to early Taoist schools and so perplexing to later commentators.

Needham continues to address the theme of the feminine in Taoism as follows:

> The Confucian and the Legalist social-ethical thought-complex was masculine, managing, hard, dominating, aggressive . . . the Taoists broke

> with it radically and completely emphasized all that is feminine, tolerant, yielding, pensive, withdrawn, mystical and receptive . . . [This was the way in which they observed Nature, and it was] inextricably connected with the feminine yieldingness which they believed should be prominent in human and social relations.
>
> . . . .
>
> Instead of the Confucian or Legalist leadership from above, we reach the Taoist principle of *leadership from within.*[18]

To further illustrate this, Needham quotes from the *Daodejing*, chapter 66:

> How did the great rivers get their kingship over the hundred lesser streams? Through the merit of being lower than they . . . Therefore the sage, in order to be above people, must speak as though he were lower than they. In order to guide them, he must put himself behind them . . . The sage does not enter into competition, and therefore no one competes with him.[19]

In evolutionary terms, the development of consciousness and the ego may well play an equally important role in the discovery—and the affirmation—of the unconscious. However, it is important to emphasize the significance of affirmation, because I will never forget Dr. von Franz's response in the film *Remembering Jung*, part II, when she was asked: "What is the shadow of Jungian psychology?"[20] The truth of the matter is, she replied, that everything that C. G. Jung discovered and used to help others later on, he first lived through, endured, and intensely explored in his *own* life. Jungians today, she went on, dispense their knowledge as medicine that they have discovered themselves, forgetting at the same time to reflect upon where *they* stand in their relationship to the unconscious. It seems to me that we still too often underestimate the full consequences of C. G. Jung's and Marie-Louise von Franz's life works as well as the immense influence and the dangers of the unconscious. All too frequently, we lapse into an unconscious identification with our egos (and thus with our main function) and are seduced by the illusory promise that *everything* can be healed.

Where is the religious attitude toward life that embraces the humility of that which is "incapable of life" to the same degree that it embraces that which is "capable of life," in the awareness that the cripple within us teaches us invaluable lessons throughout our lives and contributes, again and again through new layers of experience recurring cyclically, to the development of our personalities? It appears to me in our day and age that this question has become all the more pressing in view of our afflicted *Zeitgeist* which exorts us to favor personality development running along linear lines. In truth, we all know that we cannot move forward without occasionally stumbling. Nonetheless, who among us is not seduced now and then by prevailing contemporary modes of thought? In this connection, Jung's words in *Memories, Dreams, Reflections* come to mind: *"There is no linear evolution, there is only circumambulation of the self. Uniform development exists at most, only at the beginning; later everything points towards the center."*[21]

This insight underscores a second area of concern for me in connection with the story of "The Old Oak Tree." In outlining the principal stages of the individuation process and the relationship to the unconscious, C. G. Jung and Marie-Louise von Franz inevitably have had to make certain generalizations of a methodological nature. In the interest of formulating the complex dynamics of these subtle psychic processes, they have described the "passing through" of certain stages: the initial encounters with the unconscious, then with the shadow, later on with the anima or the animus, and finally with the culminating experience of the Self. But (as von Franz and Jung themselves indicated in their later works): if everything unfolds in circumambulation, do we not experience these stages cyclically, again and again, in varying degrees of differentiation? It is precisely this circumstance which is so difficult for us to accept. In my experience, no one permanently resolves basic issues so that they are *totally* erased from his or her mind and never again cause distress, need to be dealt with or remembered. Such issues come up in the course of life, whether one wishes them to or not, time and again, like the eternal transformations set forth in the Chinese worldview, demanding renewed dedication to the unconscious and its growth by taking on that which we would prefer to ignore in ourselves and our lives.

C. G. Jung put it this way: one cannot solve the great problems of life, one can only *outgrow* them.

It depends on our own attitude, to a great extent, whether we admit these fateful cycles of life with all their ups and downs and do not evaluate them either as personal failures or as the failures of others. For if we do so, we tend to become bitter and disappointed, hardened and aloof, or even compensatorily regress into a state of hedonistic puerdom or puelladom. One of the most moving aspects of Marie-Louise von Franz's nature, as I was able to experience it in the short time granted to me, was that her life was a genuine circumambulation which divined this profound secret of nature and respected it deeply, where it touched both her own life and the lives of others. In the final analysis, the question of the correct attitude seems to me to be a religious question and a question of the ability to love. Are we capable of realizing and acknowledging that "uselessness" has been granted to us so that we may put ourselves in the service of something much greater (Zhuangzi called it Tao, C. G. Jung the Self)—something we can take on only if we can learn to summon up unwavering honesty and, just as importantly, the crucial understanding and *love* for what is "broken" within ourselves? The answer seems to me to encompass a lifelong process which also entails a natural wrestling with our own fate, calling for considerable strength and endurance, as we gradually learn in a most unique way how to love.

I would, therefore, like to close with a few words from Laozi:

> Nothing under heaven is as
> soft and yielding as water
> Yet for attacking the hard and strong,
> nothing can compare to it.
> *The weak overcomes the strong.*
> *The soft overcomes the hard,*
> *everyone knows this, but none*
> *have the ability to practice it.*
> Therefore the sage says:
> *one who accepts the dung of the nation [at the earth altar]*
> *becomes the master of soil and sustenance.*

One who deals with the evils of the nation
becomes king under heaven.
True words seem paradoxical.[22]

And thus, our story of "The Old Oak Tree" comes a full circle with Laozi's portrayal of the proper kind of sacrificial attitude at the earth altar. Yet along with our daily circumambulations and struggles with ourselves and the world, ultimately that spark of grace from the unconscious is also needed, as Marie-Louise von Franz emphasized through her whole life. This spark may actually provide the very element to allow us to glimpse parts of Tao's essence:

Silent, immeasurable,
standing alone and unchanging,
moving without end or exhaustion,
it is the mother of the known and unknown
universe.[23]

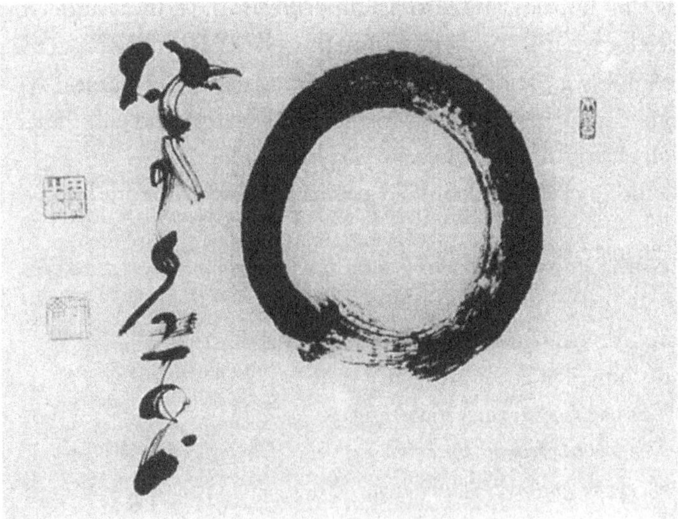

"Circle," by Yamada Kensai (1911–1974). Ink on paper. Chûô Tôkenkai, Tôkyô. Taken from H. Brinker, *Zen in der Kunst des Malens* (Bern: Scherz Verlag, 1991), p. 39.

NOTES

1. B. Watson, *Chuang Tzu: Basic Writings* (New York: Columbia University Press, 1971); and R. Wilhelm, *Dschuang Dsi—Das wahre Buch vom Südlichen Blütenland* (München: Eugen Diederichs, 1994), English edition, R. Wilhelm, *Chuang-tse: The True Book of the Southern Land of Blossoms* (Jena, 1923).
2. M.-L. von Franz, *Creation Myths* (Boston: Shambala, 1972), pp. 142ff.
3. See M.-L. von Franz, "The Process of Individuation," in C. G. Jung, *Man and His Symbols* (New York: Doubleday, 1969), p. 163; and M.-L. von Franz, *Archetypal Dimensions of the Psyche* (Boston: Shambhala, 1997), pp. 296ff.
4. J. Gernet, J., *Die chinesische Welt* (Frankfurt am Main: Suhrkamp, 1972). Zhuangzi's style is complex, a mixture of mythical, poetic, narrative, and humorous elements.
5. Watson, pp. 1–15.
6. Wilhelm, *Dschuang Dsi.*
7. Ibid., p. 66.
8. Ibid., pp. 69–71.
9. Watson, p. 62: "How much better, then, if he had crippled virtue."
10. Wilhelm, p. 71, emphasis mine.
11. Von Franz, *Archetypal Dimensions of the Psyche,* pp. 120ff.
12. K. Carr and P. Ivanhoe, *The Sense Antirationalism: The Religious Thought of Zhuangzi and Kierkegaard* (New York: Seven Bridges Press, 2000), p. 35: "In particular, Zhuangzi relied upon exquisitely composed descriptions of people who have attained a different and clearly desirable way of life. These exemplars of the Way differ in significant ways from what we might expect of other kinds of paragons: They subvert rather than reinforce the dominant social hierarchy of the day. Zhuangzi's heroes are more 'underheroes' than antiheroes . . . Almost everything about them—station, occupation, appearance and gender—make them underappreciated, even outcasts in their own society. But these very people are the ones who are able to understand and live in accordance with the *dao.* In some sense, their lowly position in the social hierarchy gives them a clearer view of Heaven."
13. B. Walker, *Lao Tzu: The Tao Te Ching* (New York: St. Martin's Press, 1995), chap. 20.
14. M.-L. von Franz, *Psychotherapie* (Einsiedeln: Daimon Verlag, 1990), p. 37; English edition: *Psychotherapy* (Boston: Shambhala, 1993). She notes that the inferior function represents the despised part but also the part that builds a bridge to the unconscious and thus carries the key to unconscious wholeness.
15. "The greatest limitation for man is the 'self'. . . Only consciousness of our narrow confinement in the self forms the link to the limitlessness of the unconscious . . . In knowing ourselves to be unique in our personal combination—that is, ultimately limited—we possess also the capacity for becoming conscious of the infinite. But only then! In an era which has concentrated exclusively upon extension of living space and increase of rational knowledge at all costs, it is a supreme challenge to ask man to become conscious of his uniqueness and

his limitation. Without them, no perception of the unlimited is possible—and, consequently, no coming to consciousness either—merely a delusory identity with it which takes the form of intoxication with large numbers and an avidity for political power." C. G. Jung, *Memories, Dreams, Reflections,* ed. Aniela Jaffé (New York: Vintage Books, 1965), pp. 325ff.

16. Ibid., p. 263: "We rush impetuously into novelty, driven by a mounting sense of insufficiency, dissatisfaction, and restlessness . . . We refuse to recognize that everything better is purchased at the price of something worse; . . . and thus we help with all our might to rob the individual of his roots and his guiding instincts, so that he becomes a particle in the mass."
17. Von Franz, *Archetypal Dimensions of the Psyche,* pp. 320ff.
18. J. Needham, "History of Scientific Thought," in *Science and Civilization in China,* vol. 2. (Cambridge: Cambridge University Press, 1991), p. 57, emphasis mine.
19. Ibid., p. 58; Needham quotes Waley's translation of the *Daodejing.*
20. M.-L. von Franz, *Remembering Jung,* part II, videotaped interview with M.-L. von Franz and Suzanne Wagner, Bollingen, March 1977; available from the C. G. Jung Institute of Los Angeles.
21. C. G. Jung, *Memories, Dreams, Reflections,* pp. 196ff; emphasis mine.
22. Walker, chap. 78; emphasis mine.
23. Ibid., chap. 25.

In Loving Memory of Dr. Marie-Louise von Franz

NORA MINDELL

The first time that I met Dr. Marie-Louise von Franz was in 1964. I was barely twenty-one years old, had just graduated from the first four years of an American university, and was in search of a different approach to the popular trends prevailing in psychology and psychotherapy in the United States at that time. I had scoured the libraries for reading material and had suddenly come across a book of C. G. Jung's which excited and surprised me because his writings exuded life, profound spiritual reality, and a vast intelligence. Shortly thereafter, a friend of mine visiting in Zürich reported that Jung had recently died and that a most unusual woman, a kind of spiritual successor, was carrying on his work together with an inspired group of other pupils.

Then I had a most perplexing dream, one of the few that I remember from my youth. In it, I was standing to one side of Dr. von Franz as she was excavating a Greek site. But instead of relics and artifacts from the past, a complex pattern of vibrating, three-dimensional geometric figures emerged out of a mandala-shaped foundation, as though they formed the skeleton of a town or a city. She beckoned to me to come closer and join in the dig.

The dream was quite obscure to me at the time, but so powerful and alluring that I found a way to visit Zürich and meet Dr. von Franz. That first encounter will remain forever etched in my memory. At the time, she occupied several rooms in the middle of the village of Küsnacht, a town on the outskirts of the city of Zürich. She gave analysis in a large room separated from a small anteroom by a room divider. In this small niche, as I briefly waited for my hour, I was accosted by a lovable bulldog named Nibby, who enthusiastically sniffed and licked me all over. (Only afterward did I realize that he was tracking the smells of my own collie, whom I hadn't brought with me to the hour. That was a mistake I quickly learned to correct in future sessions. The two dogs became fast friends, and I was able to enjoy peace during my hours, relatively speaking, when I brought my dog, Cleo.)

Then Dr. von Franz suddenly stood before me, shook my hand, and led me into her main room, where she sat me down in front of her and began to question me in depth. I was overwhelmed by a striking variety of impressions; first of all by this small, stocky, attractive woman, her intense gaze, her colorful, sophisticated level of conversation in English, and her no-nonsense, earthy manner (even evident in several food stains visible on her tailored suit; I later learned that she privately enjoyed such indications of natural imperfection in contrast to the elegant, sterile atmosphere of her childhood). Dr. von Franz was in a class of her own. One might describe her as eccentric, but that is too superficial a characterization. There was an aura of *numen* about her, and a powerful sense of brilliance, but most of all, a sensitivity and living connection to a transcendental dimension of reality emanating from her that deeply moved me, although I could only struggle to grasp it at the edges.

She was surrounded by stacks of books and an amazing array of objects (some priceless, others personal and interesting) along with some patrician pieces of antique furniture—family heirlooms, no doubt. The entire picture revealed manifold aspects of her unique personality. It is impossible to actually convey in words the many different facets that struck me in that initial hour.

Throughout our conversation, I was repeatedly touched and fascinated by what she said and by the way in which she spoke to me out of the depths of what seemed to be a deep, unseen source. At the same time, she was full of humor, curious about mundane matters in daily life, and at times refreshingly revealing about her own personal opinions. When I finally summoned enough courage to ask her if she would consider giving me analysis (fantasizing all the while how unrealistic my wish must be), she politely declined, explaining that the sanitation pipelines underlying Küsnacht had been overflowing in a recent dream of hers, a warning that she was overworked. Then she patiently went through a litany of names and remarks about possible alternative candidates. After a while, she suddenly became silent, as if she was pondering some private thought. Then she smiled broadly, declaring: "Well, I guess there is nothing for it. I shall have to take you on myself . . . But please don't let Miss Hannah know, because I promised her I wouldn't do this!"

I left the session shortly thereafter, stunned, joyful, and full of wonder and fear that she would change her mind, particularly if this lady who was not known to me did find out.[1]

Over the years I came to know Dr. von Franz not only as an extraordinary analyst but also as a revered mentor and a most dear friend. There are so many wonderful stories I could recount to honor her, one of the great women of this century, who will probably not be recognized as such because our Zeitgeist lags behind.

Among many things that Dr. von Franz taught me was to make my Latin soul aware of the fact that its emotional spontaneity (which I would enjoy giving rein to now by sharing some more recollections) longed to learn to bow and serve a deeper imperative of the objective psyche. And so I feel that I must sacrifice my urge to relate more personal stories in order to attempt a different task, clearly laid out by my unconscious when I dreamed (in relation to writing a contribution to this Festschrift) that Dr. von Franz was alive again and needed my help to clear out her attic. It was a rather challenging task because the attic contained a large living fish that she wanted me to carry down to the main room.

Fairy tales, Greek, Chinese, and African mythology—among so many other fields such as alchemy and mathematics—her life included a multitude of interests which she pursued with a depth of intelligence given to few, at the same time that she possessed a dedication to and heartfelt sense of the importance of irrational reality. Her prolific and outstandingly creative career culminated in an investigation of Jung's thesis that the duality of spirit and matter rests on an underlying unity. As she put it in her own words: "The empirical world of appearances is . . . [ultimately] based on a transcendental background."[2]

After Jung completed his initial work on synchronicity, he speculated that the next step in understanding the unitary existence of psyche and matter would be to study the just-so character of natural numbers, namely, their qualitative as well as their quantitative characteristics. He even suspected that natural numbers in their double capacity were inherent ordering factors mediating between psychic processes and empirical manifestations in physical reality.

Jung set down his concerns, intuitions, and thoughts on number in a note which was headed by a mysterious-looking equation:

$$1 = \infty N - (\infty N - 1)$$

and was followed by a particular set of remarks about the just-so properties of the first five integers.[3] This note formed one of the primary inspirations for von Franz's books *Number and Time* and *Psyche and Matter,* both stunning expressions of her extraordinary capacity to grapple with these revolutionary ideas in depth.

Even when she became ill in later years and could no longer hold a book upright to read by herself, she continued to devote herself to this study, deepening many of her ideas, expanding others, and working on new ones. I often sat at her bedside or shared the traditional four o'clock tea, during which she frequently discussed the thoughts she was mulling over.[4]

Once, while chatting about Jung's note on number, she reported a dream about a huge fish swimming around in a tank along with many smaller ones. She expressed the hope that others would "cook and serve" them one day, because the paradigms that Jung and she dealt with were ever so essential to expanding the confines of our dominant principles in modern science as well as in psychology.[5]

This was the association to my dream that led to my decision to have von Franz "speak" through this writing and present several insights that she was brooding over which are not directly included in her published works, as far as I know.

She was naturally struck by the introductory equation in Jung's note on number (which is on line 1) and explained that the symbol ∞N represented the pleroma for Jung. She pointed out that the pleroma was alluded to in the Gospel of St. John in which Christ lived in the plenitude of the father and *was* the plenitude of the father.[6] The pleroma represents the plenitude of everything, and because it is everything, it is also nothing. Like the contents of an egg, there is no chick, she added, but the chick is potentially contained in it.[7]

The Gnostics employed the term *pleroma* to describe a metaphysical state of fullness in which all psychic potentials intermingle. In this state of latent promise, the opposites are preexistent and every facet of existence is contaminated with everything else.[8] The pleromatic condition signifies deepest unconsciousness and designates the potential condition of all forms which are not yet differentiated or actualized.[9]

According to Jung, this represents the potential archetypal world as the underlying pattern out of which all creation arises. The pleroma is the primordial condition of the collective unconscious in which all paradoxes are abolished and time is eternal. In essence, it denotes for Jung the timeless, preexistent world plan or antecedent model latent in God's mind, according to which He realized actual creation.

In later conversation, von Franz pointed out that the *unus mundus* is practically an identical concept to the pleroma, but the *unus mundus* is more Neoplatonic and rational, whereas the pleroma is more complete, mysterious, and irrational.[10] The Gnostic pleroma signifies a more dynamic and creative plenitude in Jung and von Franz's estimation. It is the creative, primordial wellspring, the "mother of the world," the flower of

Hellenistic culture, a concept which strongly emphasizes the sacred divine nature of the origins pictured as the "High God" (one of many names), also called the "Nothing of Water, Air and Fire," a male god, yet a quasi-hermaphroditic being as well.

A modern parallel to the pleroma and *unus mundus* is the relativistic world-body (block universe) of Minkowski and Einstein with three space coordinates and one time coordinate forming a four-dimensional continuum which might be only potentially existent.[11] The experience of the so-called Einstein-Podolsky-Rosen paradox also suggests a potential Oneness in the realm of matter. Successful tests on such EPR-correlations have shown that particles that were once united and are separated afterward continue to behave as though they knew about the ongoing states of each other, without the presence of causal influences. (This fact holds true even when the two particles are separated by long distances.)[12]

Von Franz also pointed to information in line 10 of Jung's note which helps to unravel the mystery of line 1. Line 10 reads:

ἕν τό πἅν. ∞N − (∞N − I) = *kenosis*

ἕν τό πἅν (hen to pan) is a Greek term meaning that one is one *and* the whole; namely, one has two characteristics—it is the basic counting unit and, at the same time, it is the totality of all numbers.

Dr. von Franz explained the double function of numbers as follows: "When you count, you are bound to be dealing with the totality of the cosmos. Therefore, when you say 'I,' what you mean is the cosmos but for 'I,' i.e., the cosmos minus 'I,' because this 'I' steps out of the totality, the totality is minus 'I.' When I say 'I,' I augment the world by 'I,' which steps out of the totality . . . or I diminish the totality by 'I.'"

Playfully, von Franz went on to expound this idea by pointing to her teacup on the table and noting that her teacup had now stepped out of the totality and become an individual, distinct object. "So, when I say one teacup," she carried on, "the totality has already lost a teacup, and that is why Jung wrote: (∞N − I)."[13]

By adding infinity to the term N (which is usually used to define the set of natural numbers 1, 2, 3, 4, etc.), Jung used the new term to imply something not real but potentially existent. Out of this primordial state of oneness (∞N), a paradoxical one (I) emerges as creation begins to unfold; this process is at the same time "one among the many" (hen) and simultaneously time bound up with totality as one is the whole (pan). In a similar vein, Jesus declared in John 12:45 "And he that seeth me seeth him that sent me." To allude to this inexplicable mysterium, Jung designates one with a slash (I) and not a normal "1."[14]

Therefore, we must emphasize that as von Franz pointed out in *Number and Time,* C. G. Jung was the first in contemporary times to bring the two definitions of one together, namely the normally accepted quantitative approach in which "1" is the first counting unit and a second definition of "1" as in "∞N − I," that is, infinity minus one. The process of the "1" emerging out of the "I," that is, out of the oneness totality (that von Franz referred to above) is known as *kenosis,* a powerful symbol of a mysterious transformation process whereby God empties Himself of His Totality, for example, as seen in Christian doctrine. Although in the Gospel of St. John Jesus lived in the plenitude of the Father, according to Phil. 2:6–8 He *"ekenosed"* Himself, incarnating into a concrete form of reality.

Before creation, God was the potential all-embracing cosmos, the pure divinity. Then he *"ekenosed"* himself into Mr. Meyer. With a big chuckle, von Franz rolled her eyes at the humorous marvel of this staggering transformation.[15] Breaking out into a radiant smile she added: "That *kenosis* of God pretty much blows us away." And she concluded that this element is what motivated Jung to declare that the infinite set of natural numbers represents—if anything at all—an abstract cosmogony derived from the monad.[16]

Furthermore, as referred to by Jung in his "Seven Sermons," the primordial continuity of the *pleroma* also contains the drive toward discontinuity and differentiation.[17] In a like manner, von Franz spoke about the eternal circle in which quantity and quality are not yet separated, but you can intuit a certain potential for a specific order or structure to come into existence and start to unfold. She called these potentials the "seeds."[18] As soon as these seeds begin to enter time and become observable, something is taken away from the primal totality; the plenitude gets impoverished. This situation is the starting point for the next impoverishment to take place. But it does not simply involve a mechanical procedure of evolution. Qualitatively speaking, you cannot simply compare changes from one state to another without observing the entire situation that has previously transpired. For instance, when you take one teacup out of the totality, you then have the totality minus one teacup. But when you remove the second teacup, you remove it from a new set of holistic conditions emerging out of the first step of the "totality minus one." This means, in reality we are viewing temporarily oriented numbers, not simply numbers ordered into a stationary set of quantities. Every step in relationship to infinity influences and shapes the step to come. "Actually, I would call this process-oriented mathematics," von Franz pronounced.[19] It is a big fish, mind-boggling, because this factor demonstrates that in reality you can never exactly predict what will emerge next from the original unity. The transformation of life processes varies unpredictably from moment to moment in terms of what evolves next when you try to measure them qualitatively and quantitatively at the same time. Herein lies the nature of the irrational individuality of processes unfolding in time.

"By the way," von Franz continued, "a certain set of patterns exist—let's call them *Bewegungskonfigurationen* [configurations of movement] that you can observe manifesting in this unfolding process."[20] They constitute our most accurate pictures of reality and are similar to the concept of trajectories in modern science.[21] This term indicates the path followed by a moving object. What we observe in terms of immediate perception is the object at different points in time and different positions in space. This moving configuration, a trajectory, comes closer to describing our own ever-changing perceptions of reality, according to von Franz, in contrast to traditional Western platonic mathematics, which is more concerned with static, timeless concepts.

By way of concluding, von Franz sighed as she commented that Jung's ideas were so ambiguous and difficult they needed a breadth of heart and an unusual sensitivity of spirit to comprehend them from the paradoxical viewpoint of infinity versus the "here and now." Science had a long way to go . . . She shook her head obscurely.[22]

May I personally add that my affection for her and my dedication to attempting to follow the quest that she undertook toward unraveling the underlying mystery of the unity of matter and spirit remains enduring. I will also never stop cherishing our times together for the rest of my life. Last night we sat chuckling over a cup of tea in my dream.

English Translation of a Handwritten Note by C. G. Jung on the First Five Natural Whole Numbers (Line Numbers Added for Reference)

1 $I = \infty N - (\infty N - I)$ This formula is a
2 *petitio principii.* I can
3 only be explained by means of itself.
4 Properties: 1. Can not multiply itself by itself,
5
6 2. and can not reduce itself by division, nor can it divide
7 itself by any other whole number.
8 3. The One in and of itself does not count.
9 The number sequence begins first
10 with 2.
11 4. If 1 counts, it is the first uneven
12 prime number.
13 5. *ἕν τὸ πᾶν.* $\infty N - (\infty N - I) =$ *kenosis.*
14 2. 1. Can multiply itself by itself
15 like all other numbers.
16 2. Can only be divided by itself $2 \div 2 = I$, in
17 this respect it is an even prime number, all other
18 prime numbers [are] uneven.
19 3. The first number that counts.
20 4. The sum of $I + I = 2x\, \infty N - (\infty N - I) = \infty N - (\infty N - 2)$.
21 3. 1. Can only divide itself by itself like
22 the 2.
23 2. Is the first uneven prime number aside from the 1.

24 Prime numbers = aperiodic intervals in the number sequence.
25
26
27
28 3. Sum of 2 + I = capable of increase, divisible only through itself,
29 = <u>prime number</u> + incapable of multiplication and indivisible.
30 4. 1. The first self-multiple, namely 2^2.
31 [1.] 4 points = 3-sided pyramid. <u>First body.</u>
32 2. Equations of the 5th degree can no longer be solved
33 ± property of 4.
34 3. Sum of the first two prime numbers I + 3, i.e.
35 that which is not capable of multiplication by itself and is indivisible
36 + that which is capable of multiplication and is divisible by itself.
37 (duplication 2x + 2÷) = Axiom of Maria 3 + I o.[r?] 4 − I [?].
38 5. 1. Prime number.
39 2. Whole number 4 + I.
40 Sum of the divisibles 3 + 2.

NOTES

1. Wondering whether this woman was a devoted housekeeper, I came to learn that Barbara Hannah was quite a lot more than that. I developed a friendship with her in her later years and deeply cared for her. She was a singularly gifted personality in her own right, one of the most "individuated" people I have ever met.
2. M.-L. von Franz, *Number and Time: Reflections Leading toward a Unification of Depth Psychology and Physics* (Evanston, Ill.: Northwestern University Press, 1974), p. 9.
3. The one used by Jung here is a slash, in contrast to the conventional way of writing "one" in conventional mathematics. The note was given to Dr. von Franz shortly before his death with the comment that he was too old to continue working on it and passed the task on to her. See *Hs prov von Franz* (Zürich: Scientific Historical Collection of the Swiss Federal Institute of Technology).

4. Often I was in the company of my close colleagues, Dr. David Eldred and Dr. Roy Freeman, during these discussions.
5. Personal communication, March 5, 1994.
6. Personal communication, January 26, 1997. This notion is expressed in the Bible as Christ being God's envoy and representative on earth. See J. Becker, *Das Evangelium nach Johannes: Kapitel 11–21* (Würzburg: Gütersloher Verl.-Haus Mohn, 1991), pp. 484–494.
7. Personal communication, January 26, 1997.
8. C. G. Jung, *Dream Analysis—Notes of the Seminar Given in 1928–1930 by C. G. Jung* (Princeton, N.J.: Princeton University Press, 1984), p. 131ff.
9. Ibid., p. 593.
10. Personal communication, April 5, 1997. Jung uses the term *unus mundus* frequently (i.e., in volumes 10 and 14) to designate the matrix of the collective unconscious as the "universal seed bed" preconditioning all forms of concrete reality in psyche and matter. See C. G. Jung, *Civilization in Transition, CW,* vol. 10 (Princeton, N.J.: Princeton University Press, 1964), par. 780; and *Mysterium Coniunctionis, CW,* vol. 14 (Princeton, N.J.: Princeton University Press, 1963), pars. 325ff, 413ff.
11. A. Wenzl, *Die philosophischen Grenzfragen der modernen Naturwissenschaft* (Stuttgart: Kohlhammer, 1954).
12. The original idea was laid out in A. Einstein, B. Podolski, and N. Rosen, "Can quantum-mechanical description of physical reality be considered complete?" in *Physical Review,* vol. 47 (1935), pp. 777–780; and C. P. Enz, "Wolfgang Pauli between quantum reality and the royal path of dreams," in *Symposia on the Foundations of Modern Physics 1992: The Copenhagen Interpretation and Wolfgang Pauli* (Helsinki, Finland, June–August 1992), K. V. Laurikainen and C. Montonen, eds. (Singapore: World Scientific), p. 198. I am grateful to Daniel Zimmermann for making me aware of the two examples in this paragraph and the references in notes 11 and 12.
13. Personal communication, November 11, 1995.
14. My appreciation goes to D. Zimmermann for confirming that this "nut" was cracked correctly.
15. Personal communication, January 26, 1997.
16. C. G. Jung, *Memories, Dreams, Reflections* (New York: Random House, 1963), p. 310f.
17. Ibid., pp. 378–390.
18. Personal communication, June 9, 1996.
19. Ibid.
20. Ibid.
21. R. Karr, *Goldmann Lexikon Physik. Vom Atom zum Universum* (München: Wilhelm Goldmann, 1999), p. 90.
22. Personal communication, May 18, 1996.

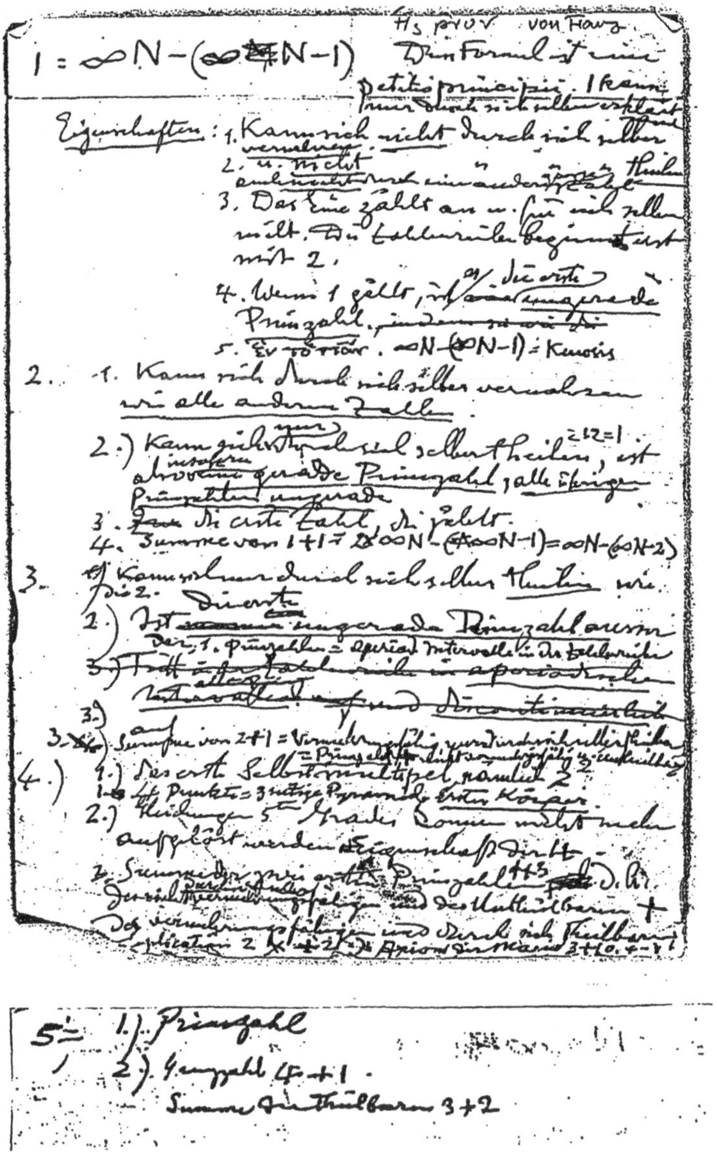

Figure 1. Facsimile of the original note. ETH-Bibliothek, Archive, Hs Prov/von Franz. Carl Gustav Jung, Notiz zu den "individuellen Eigenschaften der ganzen Zahl," 1961. Reproduced, with thanks, by permission of the ETH-Bibliothek Zürich and the Erbengemeinschaft C. G. Jung.

I Had the Privilege . . .

RAFAEL MONZÓ

I had the privilege of a personal collaboration with Dr. Marie-Louise von Franz during the last five years of her life. For this honor I would like to thank Dr. José Zavala and Dr. Dieter Baumann. And, in particular, I would like to express my gratitude to Ms. Barbara Davies who, due to Dr. von Franz's limited physical capacities during these years, assisted us in our correspondence.

Everyone who knew Marie-Louise von Franz knows how much she developed eros in her own personal life. In an article on the life and work of Dr. von Franz, Barbara Davies writes that von Franz's work will remain forever as a living symbol of the feminine and its redemption in our time.[1] In her book entitled *The Cat: A Tale of Feminine Redemption* (published after her death in 1999), von Franz interprets a Rumanian fairy tale and develops the idea that, through the realization of the feminine principle, a deep transformation will take place concurring with the zodiacal developments of our era. According to von Franz, the feminine principle of eros, with its emphasis on feeling, relatedness, intuition, and inspiration will unite with and heal the wounds created by the pervading patriarchal worldview.

In a similar vein, Dr. von Franz and I often reflected in our correspondence on the independent and spontaneous manifestations of the unconscious (as witnessed in events, dreams, and synchronicities) that were apparently related to the mysterious process of the integration of the feminine principle in the collective consciousness of our contemporary society and which seemed full of hope for the future. The radiance of the archetypal content of the feminine is constellated in our time, and it is waiting to be embodied in our contemporary culture where it is actually being realized more and more. The embodiment of the feminine is expressed in a multitude of ways both on collective as well as individual levels. We see its powerful expression, for example, in the feminist movements, in the awakening of an ecological conscience, in the spontaneous movements opposing globalization, in outspoken pacifism, in movements of solidarity with our fellow men and women, and in movements defending human rights. On the personal level, this impulse is also expressed in dreams and visions and in the individual realization of feminine values such as sensitivity, tolerance, understanding, feeling differentiation and openness, and an appreciation and respect for the small things of daily life. In male psychology, the realization of the feminine principle belongs together with the contents of the archetype of the anima, that inner feminine aspect of male psychology which, when developed, transforms the conflicts of the opposites undermining a functional relationship between consciousness and the unconscious.

One of the synchronistic-like coincidences that happened in the context of our relationship was the occurrence of a dream of Dr. von Franz's in which the king of Spain, D. Juan Carlos of Borbón, went to greet the members of the analytical psychology group in Valencia. This dream, along with other significant events, coincided with the issuing of a gold coin in a centennial commemoration of the discovery of a bust, the Lady of Elche, on the reverse side of which is an effigy of the king himself.[2]

The Lady of Elche is a stone sculpture discovered in August 1897 near an archeological site in l'Alcudia of Elche, a province of Alicante, Spain. (The village of Elche lies approximately 200 kilometers from Valencia on the Costa Blanca, the southeast Mediterranean coast.) The

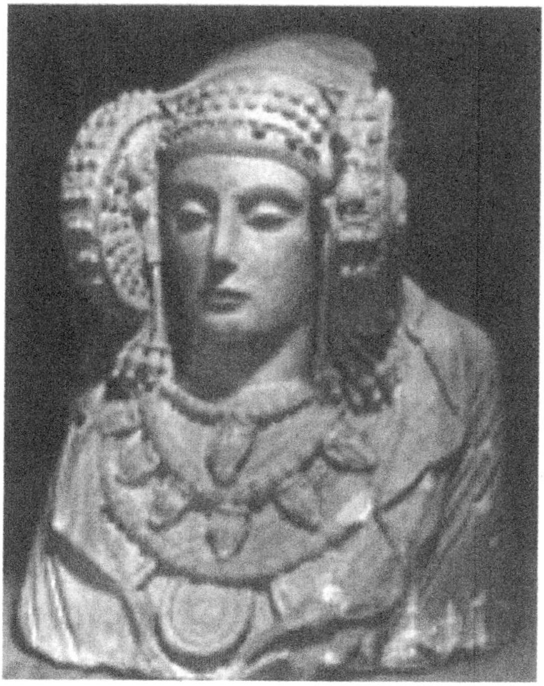

Figure 1. The Lady of Elche, an Iberian bust popularly known as the Moor Queen.

sculpture constitutes one of the most important master works of Iberian art ever to be found and appears on the one peseta banknote issued by the Spanish Central Bank in 1948 as well as on a postage stamp issued in 1969.[3] The Lady of Elche is a magnificent bust of a serene and dignified woman wearing a complex headdress with elaborate coils on each side of her face. On the back of the sculpture is a hole possibly used for the deposit of the ashes of the deceased. It could therefore be an example of a cinerary urn typical of Iberian funeral rituals. Some scholars date its production to the fourth century B.C. while others date it to the Hellenistic or Roman periods.

This enigmatic bust belongs to the Iberian culture and has been popularly known as the Moor Queen. Hypotheses regarding its mysterious origin range from the belief that it could have been the sculpture of a

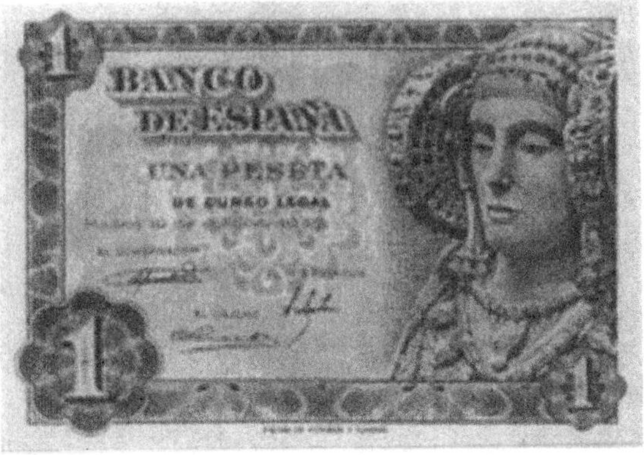

Figure 2. A one-peseta banknote.

mother goddess from antiquity such as Isis, Tanit, Cibeles, or Juno, or that it could be that of an Iberian priestess or even of a bride adorned in the ceremonial robes of that time.

Symbolically seen, these synchronistic events could represent a form of compensation from the unconscious indicating the necessity that the dominant of the collective conscious, represented by the symbol of the king, must stay in connection with the unconscious. We see these indications first in the dream, then through the psychology group, and then through the archetypal figure, the Lady of Elche, all which point in the direction of a conscious integration of the feminine principle and—*Deo concedente* (with the grace and consent of God)—toward the realization of a new symbol of the unification of the opposites.

In our correspondence on the occasion of the commemoration, I mentioned to Marie-Louise von Franz the dream of an old arborist, Antonio Masiá, a modest and humble man ninety-five years of age who had, as a self-proclaimed "physician of fruit-bearing trees," spent his life pruning the citrus orchards of Valencia. He had lived in solitude and ignorance of the world but had attained an exceptional degree of ethical reflection. He also radiated an intense aura of love. He felt that the world was far behind in matters of love, and he showed an exceptional sensitivity and respect for the dignity of women, convinced that the only thing missing in the world was equality for women vis-à-vis men. He also was deeply impressed that Pope John Paul II had forgiven his potential assassin Ali Agca. Some people had even named Masiá "the new Christ" because he said he had been born of love and was said to have gone beyond the Ten Commandments, which beseech man to "love thy neighbor as thyself," as Masiá loved his neighbor even more than himself. Antonio Masiá had finished his lifework blessed by the affection and respect of those around him. I had the privilege of listening to his inspired words as well as some of his dreams. When I mentioned Marie-Louise von Franz's dream of the king of Spain, he told me a dream of his about the king which had brought him deepest intrinsic happiness. In this dream:

> *A joyous multitude of people went to Antonio's house. The king of Spain had said that they were to express gratitude to Antonio because he had been able to summon all the rulers of the world to declare the wish for peace. Antonio held a book in his hands with the signatures of them all expressing their desire and commitment to strive for peace throughout the world. The people in the street worshipped Antonio like a savior, but he spoke to them there and told them that he was but a simple man and the only thing that mattered was to take "the Peace Book" first to the king of Spain and then to each of the rulers of all the nations of the world who owed this gesture to God, the One Creator, the author of all of their lives.*

Just a few days prior to his death, which he awaited in full conscious clarity, Antonio told me that he believed there could not have been a happier man than he, and he asked me never to forget "The Peace Book."

In Antonio Masiá we have the simple man, the *homo simplicimus,* who had been a caretaker and lover of trees, a man who remained in harmony with the vegetative world, the emotions and instincts, and who attained in his personal process of individuation a symbol of the Self and the union of opposites, which is seen in "The Peace Book." This motif was also portrayed in one of his final dreams. In the dream, he found himself standing in the orchards at home with his family, and next to them was the Great Tree that gave form to all orange trees and which united them into one single tree. He attained in his life a living connection to the Self, the archetype of totality, and as Marie-Louise von Franz says, when one is in harmony with the Self, there is an experience of peace and absolute happiness.[4] Others can judge him any way they want, they can apply destructive intellectual theories, but these cannot harm him because when one is in harmony with the Self, one becomes indestructible. Unconscious and consciousness are one, are reciprocally in peace, free and transcending the destructive attack of the emotions from within and without.

At that time Marie-Louise von Franz was concerned about the continued crisis in Yugoslavia. We spoke not only about her concern but also about the remote Yugoslavian village of Medjugorge where the Blessed Virgin Mary had been making daily appearances to six young shepherds since June 1981, bringing the message that "God is the fullness of life" and "to enjoy the fullness and obtain peace, you must return to God." To them the Virgin was announced as the "Queen of Peace," and two months later the word *mir* (peace) was seen by numerous people of the region written across the sky above the cross on top of Mount Krizevac.[5]

On an individual level, the union of opposites occurred for Antonio Masiá in the personal symbols of his "Peace Book" and in the dream of the Great Tree. On a collective level, however, it seems to me that, by necessity, symbolic expressions of the "Queen of Peace" were occurring in ex-Yugoslavia, reflecting the impulse in the unconscious evolving toward a reconciliation and union of the opposites. In a similar vein today, collective symbols may—or even urgently need to—arise in response to the present situation. In her article "Nike and the Waters of Styx," von Franz notes that new impulses are arising from the depths of the collective unconscious bringing forth new attitudes, embodying the potential to unify the opposites, and containing a creative force that may counteract the forces of destruction thus enabling eros and humanity to prevail.[6]

In but a few days after I sent my letter describing the events and dreams of Antonio Masiá, von Franz answered expressing her appreciation of what I had shared with her. In that correspondence she then drew the parallel between the Black Madonna in the Benedictine Abbey in Einsiedeln and the Lady of Elche and related a dream of hers from the previous year.[7] She wrote: "Thank you for your news of synchronistic events. Last year I dreamed that C. G. Jung, in collaboration with the 'Black Madonna' of Einsiedeln (a parallel of the Lady of Elche), would undertake something to facilitate peace in the world. And I was honored to be a witness."

This letter was then followed by another synchronistic coincidence which happened to me at the inauguration of the Museo de Prehistoria, the museum of prehistoric art in Valencia. During the festivities, a holographic reproduction of the Lady of Elche was projected; its vividness and color were so exceptional that it was as though the spirit of the lady herself was among us. (The impressive three-dimensionality of the image recalled to me a statement from Dr. José Zavala who said that Freud's vision was more two-dimensional while Jung's added a third dimension to symbolic thinking, namely, the feeling function which centers on the emotional effect and resonance that such events have on us.)

A short time later, another synchronistic event took place during the popular Fallas festival in Valencia in 1996. The Fallas is a springtime celebration in Valencia, during which gigantic, highly elaborate cardboard and paper maché constructions ("Fallas") characterizing people and figures in sundry dramatic forms (often of a satirical nature), are paraded throughout the city during four days of carnival-like celebration. The celebration has a distinct character of renewal and new life. The festivities culminate on the last day with the celebration of the *cremá* on the night of San José when they are consumed by fire to "burn off the winter." The "kings of Spain" went to Valencia on that occasion to attend the *mascletá,* one of the acts that take place in the square of the City Council. Here, a real pyrotechnic production couples ever-intensifying rhythms with the consumption of both the Fallas and such great quantities of gunpowder that the whole earth vibrates with a startling roar. According to the press on the following day, the "kings of Spain" who had attended the *mascletá* were deeply impressed by the unforgettable experience, an event that was compared to an earthquake. Alongside the article on the "kings of Spain" was, astonishingly enough, an article on the Lady of Elche which not only described her historical and archeological value but also pointed out that the Iberian culture practiced a form of mystery religion based on the vegetative cycles of nature and the annual renewal of life.[8] Now, if the Lady of Elche is a representation of an Iberian goddess, then she may be a representative of the divine kingdom of light coming from the sepulchral sphere and an expression of descent to the underworld of the earth mother goddess and the return to spring, that is, from the infernal depths and darkness of the underworld ascending to be vivified in life. Pursuing this hypothesis, the Iberian goddess would be the one to lead us back into the processes of regeneration springing forth from the earth and ascending out of darkness into new forms of life. In this sense, the Lady of Elche would be a representative of the return of the Great Goddess who has been a symbol since ancient times of the regenerative powers of the Great Mother goddesses reemerging in spring.

In the context of the intense emotional impact of the *mascletá,* that roaring inferno, coupled with the popular festivities, it seemed as though the goddess of Elche had arisen again out of the depths of the earth and realized her destiny that day by entering the household of tens of thousands of Valencians as a living symbol of the feminine Anthropos, a living archetype emerging directly out of the unconscious symbolizing the material feminine body, emotionality, and instinctiveness. (Here she is much like Sophia, her archetypal gnostic parallel who, imprisoned in matter, awaited liberation.) And on this day, she rose toward the world of light and human consciousness with the hope of integration—this time on the individual and personal level.

A similar process has been discussed by Dr. José Zavala in his interpretation of Shakespeare's Henry the Fifth.[9] Zavala discusses the motif of the fire muse that "ascends into the brilliant heavens of invention" toward a conscious integration of the masculine spirit expressing the necessity that the feminine principle and the principle of eros unite with their opposite, the instinctive aspect of the masculine spirit, fostering a relationship between the opposites.

Dr. Dieter Baumann, in his presentation on the Dialas, feminine spirits of nature, spoke to us about the present historical moment in which the feminine principle of nature wants to become human.[10] Here he sees a correspondence between the present-day constellation and the phenomenon two thousand years ago of God wanting to become man. Today the question is whether or not the world will survive and if the feminine deity will be able to transcend and become human.

In respect to the Lady of Elche, and in particular to the motif of the Black Madonna, Marie-Louise von Franz pointed out that the popular devotion—in particular to this latter image—arose in the twelfth century and has thrived to this day as an expression of the need to acknowledge, integrate, and give religious form to the dark side of the archetypal feminine divinity. This need is due to the fact that in Christianity the Virgin Mary came to idealize only the luminous side of the deity, thus robbing her of her dark, instinctive, emotional, and corporeal aspects.

In a similar vein, C. G. Jung considered the corporeal assumption of Mary the most significant Christian religious event since the Reformation. (On November 1, 1950, Pope Pius XII declared infallibly that the "Assumption of the Blessed Virgin Mary" was now a dogma of the Catholic faith. Likewise, the Second Vatican Council taught in the dogmatic constitution *Lumen Gentium* that "the Immaculate Virgin, preserved free from all stain of original sin, was taken up body and soul into heavenly glory when her earthly life was over and exalted by the Lord as Queen over all things.") This declaration, based on an oral tradition well over one thousand years old, united the celestial queen with the celestial king, the celestial wife with her celestial husband, a symbolic act that Jung commented on at length in his book *Answer to Job.* I will refer here to a few of his thoughts, as they are of great interest.

For Jung, the Assumptio was a sign of the times pointing toward the equality of women, women's rights, and how this equality had been finally and officially raised to the metaphysical realm in the figure of the divine woman. Here she was positioned next to the sacred trinity, Mary being received in the heavenly court as queen of the heavens and wife of God. This dogma gave comforting expression to the desire, the hope, and the anticipation of divine intervention arising from the depths of the collective unconscious as seen in the Assumptio of the Catholic Church as well as in popular religious movements and the frequent epiphanies of the Virgin. For Jung, these were powerful signs of the emerging archetype expressed in both the soul of the individual as well as in the collective, serving as a compensation to the rather apocalyptic world situation of that time. For Jung, this dogma completed St. John's apocalyptic marriage of the lamb and referred as well to the *coniunctio* of the heavenly bride and heavenly bridegroom prophesied in the day of judgment. This *coniunctio* was prefigured in the Old Testament by Sophia, a feminine figure of wisdom who we meet in the Song of Songs standing by God's side (in essence as his wife) before the Creation.[11] I will return to this theme later.

Jung points out that this *hieros gamos,* the sacred marriage, takes place in the heavens where nothing impure from the earthly realm can enter and contaminate this *coniunctio.* Jung felt that it is here that light unites with light, fulfilling the preordained plan of the Christian era that began in Christ and has continued onward to be completed before God can be incarnated in empirical man.

He further pointed out that when a longing for the exaltation of the Mother of God passes through the people, this tendency, if thought out to its logical conclusion, means the desire for the birth of a savior, a peacemaker, a mediator *pacem faciens inter inimicos,* a mediator making peace between enemies.[12] Although the savior has always existed in the pleroma, its birth in time cannot occur if it is not perceived, acknowledged, and declared by man. Pope Pius XII recognized this truth and, apparently moved by the spirit, proclaimed—much to the astonishment of the rationalists—the transcendental *declaratio solemnis* of the new dogma of the *Assumptio Mariae.*[13] Incidentally, he himself is rumored to have had several visions of the Mother of God on the occasion of the declaration.

Jung concludes his *Answer to Job* with a discussion of the dogma of the *Assumptio Mariae* and its expression of a renewed hope for the fulfillment of that yearning for peace which stirs deep down within the soul seeking a resolution of the threatening tension between the opposites. Everyone shares this tension and everyone experiences it in his or her individual form of unrest; the more rationalistic the point of view, the less one sees the possibility of getting rid of it by rational means.[14] The dogmatization of the *Assumptio Mariae* points to the *hieros gamos* in the pleroma, and this in turn implies the future birth of the divine child who, in accordance with the divine trend toward incarnation, will choose as his birthplace the empirical man. This metaphysical process is known in the psychology of the unconscious as the individuation process. If this process is to become conscious, one has to face the unconscious and seek a balance between the opposites. The symbols that make the irrational union of opposites possible arise out of this confrontation, are produced spontaneously by the unconscious, and are amplified by the conscious mind. The central symbols of this process describe the Self, which is man's totality, consisting on the one hand of that which is conscious to him and on the other hand of the contents of the unconscious. The Self is the whole man, the total and complete man, whose symbols include the divine child, the *filius solis et lunae,* mediator and *intermedius* of this process. "It has a thousand names," say the alchemists. And the source from which the individuation process arises and the goal toward which it aims is nameless, is ineffable.

Returning to the motif of the Lady of Elche, I mentioned to Marie-Louise von Franz that here another significant coincidence occurs. In the very same soil out of which its ancestral goddess was unearthed and, in one sense, reborn at the end of the last century, we find a centuries-old traditional celebration. The nucleus of all this merrymaking is the medieval *Festa* or *Misteri d'Elig,* the mystery of Elche so to speak.[15] Represented in the seventh-century Basilica of Santa María, the *Misteri* is a lyrical drama from the late Middle Ages centered on nothing less than the *Assumptio Mariae.* The legend behind this grand two-day celebration recounts that, in May 1266, a mysterious ark landed on the beach at Elche with the inscription *"Soc per Elig"* ("I am for Elche"). The ark contained the image of the Holy Virgin and a book detailing the liturgical festival and explaining the death, the heavenly assumption, and the heavenly coronation of the Virgin. Here we see how a collective symbol, brought forth by the unconscious, took hold in the populace, engendering the devotion to a mystery that thrives even unto our day. And that this tradition has again been revitalized by the discovery of a representation of the Lady of Elche, a tradition that has now extended well beyond the boundaries of a local festival. UNESCO recently granted this sculpture the status of Human Heritage, along with the Millennia Palm Tree of the city of Elche.[16]

Here is another curious coincidence, as the palm tree is symbolically related in antiquity to the motif of wisdom and is found in the Semitic mother goddesses and love goddesses such as Ishtar and Cibeles. Moreover, the palm tree is one of the attributes of the Virgin Mary. In the Koran (XIX:23) it is said that she gave birth to her Child under a palm and later was fed of its fruits.

Another point we need to consider is that on December 24, 1858, in the area of Moline de Segura (not far from Elche), a 144-kilogram meteor fell to the earth. This is the largest and most well-known meteor in Spain. From earliest times, the falling to earth of celestial bodies has been associated with premonitions announcing the presence of wondrous and portentous events. And celestial stones have been the cult objects of many divinities. It would be of interest here also to mention the Black Stone of Mecca, an exalted Muslim object of personal (not dogmatic) veneration built into the eastern wall of the Ka'bah, a small shrine built within the Great Mosque of Mecca. It dates probably from the pre-Islamic religion of the Arabs where it was worshiped, among diverse divinities, as the quaternity formed by Allach and his three daughters, the goddesses al-Lat, al-Manat, and al-Uzzá, represented by large stones, symbols of fertility. After Mohammed, legend then associated the stone with the fostering of brotherly fidelity and peace among tribes.[17] We will discuss this Islamic-Arab connection in more detail below.

The Virgin of Lledó, the patron saint of Castellón, represents a singular synergy uniting the chthonic pagan and the luminous Christian aspects of the female divinity. Here is one of the few testimonies in the world to the passage from a primitive goddess cult to that of the Christian Holy Mary, for in this reliquary of the Virgin there is a small niche in the interior in which a small white sculptural stone is kept, representing the female pagan goddess. The archeological dating of this figure is imprecise, although it purportedly originated in the Neolithic era. The legend of this stone holds that it is an image of the Virgin Mary found by a peasant plowing with a ox in 1366. The white stone was found under a dark stone next to a lledó tree, the medium-sized deciduous European nettle tree. Symbolically, the image of the Virgin of Lledó represents a process of transition and a unification of two different principles of the divine feminine. She expresses the emergence and ascension of the primordial feminine principle which we see represented in the small figure carved in the twilight of the Neolithic era, then sheltered in the earth (the womb of the unconscious), and after thousands of years of gestation, it was reborn, arising into the light of day, renewed as the light of consciousness.

Black statues of the Egyptian goddess Isis portrayed with her son Horus in her arms are well known. "The One with a thousand names" (as the Romans called her) was actually considered to be the Virgin Mary with child in Christian locations, and this may have led to the origin of the cults of the Black Virgin. Similar to the Virgin Mary, Isis was understanding and kind, able to grant miraculous cures; but contrary to Mary, Isis was also associated with destructive aspects of the feminine supreme being.[18]

Marie-Louise von Franz noted that the new principle would not be opposed to Christianity but would run parallel, that is, run vertically parallel to Christian dogma.[19] As an archetypal development, it portrays the ascent of moral conscience and the emotional contents of the unconscious moving along an axis that reaches down into the lower, inferior dimensions yet ascends upward to the upper dimensions uniting the feminine principle of eros with the masculine principle of logos. (We also see this theme in Danté's *Divine Comedy,* inspired by Virgil, where he had to pass through fire to reach Beatrice in her radiant splendor on the summit of the mountain.)

The motif of the vertical axis appears in the legend of the origin of the Basilica de Nuestra Senora del Pilar, which was the first cathedral dedicated to the Virgin. Legend has it that around 40 A.D. Mary appeared to the apostle James who was sitting on the banks of the river Ebro, the longest river in Spain, in what is today the city of Zaragoza in the northeastern region of the Iberian peninsula. She appeared sitting on a pillar between clouds where she requested him to build a chapel for her cult. Another example is the monumental project which, following the dogma of the Assumption, sought to complete the octagonal Miguelete, the bell tower of the Cathedral of Valencia that rises 60 meters above the city. The officials of the cathedral and Queen Elizabeth II of Spain wished to honor the *Assumptio Mariae* by completing the original plans for the tower, which called for the culmination of the Miguelete at a height of 150 meters. The Cathedral of Valencia, which houses and exalts the sacred chalice, would thus become the Cathedral of the Holy Grail. The chalice being the symbol of union among all of the cities of the world, the Miguelete of the Cathedral of Valencia would become more celebrated in the reality of the present than it was in legends of the past.[20]

In this manner, we see how the feminine, instinctive part of the spirit wants to become accessible to and assimilated by consciousness, thereby bringing to fruition a new, integrative vision that allows the feminine principle and the functions of feeling to be united with development of symbolic thinking, thereby enabling the individual to find personal meaning. This meaning then serves to heal and unify the internal struggle expressed through all types of anguish, tension, and personal conflict characteristic of daily life. Simultaneously, when on the collective level this synthesis is applied to a broad range of knowledge, it serves to endow sense and meaning to the disparate and diverse events of human history, to philosophy and thought, and to the manifestations of the arts and sciences.

In an article about C. G. Jung and the contemporary problems of women, Marie-Louise von Franz comments that in her therapeutic hours she herself has witnessed a considerable number of dreams of both Catholics and Protestants regarding the image of the Black Madonna of Einsiedeln.[21] During my very last visit with her, she related another dream in which she and C. G. Jung were preparing food in the "kitchen of the monastery" of the "sanctuary of the Black Madonna" in Einsiedeln.[22] It seemed in the dream as though the two, who had dedicated their life's work to the unconscious, were bequeathing to us an immense creative endeavor incorporating the whole affective aspect of feeling coupled with the breadth and depth of their intellectual arguments. This *opus magnum* helps bestow a voice and a path and a form to the emerging archetype from the unconscious that is opening the way to this synthesis of the opposites, this *hieros gamos.* And in so doing, they are preparing food for the "pilgrims to the Black Madonna." They have opened the doors, allowing us to integrate psychologically the contents of the unconscious so that, with the correct religious attitude (with attention and respect to the manifestations of the unconscious and personal experience), the underground God can emerge, expressed in the personal symbol so that the individual psychic content becomes accessible to understanding, to conscious assimilation and its concrete realization.

José Zavala once told me that Jung and von Franz when analyzing a dream had always posed the question: What here does nature want? They made every effort to bring no preconceived notions of what that may be to their analysis. In a similar manner, and without manipulation or force, they maintained a living relationship to nature and a living and feeling relationship to the objects around them which constitutes the very essence of the legacy they left us. They taught—and lived—the principle of encountering psychic and material reality with a strong and stable ego and of seeking detachment from emotionality and fascination without repressing or devaluing either. Thus they sought to foster the emotional eros relationship to objects, people, and nature itself. They lived and taught the objective psyche. And they understood—and encouraged—the transformation and transcendence of psychic contents by means of symbolic processes thus promoting their integration into consciousness. This was the creative work that they have passed on to us.

Their creative work integrates the affective aspect of feeling with the entire spectrum of intellectual reflection while "leaving the door open" so that, with the correct religious attitude, the underground God can emerge. This underground God is the personal living symbol, a psychic content accessible to intellectual comprehension, conscious assimilation, and concrete realization.

Whereas Freud put us in contact with a technique, Jung connected us with the unknown, inspiring us to encounter it, leaving neither technique nor doctrine but rather questions such as: How do psychic contents and events act in me? What effect do they have on me? What is the meaning for me? Thus he encouraged us to enlarge and take responsibility for our consciousness, much as the question about the suffering king of the Grail is asked in order to heal the illness.

Three months after this final visit, Marie-Louise von Franz passed away. During the funeral eulogies in Küsnacht, a significant event occurred for me. In his tribute to von Franz, Dr. Gottlieb Isler mentioned one of her dreams about the monastery at Einsiedeln that I had not known. It seems that in the summer of 1994, Marie-Louise von Franz was visited by a medium who wanted to persuade von Franz to collaborate with her, as she was convinced that the Christian and Buddhist spirits were united in the beyond, and thus the world could be saved. Von Franz did not answer the woman at the time but waited first to have a dream. That following night she dreamed:

> *She was working in the laundry at the monastery at Einsiedeln. She was told that Jung would return from the heavens for the wedding of the Black Virgin. And that she would belong to the one hundred elect that would participate in the festivities.*

Her reflections on the dream were that the unconscious was indeed preparing a type of salvation for the world, a union, not a union up in the ethereal realms of the spirit, but a union between above and below, a union of the spirit with matter. The Black Madonna was considered from earliest times to be of the earth, the Black Virgin being a goddess of nature. And now the union was actually taking place within the Christian context, a setting which she herself up until now had never accepted. The dream filled her with profound joy.

The rehabilitation of eros relatedness—coupled with the relationship to feeling and openness to transcendence—was the subject of one of Marie-Louise von Franz's last public lectures, entitled "Jung's Rehabilitation of the Feeling Function in Our Contemporary Civilization."[23] She noted here that we must counter the extreme polarities and conflicts of our age with the development and integration of the feminine dimensions of the psyche. And we must turn with hope to the psyche for symbols of a unifying nature that can bridge the gap between psyche and matter so that the two worlds can complement and supplement each other, progressively fostering psychic transformation both on the individual and on the collective level.

This theme was taken up again by Marie-Louise von Franz in her last letter to me a few months prior to her death in which she expressed her personal conviction that a rapprochement between Christianity and Islam would undoubtedly be the task for the future. She felt that alchemy would provide the means for this reconciliation. This comment about the unification of these two religions also referred to a discussion I had had with her regarding the sacred chalice of the Last Supper, worshipped in the Cathedral of Valencia, one of the most important symbols in occidental spirituality that, so to speak, ameliorates Moslem and Christian beliefs.[24] This relic reappeared in the Aragonese Pyrenees during the time of the grail legends that arose with the apocryphal gospel of Nicodemus, where it is said that José of Arimatea gathered the blood of Christ at the crucifixion in the chalice used at the Last Supper, and from there it made its way to the Occident. The poetic nature of this legend and the inherent symbolism were, for Marie-Louise von Franz, illustrative of the unconscious psychic processes preparing the way at that time and presaging the religious problem of modern man.

The sacred chalice is a proper cup to which a gold support with two handles has been added. Carved out of a single piece of oriental cornelian agate, the cup is reddish in color, approximately 17 cm high and 9 cm in diameter. The cup and its base are connected by a centered hexagonal column with a round nut in the middle and topped by two small plates, the upper one holding the holy chalice and the lower one supporting the structure's base. The two lateral serpentine-shaped handles (hexagonally carved) and the garniture of the base are of gold. The upper cup is purportedly the very chalice in which Jesus Christ consecrated the blood on the Thursday of the Supper. Archeological studies reveal the work was done in a Palestinian or Egyptian workshop between the fourth century B.C. and the first century A.D., and its history has been traced by some scholars back to the Last Supper.[25] The chalice has the

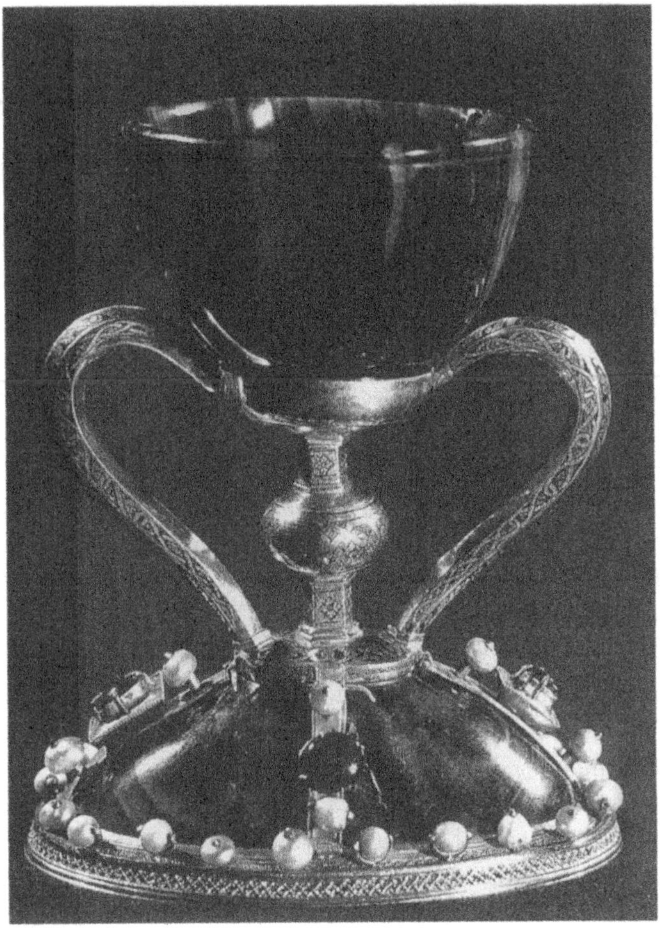

Figure 3. The chalice.

paradoxical peculiarity of being formed of two well-differentiated cup-like elements connected with two arms and a central post, all of ornate Mozarabic (Moor-Islamic) gold craftsmanship. Historically, there is nothing against the possibility of the upper cup alone—without the extensive ornamentation—having been used at the Eucharist.

History records that, shortly before his death (at the hands of the Roman emperor Valerian), Pope Sixtus II gave relics, treasures, and money to his deacon Lawrence, a native of Huesca, Spain (who was also martyred), but not before sending the Eucharistic chalice to his native city. This was around the year 258 A.D. The cup (purportedly a possession of St. Peter, who took it with him to Rome) remained in Huesca until the Moslem invasion, when it was taken in refuge to the caves of Mount Pano, the hermitage of John of Atares. The monastery of St. John of la Peña founded at this site was an important focus of the Mozarabic movement that was opposed to the Carolingian influence. The presence of the sacred chalice in the monastery of St. John of la Peña is attested to by a document dated December 14, 1134. The relic was moved to Zaragoza in 1399 by Martin, King of Aragon and Valencia. During the reign of Alfonso the Magnanimous, it was moved to Valencia. Since March 18, 1437, it has been kept in the cathedral of that city, built on the old mosque.

The lower part of the chalice consists of another cuplike form of cornelian reddish brown agate, this time inverted and surrounded by pearls, two rubylike balases, and two emeralds. This lower chalice, of Hispanic-Arabic origin from the eleventh century, is inscribed with an enigmatic text and was used as a censer in the Muslim occupied al-Andalus (Andalusia).[26] (When the Muslims entered southern Spain—which they called al-Andalus—barbarians from the north had overrun much of Europe and the classical civilizations of Greece and Rome had gone into eclipse. Islamic Spain then became a bridge by which the scientific, technological, and philosophical legacy, as well as the Judeo-Christian and Islamic theologies, were preserved to be reintegrated in Europe at the time of the Renaissance.) The chalice then constitutes not only a symbolic representation of the union of opposites interweaving Christian and Islamic elements, but actually served as an actual, physical union of the cultures as well.

This treasure belongs to the Mozarabic culture that developed in Andalusia thanks to the coexistence of Iberian Christian and Iberian Arab cultures.[27] The Iberian peninsula was in fact a cultural crossroad during the earlier centuries of the Middle Ages where Christians, Muslims, and Jews productively cohabitated for centuries. From here arose one of the most splendid civilizations in history, engendering musical, poetic, and mystic languages of incredible refinement. At its zenith in the eleventh century, it attained a cultural synthesis of an unprecedented grandeur that was the very link between Christianity, Islam, Judaism, and, of course, the Andalusian-Iberian culture. Lamentably, it was unable to endure, succumbing to the Crusades which ushered in the ensuing period of cultural and religious expulsions and inquisitions.

Within this cultural synthesis, the spirit of eros thrived for centuries. There were the Mozarabic poets in their lyrical tradition of love songs[28]; there were Muslim texts such as *The Necklace of the Dove;* there were the celebrated love stories of Cordovian Ibn Hazm (994–1063), scientist, scholar, jurist, and philosopher; or the countless poets of the Arabic Andalusian tradition, who remained autonomous and independent of the authority in Baghdad and who are considered to be the predecessors of the European troubadours and heralds of courtly and chivalrous love. Within this synthesis of traditions, the individuality of the man's anima and the equality of women were extolled. It was later that they were replaced by a collective symbolism, as in the cult of the Virgin Mary.

This synergetic tradition was then transmitted from the Iberian peninsula back to the rest of the European continent, where it was a powerful influence on alchemy and its attempt to penetrate the mysteries of nature via the principle of eros. The Cabala reached its summit with Moses de Leon (1240–1305), and the cabbalistic Zohar attained a level of spirituality equivalent to the Bible and the Talmud over a period of centuries. In the Zohar, the Shekhinah, the glory and primeval light of divine glory and wisdom is personified not only as the heavenly queen and daughter, but as the very bride of God.[29] The Shekhinah is the feminine personification of divine wisdom and, in her union with God, is at the center of the theosophical and ethical system in which the world attains harmony. The great doctrine of love of Ibn Arabi (1165–1241), a Muslim scholar born in Murcia in southern Spain, is based on a seminal vision he had as a student in which he met and received instruction from Jesus, Moses, and Muhammad. Where else but in this Arabic Andalusian era could you find the wellspring of the verses in his *Interpreter of Desires,* where he writes:

> Oh marvel! A garden amidst the flames! My heart has become capable of all forms: For gazelles, a meadow, for monks, a monastery, a temple for idols, the pilgrim's Ka'bah, the Tablets of the Torah, the Book of the Koran. I profess the religion of Love, and whatever the diction . . . Love is my religion and my faith.[30]

In respect to the manner in which the spirit of eros was expressed in the Andalusian society, it is highly significant that, after her discovery, the Lady of Elche became popularly known as the Moor Queen. From the psychological point of view, we see that within the populace the roots back to the end of the first millennium still thrived. In other words, the eros of the Islamic Mozarabic culture has remained alive for nearly one thousand years in the collective unconscious in Spain.

In that threefold culture of Spain we also find Ibn Tufayl of Cordova, the twelfth-century Spanish Arab philosopher and physician who carried on the tradition of Avempace, Spanish Arabian philosopher, physician, astronomer, mathematician, and poet. Ibn Tufayl subsequently influenced Averroes, a Spanish Arabian philosopher, astronomer, and writer on jurisprudence who furthered a nondogmatic conception critical of Islamic thought. In his work, *The Autodidactic Philosopher,* Ibn Tufayl foresees the seeds of decadence arising at that time and writes about the ethical heights attained by some members of the society which transcended collective religions, aspired to individual values, and remained open to the direct, individual experience of the unconscious by means of the quest for the personal symbol.[31] One could say that nine centuries ago Ibn Tufayl anticipated the psychology of our time.

Unfortunately, the Christian spirit imposed on Spain by the Crusades extinguished the multifaceted Mozarabic culture. Later, the Inquisition, the burning of thousands of Arab manuscripts, and the expulsion of first the Jews and then the Moors rent asunder the collective soul of these three cultures. The emerging Christian shadow configuration then swept across the Occident and ruled until our day, somehow languoring still in hope of being integrated into consciousness. Naturally, from the psychological point of view, the suppression of the shadow can be either positively or negatively influential, but such repression often has dangerous consequences. Today, in numerous cities, and in particular in the region of Valencia, annual festivities of Moorish and Christian origins celebrate a living relationship to what has become the Christian shadow.

In his memoirs, C. G. Jung speaks about his visit to Mountain Lake, the chief of the Pueblos in Taos, New Mexico, who so well described the impression that the white man has made on the Native American.[32] This chief put his finger right on the blind spot of the white man's perspective. Later, while reflecting on these issues, Jung was overwhelmed by numerous brutal images of the history of humanity. Among these, he saw the ravaging devastation at the hands of the crusaders. He saw the other face of what we describe and justify as colonization, missions, and the dissemination of civilization, that thin-eyed, thin-lipped face of the preying eagle that watches avidly and cruelly over its distant booty, a face of pirates and hijackers, robber barons and murderers: the white man on the American continents. And in the devastation of the Crusades and the Inquisition, eros and the romantic vision disappeared.

Today, this face is familiar to us, for it is this very same attitude that prevails in present-day international politics. We must only observe the fearful outcome of the latest international events which—sanctioned as a fight against terrorism under the auspices of George Bush's axis of evil—conceals, among other things, a strategy of supremacy over Iraq and the genuine covetous rapaciousness of the oil reserves of the Middle East.

In order to reestablish the syncretism and unification of these very cultures, we must search for the psychological meaning of both the great historical drama prevailing in Spain one thousand years ago and the Christian spirit that sanctioned the crusade against Islam, halting the development of the collective psyche in midstream. After the latest world events, which have shocked our lives and threaten to re-create the war between the Occidental Christian and the Islamic cultures, the words of Marie-Louise von Franz seem to anticipate the crisis, for they call for the reconciliation of the Christian and Islamic cultures, a bridging of a schism whose immediacy is paramount.

There have been some attempts to reestablish this union and some progress in this direction. One example can be found in Gotthold Ephraim Lessing's eighteenth-century play *Nathan the Wise,* in which a father bequeaths an invaluable ring and two identical copies of it to his three sons, who go to battle and then to court over which is the true ring. The key scene is one in which Nathan is forced by Saladin to declare whether Jews, Muslims, or Christians represent the true faith: he answers with a fable that is both a riddle and a plea for humility before the love of God. This allegory, possibly arising in Castile in the eleventh century, sought the fraternal spirit of the three great religions (all of which have a common father in Abraham), a spirit which seeks to unite within each of us tolerance and love without prejudice. But to attain this level of love and openness in an introverted, subjective, and personal point of view, it is necessary to reconcile the quintessential principles of Judaism, Christianity, and Islam in each of us. Jung is well known to have said that if enough people can tolerate the terrible tension of the opposites in themselves, then a third world war just might be avoidable.

Jung relates his experience of the clash with the individual shadow that he had in a dream as he was traveling in North Africa in 1920.[33] There he had the impression that time had stopped halfway. Having no occasion to actually speak to anyone about the nature of the Arab culture, he was deeply impressed by the emotional vitality of these people, a people who lived freely in affect without a great deal of reflection. The Arabs thus stood, so to speak, as an opposite pole to the European whose illusions of superiority and rationalism reign over feeling and who removes feeling and emotion from the intensity of life, thereby condemning the chthonic, emotional, and feeling aspects of the personality to (at best) a partial underground existence. In Jung's dream, he was threatened by a forceful and unexpected attack from the unconscious psyche personified in a beautiful Arab prince with whom he had to battle. Later, the prince, who had been conquered, had to sit next to Jung and read from a mysterious parchment that Jung had the impression of having written himself.

Two months after sending me her letter, Marie-Louise von Franz dreamed that she had completed her eight-volume work on Arabian alchemy. The eight volumes were set in front of her and she was exceedingly happy. Barbara Davies recalls that Marie-Louise von Franz understood the dream as saying that her lifework was now completed.[34]

During the last ten years of her life, Marie-Louise von Franz dedicated a considerable amount of her time to the writings of Muhammad Ibn Umail. Her text, *Muhammad Ibn Umail's Hall Ar-Rumuz: Clearing of Enigmas—Historical Introduction and Psychological Comment,* contains a brilliant historical survey of alchemy since Egyptian times. But above all it is a profound comment on a newly translated Arabic alchemical text from the tenth century. Ibn Umail, known in Latin alchemy by the name of Senior from Andalusia, was both an alchemist and mystic whose alchemical work is a symbolic rendering of his experience of an inner psychic process of transformation that he considered to be the highest goal in human life. Due to his extremely introverted lifestyle and his devotion toward the inner world, Ibn Umail was able to observe and describe this mysterious process with substantial symbols emerging out of the depth of his psyche. Von Franz was very pleased on the day shortly before her death that she actually first held her published work in her hands. Jung also considered that individual knowledge of one's psyche was the paramount task of life. His investigations into the psychological symbolism of the alchemical processes—meticulously elucidated in alchemical treatises—are nothing less than symbolic encounters with what Jung called the individuation process. In his memoirs, he says that, with the completion of his *Mysterium Coniunctionis,* his life's work was concluded and fulfilled.[35]

From the point of view of the historical development of the spirit, alchemy (as a medieval philosophy) was a philosophical science that compensated the attempt on the part of Christianity to repress and overcome physical nature and matter. Alchemy, on the contrary, attempted to redeem the spirit contained in matter.

In 1938, occupied with his studies on alchemy, Jung traveled to India. There he dreamed that he met a group of friends on a small island off the southern coast of England. On this island there was a castle in which a celebration of the Holy Grail was going to occur that night. But before this celebration could take place, Jung had to rescue his friends. He understood the dream as challenging his very purpose in India when he should be searching "at home" for the Holy Grail, that European sacred vessel, that *salavator mundi.* It was as though the dream was challenging him not to run away from what had been built up down through the centuries in the West.[36]

Through this dream he understood that whatever the impressions he may have in this eastern land, India was not his mission but a point of passage along his road. He nevertheless contemplated and marveled at what he felt was the secret of Islam, the supreme flower and invaluable jewel of Islamic eros, the Taj Mahal, that sublime expression of human love for another human being. Here was eros in its purest form, like a plant that could not have grown and flourished in any other land.[37] This mausoleum is enthralled in a legend that recounts that the emperor Shah Jehan contracted the architects to build this magnificent palace for his wife, the empress Mumtaz Mahal ("the exalted one of the palace"). This marriage was a real love match, and Mumtaz was her husband's inseparable companion on all of his journeys and military expeditions. She was his comrade and counselor, and she inspired him to acts of charity and benevolence toward the weak and the needy. She bore him fourteen children and died in childbirth in 1630 (only three years after his accession to the throne). Overpowered by grief, Shah Jehan was determined to commemorate her memory for all eternity and decided to build his beloved wife the finest sepulcher ever—a monument of eternal love. Thus, over a period of twenty-two years, this splendorous mausoleum of white marble was built on the riverbanks of the Yumuna in the capital. Shah Jehan planned to build a bridge of silver to connect the white mausoleum to his own sepulcher in black on the other side of the gardens and pools in front of her palace. His project was interrupted by the rebellion of one of his sons, who imprisoned him in the crypt of the Taj Mahal where he died. Thus, the souls of husband and wife are entwined in an eternal embrace.

The motif of the Grail (the sacred vessel discussed by Emma Jung and Marie-Louise von Franz in their book *The Grail Legend*) represents the vessel in which the unifying and healing essence of the feminine is integrated and contained. The Grail was the sacred object of the quest of the knights and the objective of their highest ideals. Wolfram von

Eschenbach's *Parsifal*, the earliest complete Grail romance in European prose, is rightly regarded as one of the great works of Western literature. Written in the twelfth century, the book was purportedly found among many abandoned Arabic manuscripts in Toledo.[38]

The motif of the Grail coincides with alchemical motifs such as the *unun vas, una medicina,* and *unus lapis* with which the alchemists sought to bring about the union of opposites.[39] Indispensable to the lapis, this *coniunctio* is the very goal of alchemy and the cure of all inequity. This union begins with work on the *prima materia* including the indispensable participation of the spirit of eros hermetically contained in the *vas alchemico.* The reconciliation of seemingly incompatible opposites could not occur in a natural way but rather was the fruit of intense human effort.

A legend parallel to the motif of the Grail or *vas alchemico* is found among the myths of earliest Andalusian culture in which Muslim, Christian, and Jew quested to find Solomon's Table, a wondrous table purportedly carved from emerald that was claimed to have been found in Toledo when the Arabs arrived.[40] The legend has it that it belonged to King Solomon and was taken in his day from Jerusalem to Rome and then from there brought to Spain by the Goths (fifth to seventh century). The emerald is said to be the stone of Hermes, and it plays an important role in connection with his famous treatise *Tabula Smeragdina* that relates the essence of the alchemical opus and the thirteen principles of Hermes Trismegistus, the enigmatic Egyptian god and/or wise man and author of the hermetic works. Jung says that this emerald table can be compared to the Grail, but that the table is more connected with the effort to become conscious, gathering together all dissociated parts of the personality into a whole.[41]

Marie-Louise von Franz points out that the table serves as a bearer and a base for the Grail, thus attributing a slightly different meaning, a meaning which has more to do with the human effort required in striving for wholeness, the wholeness expressed in receptiveness and in the very essence of the Grail itself.[42] Thus the table represents an aspect of collective consciousness striving for the Self.

Solomon, the son of King David, was an enigmatic king of antiquity who attained mythological status. He is best known for his poetry and wisdom (which purportedly exceeded that of all of the wise men of Egypt and the East), for building the Temple of Jerusalem, and for his celebrated encounter with the Queen of Sheba. In his *Book of Proverbs* (8:12–31), Solomon exalts Wisdom to be the very counterpart of Yahweh; she was with the Lord as he prepared the heavens before the waters, the earth, the hills and mountains were formed. Solomon ushered in a new era in Judaism, promoting peace and harmony in Israel. Many renowned Jewish thinkers see the prefiguration of the messianic kingdom in his philosophy, his love, his wisdom, and his lifework. Thus, from the psychological point of view, Solomon's table represents the intense conscious effort required to realize the union of opposites, in this case, those of Christianity and Islam.

For Jung, the union of opposites was not only a long and tortuous struggle, but a loving adventure out of whose fecundity the synthesis of the *coniunctio* arose.[43] The alchemical philosophers searched for this "living being" in the retort, that hermetic vessel, the womb which held the opposites and contained and distilled the smoky vapor, alluding to the spiritual yet highly evasive nature of Mercurius, the vital principle of the collective unconscious which can unite the opposites with eros, with love, with the feminine principle itself. This containment, this distillation, is a necessity when encountering psychic contents. It is a work that must be carried out in an individual and introverted way. And the feminine principle of relatedness—along with the feeling function—are indispensable for this process. With respect to the problem of the shadow in the individual or the collective, here a new content arises from the world of instinct compensating conscious attitudes. We must learn to accept and live with this world in the hopes that it can be integrated and assimilated. But this task can be carried out only if the psychological dimension of the feeling function is included. That is, if the psychological dimension is based in, and carried by, the archetypal principle of the essence of eros and the feminine spirit.

Returning to the motif of the Mozarabic chalice, it is important to point out again that this chalice represents the quintessence of the synthesis of two coexistent cultures, the Christian and the Islamic. And although this culture was progressively extinguished, the chalice remains today an inextinguishable symbol that would compensate the destiny of this culture, which began to unfold approximately one thousand years ago. A glimpse and a premonition of this destiny is seen in the *Cantar del mio Cid*, a poem written in the mid twelfth century about the universal Spanish hero El Cid, the Castilian Rodrigo Diaz de Bivar, who accomplished the remarkable feats of capturing the rich Muslim kingdom of Valencia and holding it as his own and of being the first of the Christian leaders to defeat the Almoravides, a warlike band of zealots from North Africa. The poem concentrates on his relationship with King Alfonso VI of Leon-Castile. Like many feudal epics, *The Lay of El Cid* portrays the breakdown of the vassal-lord relationship due to some shortcoming of the lord and the manner in which the vassal attempts to deal with this situation, and reaches a climax and resolution in a detailed account of a formal trial. But what is most interesting to us is that King Alfonso appears in the poem without the company of his queen, psychologically indicating that the dominant Christian collective consciousness that would invade and conquer Spain—and the rest of Europe—would have no relationship to the feminine. It would not be able to meet the collective task of unifying and redeeming the opposites, but once unchained, would extinguish the synergetic union of peoples and religions of the Mozarabic culture and radically promote the confrontation between cultures, which would turn out to be irreconcilable.

The reconciliation between the Christian and Islamic cultures in contemporary times will never be carried out on the intellectual or rational level alone. To restore or reintegrate the feminine principle, it will be indispensable to include feminine eros, which, as Marie-Louise von Franz pointed out, is a task that begins in each of us and unfolds in an individual and subjective manner. Within the context of analytical psychology—the modern key to the alchemical and Mozarabic cultures bequeathed to us by C. G. Jung and Marie-Louise von Franz—we can foster and promote this task which, by means of psychological insight, can facilitate the understanding of history, just as historical events can, in turn, throw new light on the question of individual psychology.

I want to express my personal, deep-felt gratitude to Marie-Louise von Franz for helping me grapple with and understand these materials, for her warm encouragement, for her intellectual stimulus, and for pointing out psychological and historical parallels and amplifications that enabled me to continue my investigations. And—*Deo concedente*—may these reflections help to encourage and support others in a similar way.

NOTES

1. Barbara Davies, "Zu Leben und Werk von Marie-Louise von Franz," *Jungiana*, no. 8 (Küsnacht: Verlag Stiftung für Jung'sche Psychologie, 1998).
2. The author uses the word *synchronicity* to mean two relatively coinciding events which correspond in meaning but which have no casual connection. This reflects the more popular usage of the term which refers not to an actual synchronicity per se, but to the principles of acausal orderedness and the *unus mundus*, the underlying principles of synchronicity. Jung and von Franz define synchronicity as a special instance of the *unus mundus* in which a conjunction of psyche and matter appears as a creative act—and here is the critical point: in a singular moment in time demonstrating a spontaneous manifestation of inner and outer realities which coincide in their meaning. See M.-L. von Franz, *Number and Time: Reflections Leading toward a Unification of Depth Psychology and Physics* (Evanston, Ill.: Northwestern University Press, 1974), pp. 6ff, 11f.—*Ed.*
3. Rafaelo Ramos, *La Dama de Elche* (Valencia: Albatros, 1997), p. 37.
4. Marie-Louise von Franz, *Alquimia: Introducción al Simbolismo y a la Psicologia* (Barcelona: Luciérnaga, 1991), p. 246.
5. *Mensajes de la Virgen de Medjugorj* (Barcelona: Ed. Obelisco, 1995).
6. M.-L. von Franz, "Nike and the Waters of Styx," in *Archetypal Dimensions of the Psyche* (Boston: Shambhala, 1997), p. 263.
7. The Benedictine Monastery and Cathedral in Einsiedeln harbors a statue of the Black Madonna, a Catholic icon to whom pilgrimages are made throughout the year. The Black Madonna receives adoration and prayers in particular from childless women seeking assistance in conception and childbirth.
8. *Las Provincias*, Valencia, March 15, 1996.
9. José Zavala, "Simbolos en el prólogo de Enrique V d' William Shakespeare," seminar of the Analytical Psychology Group of Valencia, April 1996.
10. Dieter Baumann, "The Dialas: The Voice of Natural Feminine Spirits in the Region of Grisons, Switzerland," the Analytical Psychology Group of Valencia, IX Meeting, Summer 1994.
11. For Jung, Sophia represents the fourth stage of the development of the anima after

Eve, Helen of Troy, and Mary. In the man, she would be a guide to the inner life bringing a conscience to contents of the unconscious, fostering the search for meaning, and being the creative spirit in the life of an artist, scientist, and the like.

12. C. G. Jung, *Answer to Job* (1952), in *CW,* vol. 11 (Princeton, N.J.: Princeton University Press, 1958), par. 748.
13. Ibid., par. 251n. Jung had foreseen the coming declaration of the *Assumptio Mariae* ten years earlier as an inevitable conclusion of the Catholic doctrine of *conclusion probabilis* followed by the *conclusio certa.*
14. Ibid., pars. 754ff.
15. "L'organiasacio de la Festa de Elig a traves del temps," Generalidad Valenciana, 1997.
16. The statue of the Lady of Elche was granted this honor in May 2001, the Palm Tree of Elche in November 2001.
17. The Romanesque Monastery in Montserrat, Catalonia, is also worth mentioning as one of the most popular shrines to the Black Virgin. The monastery itself was built at the base of spectacular mountainous rock formations and has been the site of pilgrimages for thousands of years.
18. Brigitte Jacobs, "From the Egyptian Goddess Isis to the Christian Mary," *Jungiana.*
19. I wish to thank Dr. José Zavala for this information.
20. Juan Angel Oñate, *El Santo Grial: Su historia, su culto y sus destinos* (Valencia, 1972), p. 73.
21. *Jungiana,* no. 6, 1996.
22. I am indebted to Brigitte Jacobs for this information.
23. "C. G. Jungs Rehabilitation der Gefühlsfunktion in unserer Zivilisation," published in *Beiträge zur Jung'schen Psychologie: Festschrift zum 75. Geburtstag von Marie-Louise von Franz,* J. F. Zavala, G. Ruska, and R. Monzo, eds. (Valencia: Victor Orenga, Editores, S.L., 1980).
24. Antonia Beltrán, "El Santo Cáliz de la Catedral de Valencia," Zaragoza, 1960.
25. Salvador Alea Antuñano, "The Mystery of the Holy Grail: Tradition and Legend of the Sacred Chalice." Antuñano is professor of ethics and sacred scripture at the Francisco de Vitoria University Center in Madrid. A photo of the chalice can seen at: www.rosslyntemplars.org.uk/holy_grail.htm.
26. The inscription, in Sufic Arabic, could be translated either as LIL ZAHIRA, "the most flourishing," or LI-LZAHIRATI, "for that which glitters."
27. Leopoldo Penarroja, *Christianos bajo el Islam* (Madrid: Gredos).
28. Alvaro Galmés De Fuentes, *Las Jarchas Mozárabes* (Barcelona: Critica, 1994), p. 120.
29. Gershom G. Scholem, *Major Trends in Jewish Mysticism* (New York: Schocken Books, 1961), p. 230.
30. Ibn 'Arabi, *Tarjuman al-Ashwaq* (*The Interpreter of Desires*), translated by Claude Addas and Peter Kingsley, in *The Quest for the Red Sulphur: The Life of Ibn 'Arabi* (Cambridge: Islamic Texts Society, 1993), p. 211. A similar idea is expressed by the

Sufi master Bawa Muhaiyaddeen: "You are a Christian because you believe in Jesus, and you are a Jew because you believe in all the prophets including Moses. You are a Muslim because you believe in Muhammad as a prophet, and you are a Sufi because you believe in the universal teaching of God's love. You are really none of those, but you are all of those because you believe in God. And once you believe in God, there is no religion. Once you divide yourself off with religions, you are separated from your fellowman." See also Miguel Asin Palacios, ed., *Amor Humano, Amor Divino: Ibn Arabi* (Córdoba: El Almendro, 1990).

31. Ibn Tufayl, *The Autodidactic Philosopher,* Trotta, ed. (Valladolid, 1995).
32. Seix Barral, ed., *Recuerdos, suenos y pensamientos* (Barcelona, 1964), p. 254.
33. Ibid., p. 249.
34. *Jungiana,* no. 8, 1998.
35. Barral, *Recuerdos, suenos y pensamientos,* p. 254.
36. Ibid., p. 287.
37. C. G. Jung, "The Dreamlike World of India" (1939), in *CW,* vol. 10 (Princeton, N.J.: Princeton University Press, 1964), par. 990.
38. Pierre Ponsoye, *El Islam y el Grial* (Palma de Mallorca: Olaneta, 1984), p. 19.
39. Barral, *Recuerdos, suenos y pensamientos,* p. 289.
40. Ibn Al-Kardabus, *Historia de Al-Andaluis* (Barcelona: Akal, 1986).
41. Emma Jung and Marie-Louise von Franz, *The Grail Legend,* chap. 9.
42. Ibid.
43. C. G. Jung, *Mysterium Coniunctionis* (1955-56), *CW,* vol. 14 (Princeton, N.J.: Princeton University Press, 1963), pars. 104–348.

Nibby

A Deeply Loved But Very Difficult Master

HANS NIGGLI

Dr. med. vet. Hans Niggli
Sonnenfeldstrasse 28
CH-8702 Zollikon
February 13, 2002

Dear Dr. Kennedy,

Yesterday, as I was celebrating my seventy-seventh birthday, the letter from the Psychology Club of Zürich arrived in regards to the Festschrift for Dr. Marie-Louise von Franz.

I became acquainted with Dr. von Franz over thirty years ago and had the honor of being her faithful companion during many years of medical treatment. Dr. von Franz had an extraordinary understanding of her male English bulldogs. As you can see in the two letters that I have enclosed, Nibby was a deeply loved but very "difficult Master." I am personally very interested in the psychology of complex animal personalities. That English bulldog was truly not easy. He played first fiddle in that household, was extraordinarily self-conscious, and he could assert his presence at any time.

Already in his first consultation at my practice he adamantly refused to be lifted onto the treatment table. As I avoid forcing an animal to do anything whenever possible, I had the idea of building a staircase of sorts up to the table out of the cushions of the chairs in the waiting room in order to give Nibby the possibility of climbing up onto the table himself. I then said to him: "Lord, Barron, may I request your presence . . ." I must emphasize that I have never devoted such procedures to any other animal. But Nibby was a great personality who then reciprocated this courtesy with amiable compliance and friendliness. Marie-Louise von Franz and I enjoyed how much this animal appreciated our obliging manner. And thus I was able to avoid a confrontation with Nibby during many consultations.

The 19th of October, 1973, was a day I will never forget. Dr. von Franz brought Nibby to me in the practice as he had become very animated during the previous night on account of a neighboring dog in heat. I examined him: his body temperature was 38.9°—which was normal—his pulse at 120 was the same. The auscultation of the heart with the stethoscope was inconspicuous. Suddenly Nibby became terribly agitated, collapsed in my arms, and unfortunately I could then only ascertain that the animal had died. Across from us, Dr. von Franz sat quietly and apparently not flustered. The next day, she wrote me a few encouraging lines assuring me that I must not reproach myself. She noted that she had fully experienced the death of her friend yet must admit that she much preferred this sudden death where, without suffering and without flaring up in his oftentimes overly excited manner, Nibby could die a completely natural death.

On my advice, five years later Dr. von Franz acquired another English bulldog, this time a female, the females undoubtedly being more understanding, gentle, and capable of adaptation than their male counterparts. Dr. von Franz truly enjoyed this dog. Unfortunately, this female had heart problems when she was nine years old. Apparently, after many months of complications, she suddenly died of a heart attack in the night of the 16th of December, 1987.

I will never forget the encounters with Dr. von Franz and her friend Nibby.

With kind regards,
E. B. Niggli

(date unknown)

Dear Dr. Niggli

Before I pay your (very modest) bill, I wish to thank you wholeheartedly for your patience with Nibby. He is well again and in high spirits apparently because he has no more pain. I do not know what I would have done with him if I had not found you. You are a "magical physician" with difficult dogs.

In case you and your wife are in Bollingen next summer, please pay us a visit. Behind our house there is a beautiful forest where many horseback riders enjoy themselves. We are there in July, August, September and up through the 20th of October.

Warm greetings and many thanks! from your
Marie-Louise von Franz

Lindenbergstrasse 15
8700 Küsnacht

(date unknown)

Dear Dr. Niggli,

I do not want to neglect thanking you for your very kind understanding of our "complicated Master," our English bulldog. His ears are still O.K. He is a very much loved, old and "difficult Master," and I am very happy that you understand him so well.

Sincerely yours,
Marie-Louise von Franz

P.S. Nibby ceremoniously raises his paw.

Sometimes Individuation Must Take the Place of the Church

GERTRUDE OGGENFUSS

Marie-Louise von Franz once said that "sometimes individuation must take the place of the church." According to Mr. Emmanuel Kennedy, she made this comment after she had written a lecture about individuation and Christianity and subsequently dreamed that a church had to be destroyed so that a tree could grow at that location. The audience at the lecture where she reported this dream was apparently shocked. This in turn clearly indicates that the theme is controversial.

I was told about this lecture because on October 20, 1991, I had a very similar dream:

> *I was sitting in a churchlike building built around a palm tree. Apparently somebody had tied an elephant onto the building and then encouraged it to pull the building forward. Suddenly, the building broke into two pieces from the roof down. It looked dangerous, but I remained quietly sitting on a church pew. Both sections of the roof fell slowly and*

simultaneously down toward the back. The palm tree remained precisely above me. One now had an open view of the heavens.

I assume that Marie-Louise von Franz's dream was a confirmation of the thesis that she presented in her lecture as well as the quintessence of the whole theme. In my case, the dream wanted to show me a personal situation in regard to an important issue in my individuation, namely, the opposition between individuality and collectivity and in particular my attitude toward these two.

The dream came two years after the commencement of my analysis, that is, in the "beginning phase" so to speak. However, in these initial two years I had become well enough prepared by previous experiences of the entirely new and completely unfamiliar paths of thought characteristic of Jungian psychology—which I experienced as positive and healing—thus I was able to accept the message of the dream. But I know that at that time I was by far not conscious enough of what this would mean to me.

Similar dreams can be found in Jung's *Psychology and Alchemy*, in the chapter about mandala symbolism. For example, a theologian dreamed that:

He entered into his church at night. There the wall behind the choir had collapsed. The altar and the ruins were overgrown with vines hanging with grapes, and the moon shone through the gap in the wall.[1]

And later Jung refers to the dream of a man who was occupied by religious matters and who dreamt that:

He comes upon an immense Gothic cathedral, almost completely dark. High Mass is being celebrated. Suddenly the whole wall of the aisle collapses. Blinding sunlight bursts into the interior together with a large herd of bulls and cows.[2]

All four dreams deal with the same theme. My dream gives me a feeling of a connection with other people who have had similar dreams although I know that the dreams I have mentioned have other motifs as well. For me, it showed the one-sidedness of my standpoint and alluded to the need to become conscious of the problem of the opposites that has been concerning me for years. Collectivity, convention, and tradition—in particular, with respect to religion—always counted in my life as the highest ranking values, while individuality was held suspect.

If I try to look at my dream in the context of the title of this essay, I can naturally only do so in Jungian terms. I will cite a few quotations even though I actually should start with quotation marks before the first word and close them after the last. In other words, everything that I write about I have learned from C. G. Jung and Marie-Louise von Franz. I would actually prefer just to present quote upon quote, because what I say with my own words is, comparatively speaking, rather banal. And yet I must try to do so just the same since Jung said quite clearly that one can only pay the debt for individuality with one's own creativity.

Individuality and the church as an institution stand juxtaposed to one another; one could say "collectivity versus individuality." In any event, this opposition expresses a deep religious problem. The sheer force of tradition can be so powerful that a secret doubt is not even noticed. The traditional forms are indeed more comfortable to maintain even if they have become hollow. That secret doubt would actually be infinitely valuable. Jung said, in his book *Dream Analysis,* that "doubt is the very crown of life because therein truth and error come together. Doubting is life, truth is sometimes death and stagnation. When we doubt, we have the greatest chance to unify the dark and the light sides of life."[3] In her introduction to the Eranos Conference of 1949, Olga Frobe-Kapteyn said it very beautifully: "Only the uncertain path, the path with no guarantees, offers us the possibility of reading the signs. . . . The uncertain path is the promising, the fertile, and at the same time the only path which remains open and receptive to truth."[4] At the time of my dream, I did not have the courage to shake the "official" version of the truth which, after all, is two thousand years old. In my dream, it is the elephant that shakes the structures . . . and with success. I recall having read in Jung's works that at times something good has to be destroyed for the sake of something better. The collapse of the church here apparently does not mean the destruction of the authority of the church per se. (In "Archetypes of the Collective Unconscious," Jung discusses the extinction of the power of the church and writes that it is like "a house whose walls have been plucked away, exposed to all the winds of the world and to all dangers."[5])

My own one-sided, conventional attitude should actually shock me, should become for me conscious, in order to be expanded by its opposite. I ask myself here why I am not shocked in this dream. Would it not be natural to have been shocked? I believe that my lack of reaction shows my religious attitude at that time. I had a faith that blindly accepted everything that comes from above without contradiction. And thus I did not regard my own nature, neither did I integrate it. In fact, I repressed it. Here it appeared in the form of the palm and the elephant and showed me that they are stronger than what I would ascribe as "religion." It only took a bit of shaking for the roof of the church to collapse. This power I now have to confront. I think that it is above all the nature of the feminine that must, justifiably, receive its due.

In Marie-Louise von Franz's book, *The Visions of Niklaus von Flüe,* one sees this aspect. There she writes: "The last vision of Brother Claus clearly shows that it is not the intention of the unconscious to destroy Christian symbolism but to extend and augment this symbolism with that of the feminine and that of the common man."[6] This quote seems to me to be the quintessence of my dream. The feminine-motherly quality of the tree and the palm are elements that I must not underestimate. This is similar to a motif in my first dream of analysis where the potato plant played a main role. Here, the fruit and the leaves of the potato are just below and just above the surface of the earth. On the path of individuation both of the dimensions seen in the palm tree must be extended.

I believe that, in the meantime, the necessary process is underway. There have been dreams that have taken up this theme again. However, due to my own personal work on myself, the process of individuation is now beginning to really grow. To show a bit of this development, I would like to mention a dream from September 29, 1997, that came approximately in the middle of the period of time between 1991 and 2002. In the dream,

> *I went to a church. In the front stood the pope, fully alone. None of the people passing by noticed him. I also did not turn to him.*

The experience of the divinity in nature is apparently more highly esteemed by the Self than that which is experienced traditionally in the church. In my dream of the palm tree, the divinity of nature would seem to be highly valued, although for other people the church can be a synonym for individuation. For me, individuation involves the integration of newly acknowledged values, that is, those of nature and of instincts and drives. These belong unconditionally to wholeness. This means that I must grapple with these aspects of nature in order to approach my own truth, and in my pursuit I must accept and carry both my errors and my uncertainty. It apparently also means to take up my own guilt since, as Jung said, there is no expansion of consciousness without guilt. This third path which passes down the middle of the extremes is no comfortable one, but it is undoubtedly a more fulfilling one, neither hollow nor commonplace.

Apparently, the path to a new attitude can only be prepared by a radical event, for example, the collapse of a church roof. That this is actually a positive act I first discovered only through the interpretation of the dream. My ego-consciousness naturally believed at first that the collapse of the roof was an error. I thought that this should not have happened. But now much later, I experience that my horizon has been expanded and that nature is coming to her own right, thus a balance is created which belongs to becoming whole and to individuation per se. Church and religion must be brought into a unity with nature and the nature of men and women. Here Jungian psychology makes an inestimable contribution.

I have the task of sacrificing a large piece of tradition and convention in order to discover myself and to live in accordance with my own nature. Because it is a dream, it means that this is a demand of the Self. I must now ask why it is making this demand of me. There are in fact various reasons. I must recognize the one-sidedness of my standpoint. I need to acknowledge the opposites within and avoid identifying with one or the other. I should strive to recognize resistances and thus overcome them. And I have to struggle to attain the union of the opposites, that is, to expand tradition and convention with renewed, independent, and natural thought.

In the first twenty-one years of my life, I lived in a very Catholic setting, and I actually lived with nuns the last six of those years. This religious convention became for me a life-conditioning factor where fundamental questions were hardly allowed and doubt was sin. I remained attached to this institution long after I had left, and I let myself be constricted and spoon-fed. As Jung writes in his article, "On the Nature of the Psyche," I was wedged into a "collectively accepted system of religious statements neatly codified as dogmatic precepts" in the precincts of collective consciousness.[7] Jung goes on to say:

> If the subjective consciousness prefers the ideas and opinions of collective consciousness and identifies with them, then the contents of the collective unconscious are repressed. . . . The more highly charged the collective consciousness, the more the ego forfeits its practical importance. It is, as it were, absorbed by the opinions and tendencies of the collective consciousness, and the result of that is the mass man, the ever-ready victim of some wretched "ism." The ego keeps its integrity only if it does not identify with one of the opposites, and if it understands how to hold the balance between them. This is possible only if it remains conscious of both at once. However, the necessary insight is made exceedingly difficult not by one's social and political leaders alone, but also by one's religious mentors. They all want decision in favor of one thing, and therefore the utter identification of the individual with a necessarily one-sided "truth." Even if it were a question of some great truth, identification with it would still be a catastrophe, as it arrests all further spiritual development. Instead of knowledge, one then has only belief, and sometimes that is more convenient and therefore more attractive.[8]

It is apparently impossible to become independent and stand alone with a collective setting such as the Catholic church. Jung writes, in

The Symbolic Life, that he has never found "a community which would allow 'full expression to the individual within it.'"[9] As mentioned, certain values must be retained. The tree appearing in place of the church in my dream indicates that another form of mothering should be preserved. I assume that it is the quality of protection, shade, and nutrition provided by the tree. It is the natural aspect of mothering, not an artificial wall which holds a person fast and hinders development.

The collapse of the church roof in the dream effectively extends sight and opens one up to light and fresh air. My life is thus enriched. I can only ask the question, since it is the church roof that has collapsed, should I give up my faith? But what does "faith" mean? I cannot express it better than C. G. Jung, who writes in his *Symbols of Transformation:*

> "Legitimate" faith must always rest on experience. There is, however, another kind of faith which rests exclusively on the authority of tradition. This kind of faith could also be called "legitimate," since the power of tradition embodies an experience whose importance for the continuity of culture is beyond question. But with this kind of faith there is always the danger of mere habit supervening—it may so easily degenerate into spiritual inertia and a thoughtless compliance which, if persisted in, threatens stagnation and cultural regression. This mechanical dependence goes hand in hand with a psychic regression to infantilism. The traditional contents gradually lose their real meaning and are only believed in as formalities, without this belief having any influence on the conduct of life.[10]

In this area of religion fall the opposites good and evil. To exaggerate a bit: earlier I thought that it was good to choose tradition, and in particular religious tradition. When, in Jungian psychology, one finds oneself confronted with the problem of good and evil in a new manner, then the roof of the church really does begin to shake and fall apart. Since not only that which must be destroyed is destroyed, but new values were also shown, I did not become panicked in the dream. The open view of the heavens—as well as the palm—are substitutes for that which is lost.

This quote—"Sometimes individuation must take the place of the church"—expresses the deep conflict between convention and individuality. Deep conflict also indicates deep resistance. How do I deal with it? I must attentively turn to this question time and again. And this is close to Jung's definition of *religio* in *Mysterium Coniunctionis,* which he defines as a careful consideration of what happens, "a continual flow of interest [by ego-consciousness] toward the unconscious, a kind of constant attention . . . which might also be called devotion."[11] This would be practically the opposite of religious confession.

I am reminded here of Jung's experience of the Basel cathedral as a youth in which he allowed himself to think the unthinkable thought: the roof of the church burst asunder due to a reason that probably no other human being would have accepted—a large pile of excrement thundered down upon the roof from God's heavenly throne—a truly monstrous image. But where would we be today if he had been closed to unconventional thought?

If the church is substituted by individuation, and if this is done in the service of the Self, then this is a liberation from coercive constraints that block the path to the development of a true individual. The quote at the beginning of this essay holds the problem and the answer. I do well to follow that individual path. My dream and Marie-Louise von Franz are my guides.

NOTES

1. C. G. Jung, *Psychology and Alchemy* (1944), *CW,* vol. 12. (Princeton, N.J.: Princeton University Press, 1953), par. 179.
2. Ibid., par. 180.
3. C. G. Jung, *Dream Analysis: Notes of a Seminar given in 1928–1930,* William McGuire, ed. (Princeton, N.J.: Princeton University Press, 1984), p. 89.
4. Olga Frobe-Kapteyn, ed., *Eranos Jahrbuch* (Zürich: Rhein Verlag, 1950), p. 6.
5. C. G. Jung, "Archetypes of the Collective Unconscious" (1954), in *CW,* vol. 9i (Princeton, N.J.: Princeton University Press, 1959), par. 23.
6. M.-L. von Franz, *The Visions of Niklaus von Flue* (Einsiedeln: Daimon Verlag, in preparation), S.109.
7. C. G. Jung, "On the Nature of the Psyche" (1954), in *CW,* vol. 8 (Princeton, N.J.: Princeton University Press, 1960), par. 426.

8. Ibid., par. 425.
9. C. G. Jung, *The Symbolic Life. CW,* vol. 18 (Princeton, N.J.: Princeton University Press, 1977), par. 1676.
10. C. G. Jung, *Symbols of Transformation* (1952), *CW,* vol. 5 (Princeton, N.J.: Princeton University Press, 1956), par. 345.
11. C. G. Jung, *Mysterium Coniunctionis* (1955–56), *CW,* vol. 14 (Princeton, N.J.: Princeton University Press, 1963).

A Dream with an Owl

MARTA SUSANA PÉREZ

Dear Mr. Kennedy,

I'm enclosing herewith a small contribution for the Festschrift honoring Dr. Marie-Louise von Franz. The paper tries to convey the impression, dreams, and feelings of a little group of friends who live in Argentina and have been studying Jungian psychology since the 1970s. Hoping your efforts will be fruitful and full of meaning, I remain yours very sincerely,

Marta Susana Pérez

As a little group of friends who are not analysts, we've been studying for years C. G. Jung's psychology, moved in spite of our individual differences by a common need of giving form to ourselves. The first book was the Spanish version of *Man and His Symbols.* It was there that we met for the first time Marie-Louise von Franz and immediately respected and admired her. These feelings did not cease to increase all along these years, all the more as we began translating and reading in common her works. It was thanks to our contact with Dr. Monzó and the Valencia group that we became acquainted with some anecdotes and details concerning her personality that brought her nearer us.

However, many years before this contact, even before we came to know about her last illness, one of us had this dream:

> *Dr. von Franz comes to Zavalla. I meet her in the village, talk to her, and she tells me that she is very ill, that she isn't even able to walk anymore.*

This dream was very significant to the dreamer, for her presence in his dream in a personal contact with him, and in the village where he was living in reality, was a sort of corroboration about the seriousness of his efforts concerning the work on himself.

Another member of the group, a woman, dreamed once that

> *Dr. von Franz had a woman analysand and told this one that she (the patient) had to make contact with an Arab woman, but at the same time with her own husband and with her lover, who were opposite between themselves.*

Apart from the personal value the dream had for the dreamer, this woman did not know, at the time she had this dream, that Dr. von Franz had written a book about eros in the Arabic alchemy.

Another woman of the group dreamed once that

> *Marie-Louise von Franz and Barbara Hannah were in relation to an owl, and oddly enough, it seemed in the dream that they themselves were owls.*

The owl was a recurrent motif in the woman's dreams and pointed to the feminine and the ability to "see in the darkness."

We all felt very impressed in reading Marie-Louise von Franz's marvelous interpretations of fairy tales. There was one of them especially, "The Girl Without Hands," that more than once had a synchronistic effect on the reader: it arrived "just in time," saying "the right word," for what the reader was unconsciously expecting, all the more if his or her actual circumstance was especially difficult or full of conflict, and consequently, of emotionality.

Although we knew through Dr. Monzó that she was seriously ill, the news of her death caused us a great distress. Moved by a feeling toward her, in February 1998 we decided to read in common various passages of her work, as a sort of private and intimate homage.

Words can convey only a part of feelings when they are deep enough; however, we want to render with this paper a humble tribute to what she and Jungian psychology mean in our lives.

Pagan in the Head—Christian in the Heart

GORM RASMUSSEN

In the early spring of 1991, I had the pleasure of visiting and interviewing Marie-Louise von Franz for the Danish Broadcasting Corporation's radio. She was already very ill and frail, so it was a truly magnanimous gesture to allow me to come.

I remember vividly the sticker on the mailbox outside the villa in Küsnacht. Printed in large and very determined letters, it said, "no advertisements." The words reminded me of something she had written somewhere about the damaging effects of advertising and propaganda. It was clear that both would be wise to keep away.

I rang the doorbell, and after a long wait I heard labored footsteps, and finally the door was opened by the lady herself, a white-haired woman with a stooped neck and shaking hands.

Her fragility made a distinct impression on me, as the only picture I had of her was from the newspaper article that had set me on the track of this interview: a review of her book, *The Interpretation of Fairy Tales*, published in its eighth impression in 1987.

In the program I made after my visit, I described her roughly like this: "She is old now, seventy-six and in poor health. A tiny little woman with a strong and defiant look in her eye. I have seen that look before in a newspaper picture, sharp but not stabbing, observant but not obtrusive. I thought to myself, she can see through you and read the shirt size on the back of your neck if she wants to. Faced with a look such as that, you say to yourself, no room for idle chat here, and no chance of lying."

I would characterize my visit as a friendly diplomatic mission, the reason behind which were her comments on our principal international literary trump card, H. C. Andersen. The following is from chapter nine, the question-and-answer session of the lecture given at the C. G. Jung Institute in Zürich in the winter of 1963, which forms the basis of her book.

> Question: What pattern does a literary author of fairy tales such as Andersen follow?
>
> Dr. von Franz: Well, Andersen is certainly a great author, but in my opinion he is very neurotic, and I cannot read his stories because his neurosis disturbs me so much that it is like a knife scratching on a plate. I am sensitive to his sentimental, morbid stuff. His main neurosis is not his problem alone but that of the whole of Scandinavia: a terrific sex problem due to an imposed, rigid Christian prudishness with a very wild pagan temperament beneath.

I liked that for several reasons. Many years of chasing around in the freelance wilderness after prey has taught me that, in my line of work, the stack of bills in the post is always bigger than the stack of advertisements, so you might as well go and chase after things you actually want to do, and I immediately saw the chance of getting the radio station interested in the interview (and they were very generous).

Also, much of my youth in the antiliterary, politics dabbling and chill-out 1970s had been spent reading psychology, antipsychiatry, Fromm, and not least Jung, and analysis from which I have benefited much.

I didn't say anything to her about this as I readied Switzerland's classic contribution to radio technology, the Nagra tape recorder, but I did stress how fond I was of those characteristics of the Scandinavian problem and the wild pagan temperament.

She looked at me with eyes wide open, but it's true—what man of average vanity would not like to be a civilized berserk—and what's more, it fitted in with Andersen.

It had occurred to me before my visit, during some erratic and somewhat unstructured reading of his works, how precise much of her characterization was. Why then this hypersensitivity to H. C. Andersen, and from an analytical psychologist?

> Marie-Louise von Franz: This is a conflict for me, and therefore maybe he has touched a personal problem. What I saw in him is that he is a mummy's boy of a poor washerwoman, obviously was brought up in a Christian way to be a good boy, and he was a good boy, even a goodie-goodie boy.
>
> He never slept with a woman, he stayed, in his obsession with his mother, true to his mother's principles, and as such, all masculine tendencies of a stronger or more brutal character were suppressed, and sex was suppressed, and therewith much of life. I see him as a tragic figure. I think that it can best be seen in "The Little Mermaid." The unlived life is depicted as the little mermaid, and she is a pagan, she is forbidden access to the Christian world and later disappears into the sea. And that touches on a problem much deeper than Andersen's own mother complex, the problem of the whole of Germanic northern Europe.
>
> We have been Christianized too soon; in the Mediterranean world, paganism was tired and worn out, and Christianity superseded it at the right moment as the next step in development.
>
> But we of the north were still barbarians, and paganism was still a meaningful way of life, which was interrupted by the missionaries. The missionaries called it devil worship and superstition, and Christianity was forced upon the people by converted kings. This creates a definite conflict in our minds. We have a Christian, reasonable, civilized consciousness and a subconscious pagan soul, which has, so to speak, been thrown into a sea of unconciousness.

> And it is still there and wants to be drawn back to life. In Andersen, it has taken an extreme form, because he has been just his mummy's good boy, decent, honest, and so on, just what Christian morality demands. And all life's pagan opportunities—the experience of sex, leaving his mother, having a family, having to fight life's battles—were all sprung over. It's this that we all suffer from a little.

One of the most staggering things about Andersen, and there are many, is his own insight into this precise problem. Exactly how much would become apparent later as I continued reading on my arrival home. If not, I might have sat and maybe from sheer embarrassment "scratched the plate too much."

When he was in his fifties, he wrote the book that he himself considered his principal work but which nowadays is considered one of his weakest, the novel *To Be or Not to Be.* He wrote of the project in a letter: "I would like there to be peace and reconciliation between Nature and the Bible. If I can resolve this, then the divine all-devouring monster of materialism will die too."

The theme is thought-provoking in relation to Marie-Louise von Franz's words. And so is the title he originally considered using for the novel, "Pagan in the Head—Christian in the Heart." And precisely that is, apparently, not a problem for him to be. His fairy tales are overflowing with examples of pagan myths, crowned with the halo of his Christian piety. Pagan in the head—Christian in the heart. One is tempted to ask, What about the rest of the body?

"He should have gone to a brothel" was Marie-Louise von Franz's opinion.

I struggled on Andersen's behalf, offering up all the arguments I could think of for his greatness, telling her that he was the world's most translated fiction writer, giving examples of his own insight into all of it, and so on and so on. I must have sounded a bit like a football fan waving an H. C. Andersen flag.

She probably found it quite amusing, but it made no difference. "Let's just see if he lasts, time will tell" was her conclusion.

She would, of course, rather pass her own judgment on the world's problems and tell of the enlightenment she found in the old folk stories.

Marie-Louise von Franz: These are clear examples because they are games that simple natural people play out in their own fantasy. They have no idea what they are telling. They just let their poetically creative fantasy run wild.

Whereas an author normally will have a lot of aesthetic aims and theories and interpretations of his work, the common man who tells an old story, which his mother told him, will just tell it as it is. If he embellishes a little, as sometimes happens, he will do it from naïveté. And here you can find quite wonderful examples of how to associate with the devil. First you are in his service for seven years; then, in the end, you find a way to prevent him from stealing your soul. A totally different attitude toward evil. There are many good stories where there is a simpleton who is good at lying and in the end becomes the king. Good and evil are regarded far more comparatively.

The Christian outlook not only represses material things and Mother Nature, it also represses the evilness. Jung wrote a lot on this subject in his book *Aion,* that the early fathers of the church taught that evil has no substance. It is a *privatio boni,* a lack of good. So if you kill people, for example, in a concentration camp, it is not evil, more a lack of goodness. When you look closely, you can see just how cynical that is.

The Christian point of view has a far too optimistic and childlike attitude toward evil, and Andersen was compelled in that direction by his typical mother complex. Everything will end well, and he will walk into Paradise carrying a white flag, and the devil doesn't exist or will disappear. This is our disease, and if you overlook the virus, then it will spread. And if you overlook evil, then it can blossom. Just take a look at the Gulf War. Now here is the question: What do you do when faced with absolute evil? Go up to Saddam Hussein, brush him on the cheek, and say, "Dearest, I love you in the name of Jesus," and see what happens.

This was during the first Gulf War, the oil war, and that also was put into perspective:

The monotheistic religions, or at least our own—Christianity, Islam, Judaism—are all patriarchal, and they suppress not just paganism, they also suppress femininity. So for us, paganism and our femininity are coupled together, can you see, paganism worships Mother Earth as well as the father spirit, praises the earth, material things. In the same way, paganism's magic is carried out using material things. You write a sign on a piece of paper and secretly carry it in your pocket as protection against evil. There is always some material thing. The only remotely material thing in Christianity is the communion, altar bread. There is nothing else left. The pagan religions are full of material traits and rituals, because they worship natural and material things. So you see, it's the patriarchal religions like Christianity, Islam, and Judaism that habitually spoil nature, take profit from nature, and are inextricably coupled to the problems of the environment and pollution.

In the patriarchal religions, you find the Master of the Datamatter, Master of Facts. In paganism, we find the child of Mother Substance; one has to respectfully honor Mother Nature and ask for her gifts instead of stealing them.

You see how deep the problem goes . . . We are up against it now, Mother Matter is very angry, might finish us all off, because we have despised Mother Matter and Mother Nature, now what goes with it.

We covered a lot of ground. I was amazed how naturally she talked of paganism as though it were still a powerful force. I also heard about the differences between the Nordic Odin and the Germanic Wotan and the connection of the latter to Nazism and received learned references to pagan legends, Asiatic religions, Greek mythology, and a good deal more. And the whole time, that inquiring look—was I paying attention? As well as I could, while keeping an eye on the Nagra and her ever-increasing tiredness. I threw in my questions and stuck the lid on as tight as I could on Andersen. He just kept simmering in the pot, trying to get a word in edgewise. How much he in some way managed to I only found out after I got home from the trip and continued my reading.

The day before my meeting with Marie-Louise von Franz, I had been down to take a look at Jung's tower, "the castle" on the edge of the lake at Bollingen. I skulked around like a prowling barbarian, at last knocked on the door, and Jung's grandson, Dieter Baumann, opened. At the sight of the Nagra, he burst out with a raging, machine-breaker look, "Turn that off."

And then he welcomed me and ushered me around in a hospitable and friendly manner. He told me about the castle and not least about the stones outside, on which Jung himself had chiseled sentences and small pictures. One in particular caught my attention. He read out the immensely learned Latin text, whose principal content was that Christianity and paganism will never be able to swallow each other up, so we will have to find something new. That was exactly what Jung was thinking of when he found a dead snake with a dead fish in its mouth on the banks of the lake. And it was that which gave him the theme for the picture in the stone.

As Marie-Louise von Franz explained the next day:

> The fish died and choked the snake. Yes, and this is an expression of the problem between Christianity and paganism. We need something new to grow out of Christianity, the innocent, fishlike Christianity. A fish is a very unconscious creature, but Christianity needs to be more conscious. It is too childish and naïve: Jesus Christ's little lambs, and being sweet and nice, and then everything will be alright. I'm exaggerating a bit and coloring things in black and white. They don't need to give up Christianity but live it in a more conscious way. Not so childish.

Not like H. C. Andersen, one could add.

He would have liked the tower in Bollingen, the interior décor—which in style was not so far from his own period, even though 2005 will be two hundred years since his birth—and the pictures on the walls, not least the picture Jung painted of Philemon, his personal guru. Philemon is one of the two old people that Mephistopheles gets rid of for Faust, and on his orders, in the play by Goethe. He burns them and their little hovel because they are spoiling the view from Faust's copious palace. With this mortal sin on his conscience, Faust is doomed and Satan's certain prey, but the angels save his immortal soul. This episode had an important influence, as did the whole play, on H. C. Andersen in *To Be or Not to Be,* or, as it was originally called, *Pagan in the Head—Christian in the Heart.* Goethe's Faust gives him, or at least the heroine Esther does, a whole list of examples and proof of God's existence, the good and gracious God's existence. He didn't believe in the devil at all.

Andersen must have passed by Bollingen on one of his many trips to Switzerland. He must have sailed past. Switzerland, and especially the landscape, played a part in several of his fairy tales; one of the longest, most reworked, and least known, "The Ice Maiden," takes place there and is based upon an actual event, a tragic drowning accident in 1856 on Lake Genfer. The fairy tale is about a young hunter, Ruddy, who as a baby is kissed by the spirit of the glacier, the Ice Maiden, but he escapes. He becomes the best hunter in all the Alps. He is never dizzy (he learns this from the cat), he knows no fear, and he understands, as does Andersen himself, how to bridge the class barrier. He wins the favor of the rich miller's daughter, Babette, and now he needs the approval of her father. This is difficult, but even here he succeeds. Everything succeeds, but then the Ice Maiden kisses him again.

> "Mine! mine!" sounded around him, and within him; "I kissed thee when thou wert a little child. I once kissed thee on the mouth, and now I have kissed thee from heel to toe; thou art wholly mine." And then he disappeared in the clear, blue water.
>
> All was still. The church bells were silent; the last tone floated away with the last red glimmer on the evening clouds. "Thou art mine," sounded from the depths below; but from the heights above, from the eternal world, also sounded the words, "Thou art mine!" Happy was he thus to pass from life to life, from earth to heaven. A chord was loosened, and tones of sorrow burst forth. The icy kiss of death had overcome the perishable body; it was but the prelude before life's real drama could begin, the discord which was quickly lost in harmony. Do you think this a sad story?

Yes, I think that's what you can call it; but for H. C. Andersen, it's happy. A devastating attack on the young couple's love for each other is anticipated in a dream, and the young widow bride is resigned to being left alone as a old spinster and eternal virgin and accepts that all that happened was for the best.

> There is a rosy tint on the mountain snow, and there are rosy gleams in each heart in which dwells the thought, "God permits nothing to happen which is not the best for us." But this is not often revealed to all, as it was revealed to Babette in her wonderful dream.

H. C. Andersen had lived with the belief that a feeling of total happiness was a warning of death, and the conflict between paganism and Christianity comes into play here as it does in a few of his other stories.

The ice maiden's kiss and the cold kiss in the much better known Snow Queen fairy tale are the only truly erotically described and erotically impressive moments in Andersen's work.

As Marie-Louise von Franz continued in her answer to the discussion at the Zürich fairy-tale seminar I quoted earlier:

> Andersen had this collective neurosis to an extreme extent. He never married and was never able to touch a woman. He died a virgin, but was so swamped by sexual fantasies that he nearly went mad and on his deathbed raved and spouted obscenities. But it can be said that insofar as his conflict was not his alone but a conflict of the whole of the North, that would account for the success of his fairy tales.

I never managed to convert Marie-Louise von Franz to H. C. Andersen. No advertising! No, no, that was not the intention.

By the way, he has no need for that. Again and again in his works, he refers to the prediction that the old neighbor woman, Mrs. Bunkeflod, in his childhood town of Odense (Odin's sanctuary) gave about the poor, gifted little boy Hans Christian, that it would some time be illuminated in his honor. He persevered, and it came to pass. (And see now all the international commotion about the two hundredth anniversary of his birth in 2005.)

But I came to meet her; Andersen was just a pretext.

In truth, her eyes were darker than the newspaper picture had shown. The strength in them was of a different character to that in the snapshot, one of lightning sharp intellect, eyes that can turn and see right to the essence of things. The intensity was, don't misunderstand me, like that which you see in the eyes of very small children. They don't blink for anyone or anything; they are, to quote the American author and doctor William Carlos Williams, "naturally aristocratic."

She said of her own methods: "I consider my task to be to pull people I respect to zero and say we know nothing, Jung taught us nothing. See what is happening in your own soul, and let's discuss that."

A whole hour's interview here in the Swiss spring, in a villa on the mountainside in Küsnacht, must have been a huge physical exertion. "One last question," she whispered, and I mentioned the fairy-tale researcher Bengt Holbek and his definition of a legend (and the role of the storyteller) as a soul opener. And as she answered and reflected on her own country's, the Swiss, fairy tale, church bells began to chime somewhere in the far distance.

> We have a lot of sagas, and in ninety percent of them supernatural powers are featured. A man is on his way home and when he arrives at a particular bridge, a little man appears and tells him something and he then falls down and dies. Sinister stories and stories with parapsychological ghosts, small dwarfs that appear just before someone dies, church bells that ring without anyone ringing them. Here you find the whole world, the world of the dream and the night.
>
> I don't remember which country, I think it's one of the Slavic countries, there, when they begin to tell a fairy tale in public, they start with "Last night I dreamed that," and then they tell the story.

The "Stone Tower im Moos" in Bollingen

CHRISTINE RAYMANN

My mother served many years as a substitute postal service official in Bollingen. During my school years, I was allowed to join her at work on Wednesday afternoons and on my free days. I got to stamp letters, attach stickers, hop around in mail sacks, and put letters in mailboxes on the delivery route.

In Moos, on the edge of the forest above Bollingen, I discovered this stone tower. I asked my mother what this tower was all about, and she told me what she knew. But my fantasy developed its own picture, namely, a tower from the Middle Ages, a sort of watchtower, where a crotchety old woman lived without water and electricity. Its position on top of the hill and the fact that the tower was so simply furnished fascinated me from the very beginning.

Later, I often rode my pony to the "Little Stone Tower." I never met anyone and only seldom caught a glimpse of the inside as most of the time the wooden shutters were closed.

Almost twenty years after I first saw the tower, I was walking my dog up the hill and thought to myself how nice it would be to be able to live here. The wish to see just once the inside of the tower grew stronger and stronger. I asked my mother whether she knew who the tower now belonged to, as the old woman had passed away. She sought out the address of the doctor who now owned the property. Dr. [Manolis] Kennedy was very friendly to me on the phone and told me the story of the tower and, above all, that this crotchety old woman was in truth a world-famous psychologist. I was astounded about the actual people and occurrences around my "Little Stone Tower." We spoke for a long time on the phone. I have never recovered from my astonishment.

Unfortunately the tower did not belong to [Dr. Kennedy], but he gave me the name of the new proprietor whose number I then phoned. The doctor's wife was also extraordinarily kind and invited me to visit the stone tower next summer. I look forward to this coming summer like a child looks forward to Christmas.

With kind regards,
Christine Raymann

Searching Continually for Meaning

VICKI REIFF

I was thirty-two years old when I began helping out in the Lindenbergstrasse household. Maria (who had been Marlus's family housekeeper since she was a young girl) had become too ill to continue. Alison Kappes was already working part-time there and needed some help. I was then asked to be that help. I would be there for more than seventeen years, until Marlus died in 1998. These years were an immeasurably valuable and meaningful part of my life. I experienced love, generosity, kindness, humility, humor, compassion, and wisdom. I was challenged, supported, and educated into the reality of living a life rooted in the inner world.

It is difficult to capture all the experiences and memories in seventeen years that have been woven together to form the feeling I have for Marie-Louise von Franz. However, I do think that I could focus on three areas: Marlus's genius sense of humor, her connection to so many different kinds of people, and how she lived a life unquestionably in relationship to the unconscious.

However, I cannot begin to mention Lindenbergstrasse or Marlus without first writing something of her dear friend, Barbara Hannah.

Alison and I have always, and will always, refer to her affectionately as "Miss Hannah." I think the first thing that impressed me in making the acquaintance of Miss Hannah at ninety years of age was that she was at such peace with herself. She was vivacious, had lived a full life, and had no bitterness whatsoever. She genuinely lived Jung's psychology and, in my eyes, was *the* example of an individuated woman. She was deeply related and most of all helped teach me what eros is. And she was terribly protective of Marlus! Miss Hannah would never hesitate to knock on Marlus's door to end an hour that had gone too long or to call her to eat lunch before it got cold. She would also not hesitate to block the entrance, intimidating the "uninvited" appearances of certain individuals. Now, this is an image that I will never forget: Miss Hannah at ninety years dauntlessly stopping visitors at the front gate.

Having a negative mother complex myself, I can be overly sensitive to criticism; however, this was never constellated with Miss Hannah. She had so united the opposites within herself that her criticism or challenges were never wounding. I was only left with the motivation to improve myself and get it right the next time. "My dear," she would begin, "you've done something dreadful" (like opening and pouring several packages of Jacob's fresh coffee into the tin at once!). "I don't mind that you made a mistake, everyone makes mistakes, but it would be tiresome if you did it again!"

I had come to Zürich to study at the C. G. Jung Institute, and I was somewhat fearful of the task ahead until the day I found Miss Hannah reading *Memories, Dreams, Reflections.* She looked up at me and said, "My dear, I am reading this book for the tenth time and I still learn from it." Yet another time, I found her reading *Answer to Job.* Again she commented, "My dear (she called me that a lot), I am now reading this book for the twelfth time, and I think that I am finally beginning to understand it!!" She was a humble and honest person, helping me relax and overcome my fear of beginning my studies. I was naturally nervous when I submitted my application to the Jung Institute until Miss Hannah put the process into her perspective (she was not particularly enthusiastic about everything at the Institute). She commented: "Well, if they don't accept you . . . that is only a compliment."

As I have written, Miss Hannah had a natural gift of feeling and relatedness with herself and with others, a wonderful eros. Of course, her poor sensation function was not only infamous, but also a major source of laughter in the household. For example, Miss Hannah could never ever find her slippers in the morning. She told me that I was the "best finder" because I somehow always managed to find them. I didn't have the heart to tell her that they were under the bed, just at the edge! Another time, while doing the spring cleaning at Bollingen, I found a huge sum of money left forgotten on her wardrobe. In addition, a friend of mine borrowed a book from Miss Hannah, *The Old Testament.* When he opened it to the chapter on Sophia, he also discovered a large sum of money! Then again, what Miss Hannah lacked in sensation was compensated for by her uncanny sense of intuition. While driving through Küsnacht one day, she knew the exact moment to apply the brakes, just seconds before an unseen child ran between two parked cars into the street in front of her.

Speaking of driving, I will always have the image of these two very unique women driving in the small, ancient, green VW Polo with Marlus behind the wheel. Marlus loved to drive over Swiss alpine passes. Her favorites (if I remember correctly) were the Albula and the Susten. Marlus was a slow driver, much to the frustration and displeasure of the drivers behind her, who would flash their lights or honk the horn for her to speed up. This would only result in a mischievous reduction in her speed! And all this while Laura, the English bulldog, would sit in the backseat having her own personal *Auseinandersetzung* with the cushions—ripping, tearing, growling, and shaking herself back and forth. By the time Laura died, the Polo no longer had a backseat. "That wicked animal," Marlus would call her.

Marlus had an incredible sense of humor. She loved to hear a good joke and tell one as well. Her favorite joke was about the pious man who went to heaven (I've included it below). However, her sense of humor also came through in so many different incidents and moments, a few of which I can tell you here.

For example: after a misunderstanding between us, I went to speak with Marlus. Naturally, my negative mother complex was quite present.

Marlus was open, honest, and humble. She described how, still at her age, she was battling with her own negative mother complex. She recounted the story of her birth: the delivery had begun before the midwife arrived, and Marlus was wrapped dangerously in the placenta. Her mother was helpless, and the infant could have died if the midwife hadn't arrived just in time to save her. A few days after our conversation, I was helping Marlus get undressed for bed. (Because of her Parkinson's disease, this was not something she could do alone.) Her red sweater got caught over her head as I was trying to take it off. My body tensed and I felt the panic beginning! Marlus surely felt this, too, because she cried out, "Oh no! It's the placenta!!" Then she laughed like mad, causing me to laugh, and the sweater slipped easily over her head. Her humor often carried a deep relatedness and sensitivity to the others around her, especially in the basic condition of being wounded.

Another unforgettable humorous incident occurred before Miss Hannah died in the summer of 1985. Marlus had gone alone to Bollingen for two weeks while Alison and I looked after Miss Hannah. (After breaking her hip, Miss Hannah was unable to climb the stairs at Bollingen.) My husband and Sal Celi had gone to pick up Marlus and drive her home with Laura. We were all sitting upstairs in Miss Hannah's study drinking afternoon tea. Sal discovered a tick on Laura and pulled it off. He placed it in a small bowl on the table (which he mistakenly thought was an ashtray). Unfortunately, this was Miss Hannah's "meds" bowl and contained all her pills for the day. The rolled up tick appeared to be just another pill in the bowl. Upon realizing his mistake, Sal wanted to take the tick away, but Marlus stopped him, then began to laugh and laugh until tears rolled down her face. Miss Hannah, whose hearing was terrible, sensed that the joke was at her expense. Marlus enjoyed herself immensely (and we did eventually throw the tick away).

I often saw her laugh so heartily that tears would roll down her face. My husband had an hour with her once and wrote a card to thank her. I was sitting at lunch with Marlus and Miss Hannah when she opened the card. At the end of the card, he wrote: "Please give my greetings to Miss Hannah and a pat on the rump to Laura." He signed the card then added a postscript: "Please don't confuse these two greetings . . . I have enough problems as it is!!" Marlus had been eating when she read this. She spit out her food and laughed so intensely that tears streamed down her cheeks.

Marlus absolutely enjoyed hearing animal stories. She especially loved the story of one of her student's cat: the man was late for work one morning, eating his breakfast in a hurry, and forgot to feed his cat. The cat was quick to get her revenge and deposited her feces in her master's shoe before he could leave for work! Her master's foot, not his eyes, discovered the mess.

She also took immense pleasure in watching Laura chase me every day out of the door. Laura never attacked anyone when they came into the house, but loved to do so when they were leaving. When I would leave after lunch, Marlus would hold Laura back just until I was almost at the door, then release her so Laura could have the good fun of charging down the hallway and biting at my feet before my escape. This became a daily ritual.

Marlus never lost her wonderful sense of humor, even with the onset of her illness and the suffering it brought. When she could no longer climb the stairs to her bedroom or sit in her analyst's chair, her bed was brought down to her study. I joked with her that with a couch in the study, she was turning Freudian. She quickly retorted, "neo-Freudian, because in this case, the analyst lies on the couch!"

Another most gratifying aspect of being at Lindenbergstrasse was the continual flow of visitors. Marlus generously gave of herself, her time, and her wisdom, touching a remarkable spectrum of individuals from many different cultures and areas of life. She once remarked that "if I didn't have contact with someone because of his or her shadow, well, there would be no one left." A vast variety of people crossed into her consulting room seeking hours with her: the psychologists, colleagues and students, medical professionals, educators and scholars from all fields, engineers, theologians, musicians and artists, business people, housewives and folk from the village. They included, for instance, Swiss, English, American, French, Spanish, Brazilian, Italian, German, Japanese, Swedish, Mexican, and Greek.

In addition, there was the constant flow of gifts, thank you cards, and telephone calls. The "pineapple man" always brought a fresh pineapple to his hour on Tuesdays. The "honey lady" brought a jar of Marlus's favorite hard honey on Wednesdays. Then there were the gift baskets, the Sprüngli and Teuscher's pralines and truffles (her favorite), and an abundance of flowers of every imaginable kind! Each gift never failed to touch Marlus or be greatly appreciated by her. As were the countless letters, cards, and telephone calls that came in, not to request an hour but simply to express gratitude for something she had written. One typical call came one afternoon from a young man in Germany. He had just finished reading *Puer Aeternus* and was so profoundly moved that he was impelled to telephone in order to express his deepest gratitude "for opening my eyes and changing my life." I often had the impression that these simple expressions of thanks were the most touching to Marlus. She frequently remarked that "not everyone should become an analyst, but rather take what they learn from their analysis back into their lives and try to integrate it."

Marlus's ability to make this contact with such a diversity of people comes from the third area I would like to touch upon, that being her profoundly genuine relationship to the unconscious. She related to that source in each and every individual. And this was the most meaningful and nourishing aspect of my years at Lindenberg—having the great fortune to experience directly her unqualified connection to the reality of the unconscious. She once remarked that "it was like walking with one foot in each world" and that was exactly how she lived.

When I became pregnant in 1986, a doctor told me that I would need to give away my three cats, who I loved very much. He succeeded in frightening me. Marlus reassured me, insisting that I should ignore the doctor—my dreams would tell me. I responded that I was so rattled, it was hard "to believe." Marlus gave me a look that penetrated through me. I will never forget it. Then she stated flatly, "Then may God have mercy on you." I was flat-out humbled. I felt myself to be little more than two inches tall! Twenty minutes later, she came into the kitchen, took my hand lovingly, and pulled me back to myself. "What has gotten into you? Stop worrying!" She did this with such love and acceptance of my stupidity that I could stop my blind fear and rationality. I kept my cats and gave birth to a healthy child, as my dreams said I would. For Marlus, the dreams were *the* reality.

Whenever something would happen in the house, for example, a picture had suddenly fallen off the wall, Marlus would ask me to note the time and date that the incident occurred. This kind of example was typical of her unrelenting, always-present attitude relating to the presence of the unconscious. I saw this in Marlus even following Miss Hannah's death. After the funeral of her dearest friend, she stated in her stoic manner: "Now I have to find the meaning of why I was left behind." She directed herself continually toward the search for meaning.

I have many fond memories that I could go on with—small moments—like how she enjoyed her Cinzano before her meals and once told Miss Hannah, who was thinking of giving up her Dry Sack sherry, "not to castrate your pleasures"; or how she liked to leave her study and go outside to clean the leaves off the stairs or stack the wood at Bollingen herself; or how much she loved her frog pond at Bollingen. (I was forbidden to use any harsh cleaning fluids for the spring cleaning in order to protect the frogs' waters.) Another touching moment was in December 1996, just before Laurens van der Post's death. He was in Zürich to show one of his films. He was scheduled to visit Marlus at Lindenbergstrasse but due to his failing health was unable to come. They spoke to each other on the telephone. Mr. van der Post was struggling to speak and Marlus was struggling to hold the telephone receiver in her hand. She managed to say to him that "two old Bushmen don't have to see each other to be together."

It is difficult to convey how almost every area of my life was touched and transformed through my experiences of Marie-Louise von Franz and Barbara Hannah. However, two simple dreams I had during my years at Lindenbergstrasse might express what the relationships meant to me. In one dream, Marlus was turning on lights for me. In another dream, I was at Lindenbergstrasse and looked out the window. I saw a garden which was vast and magnificent with lucidly green grass and the strongest oak tree that I could ever imagine!

I would like to conclude with one last story. One morning, Marlus met me at the door excited to tell me the dream she had had the night before. It goes more or less as follows: "I dreamed of an old soldier who was receiving a medal for his years of dedicated service and then could retire with honors." I believe this dream shows the essence of the fighting spirit of Marlus's life, a spirit that served humanity with boundless devotion and generosity. In deep gratitude, Marlus, I salute you!

The Joke of the Pious Man

A pious man died and went directly to heaven. When he got there, he was given yogurt for his meal. Just yogurt, he thought? Well, maybe because it was the first day. However, the second day he was given yogurt for breakfast, yogurt for lunch, and yogurt for dinner! What was that about? I lived a good life and all I get for it is yogurt? Impossible!! After several more days of yogurt and more yogurt, the pious man looked down into hell to see all the sinful people eating banquets of wonderful foods. He was outraged and decided to complain directly to St. Peter. He went to see St. Peter. "What is this?! I live a good, long, pious life and all I get is yogurt?" St. Peter regarded the man and responded: "Well, you know, it doesn't pay to cook for just two!"

For the Festschrift in Honor of Marie-Louise von Franz

ALFRED RIBI

My memories of Marie-Louise von Franz first and foremost involve deep gratitude. She gave my life its decisive impulse. I cannot find the words to explain the reasons for this gratefulness, I can only allude to them below.

When I began my analysis with Marie-Louise von Franz in 1963, I had already read most of the Collected Works of C. G. Jung. It had occurred to me that the analyst himself (or herself) is the healing agency and thus he himself must undergo a training analysis. I came to von Franz with this attitude, thinking that I was pretty much normal and had no problems, and brought her my dreams, which I had already interpreted with the usual catchwords from Jung such as animus, anima, shadow, and Self. Marie-Louise listened to these dreams and added most modestly: "Maybe one should also look at these dreams as. . . ." I am very grateful for her patience. She led me gently to my own problems in such a way that I could slowly understand that my dreams were really talking about my issues and that I actually had problems. We worked many years on these problems. Later the analytical relationship developed into a personal friendship.

At the age where she could no longer leave the house on her own, I often had the honor of taking her for rides in the car, and I had the opportunity to cook for her and to experience her in her private life. These undertakings were very valuable, as I was able to experience Marie-Louise not necessarily as the analyst but how she lived day to day.

In my own analysis, I often asked her how she experienced Jung. She spoke a lot about him, which was for me very important, for this was the way that the man behind the Collected Works became visible. His works convinced me only because his life was lived according to the texts he wrote, and thus it was so important for me to be able to grasp the man, C. G. Jung, himself. This Marie-Louise communicated to me in seemingly endless numbers of conversations. When Ludwig van Beethoven moved from Bonn to Vienna to study with Joseph Haydn, he wrote to his friends that he had "received the spirit of Mozart from Haydn's hands." I received Jung's spirit from the hands of Marie-Louise, and for this I will be grateful to her for the rest of my life.

My Personal Memories of Marie-Louise von Franz

REMO ROTH

Since her death on February 17, 1998, there has been a lot written about Marie-Louise von Franz. Therefore I would like to limit the following explanations to some of the more important aspects of our personal relationship.

Some months after the publication of her [second to] last book, *On Dreams and Death,* in the autumn of 1984, Marie-Louise fell ill with Parkinson's disease. After this, she told me several times that she had the distinct feeling that the illness was a direct effect of writing the book.

She never went into details, but I felt she had not yet found the individual solution to the problem of the developing of the so-called subtle body (the diamond body in Eastern esoterics) for life after death. This was one of the most important topics in her book, and I saw that she continued to deal with this subject intensively.

Marie-Louise suffered her severe illness with stoic patience for thirteen years until she was released by death. In spite of the fact that she was hardly able to speak at the end of her life, her alert and critical mind was ever present. It was therefore a great pleasure for me when I realized that, despite her disease, she continued to be interested in my creative work—research on the application of Carl Jung's synchronicity theory to psychosomatic and somatic illness—which is itself based on the phenomenology of the subtle body.

She often gave me symbolic hints about the direction of my research based on dreams I sent her by mail or told her during personal meetings. It was exactly the fact that her advice was given in *symbolic* language, formulated in extremely short statements, that allowed me to have the space for my own creative ideas.

Through this behavior, developed out of her intense, conscious suffering, Marie-Louise supported my individual freedom of research. And this made possible my body-centered imagination or symptom symbol transformation techniques for psychosomatic and somatic disease. To my great pleasure, I could also see that she began to experience for herself this body-centered method for the creation of the subtle body, which is based on a combination of active imagination and creative insights of Paracelsus and seems to be a modern interpretation of Gerhard Dorn's *unio corporalis.*

But the last thirteen years of her life were not only stamped with the role of the *femme inspiratrice* for close friends. When one tried to see Marie-Louise with the "inner eye," one could feel that she had finally found an imaginative technique for developing the subtle or eternal body, the goal of Paracelsus's *vita longa,* for the life in the beyond. According to the church father Origenes, this is the main challenge in this life on earth (as she describes in her book). And only through this transformation of the physical into the subtle body is *individual* life in the beyond possible.

The closer Marie-Louise's physical death came, the more intensely I felt that she succeeded in developing the subtle body for her individual life in the beyond, a development which she described in her book, *On Dreams and Death,* amplifying this point with historical examples. It was exactly this unique, individual, and absolutely introverted transformation, her psychological realization of Gerhard Dorn's body-centered *unio corporalis,* which is intellectually practically ineffable, that was the final chapter to her opus in this world.

One was able to perceive this development also in regards to the transformation of her physical presence. Her body—always reminding me of that of a peasant woman—changed over the course of time into the body of an elflike being. In so doing, it took on—especially toward the end of her physical life—an aura inexplicable by natural science.

One of the goals of alchemy was the production of the philosophical gold or stone (lapis). As gold, the lapis possessed such intense "radiation" that all matter around it was also transformed into gold. The same idea was the so-called *multiplicatio* of the lapis: a "radiation" coming out of the lapis which influenced the whole universe in a positive manner. In the case of the alchemical opus applied to the physical body, this goal was nothing less than the creation of the above-mentioned subtle body as the guarantee for individual life after death.

Precisely this *corpus mysticum* (the mystery of the body) was the opus of the medieval priest-physician Hildegard von Bingen eight hundred years ago. Her lifelong physical suffering was the *prima materia* for her visions, now famous today (see C. G. Jung, "Flying Saucers: A Modern Myth of Things Seen in the Skies" (1958), in *CW,* vol. 10 (Princeton, N.J.: Princeton University Press, 1964), par. 765). I am deeply convinced that by means of her individual development of the insights of Carl Jung in her opus of suffering, Marie-Louise von Franz found a modern extension of Hildegard's work.

Marie-Louise von Franz and Her "Apero"

MARY SCHEINOST

For the last two and a half years of Marie-Louise von Franz's life, I was involved in her care, or perhaps better said, being there for her when she needed someone or something. My involvement was through a friend and co-worker, Mrs. Annemarie Wöbel, who also worked for von Franz.

This was my second experience being with a person in their home. I quickly learned that, after many years working as a registered nurse in a clinic, all my medical knowledge and nursing skills could be thrown out the window.

M.-L. von Franz knew what she wanted and was forceful in not accepting what I thought "might be good for her." To learn to be there for someone instead of always doing something for a patient was a good learning experience for me. The beginning months were difficult for both of us, and more than once I thought someone else would be better for her than myself.

Her great sense of humor and genuine interest in people, myself included, are two of her many qualities that come first to my mind.

She wanted to continue with her life even as everything became more difficult. For example, three days before she died, with difficulty she was able to get up from her bed to eat a small amount of food in her bedroom. In a strong, reproachful voice, she said, "Mary, my apero!" I had thought she wouldn't want one and had neglected to ask.

This was a valuable time for me in Küsnacht and Bollingen, where I grew very fond of her, and I am grateful for being able to have been there with her and for her.

Marie-Louise von Franz

An Example of Complete Loyalty

GERTRUD SCHELLBRETT

Marie-Louise von Franz was a loyal person, loyal to me as a friend and loyal to my daughter as a godmother. She often visited her godchild, who was ill, or invited her to her house in Küsnacht. She took her role as godmother very seriously. Marie-Louise took *everything* seriously.

In the university where we studied together, she was overly arduous. But the one thing she took more seriously than anything else was her studies with Jung. She was in love with Jung's psychology, studied it with great zeal, attended all of his lectures at the university, and was very loyal to its basic principles.

She did not like groups, so very often the two of us went by ourselves to ski in the Alps. She always brought along the *I Ching,* never parted herself from it, and consulted it frequently.

Jung made the right choice with von Franz. She was the right one for him not only because she helped him with Old Greek and Latin but also because she was the more imaginative of the two. She had far more ideas than Jung. She profited from Jung, but he also profited from her.

Dream of a Lit Up Cathedral Buried in the Mountain

FRANÇOISE SELHOFER

20, Chemin de l'Etang
1219 Geneva
January 8, 2003

Dear Dr. Kennedy,

Since I received your letter regarding the Festschrift—a letter that I would like to thank you for—I have been waiting for a dream, a sign, a "north-sea fish." Yesterday evening I set your letter to the side—the deadline was now past—and this morning I awoke having had this impressive dream.

> *I pick up a book by C. G. Jung in my library and am astounded that I have never seen the pictures in it before. One sees a mountain with a tower perched on a precipice. It is supposed to be the north tower of Jung (possibly in Bollingen?). Yet when I approach*

this tower (I am now in this landscape), I see that it is part of an immense church buried in the mountain. As I climb upward (half mountain, half tower), the entire building slowly appears: it is an old cathedral. The round tower that I am climbing looks now like the top of a bell tower although the bell is missing. When I look down, I can see many people down in the nave of the church working to dig it out and restore it. Then I am down below. A young worker says to me that we should go no further as one should not trample the earth with one's feet. The bottom of the nave is still covered in a beautiful brown earth much like a large bed in a garden. The young worker smiles at me, and I feel very comfortable with him. Later I see young students and children that are preparing themselves for a production. A banquet is also being prepared. Then Dr. von Franz arrives. I can only greet her briefly as many people are accompanying her into the cathedral which is now fully lit up. I remain outside and feel very sad. I know that it is now too late to contribute to the Festschrift, the book must have already gone to press.

The theme of the divine concealed in the earth is beautifully developed in Marie-Louise von Franz's book, *C. G. Jung: His Myth in Our Time.* Her dream in which she traveled down to the center of the earth to encounter the face of God touched me deeply and has followed me for years. The birth of Aphrodite at the end of her dream is, for me as well as many women, a symbol of the renewal of the feminine. Now it is thanks to the influence and the works of Marie-Louise von Franz that, seventy years later, there is a "cathedral" in which one can actually extol the hidden god (that is, the hidden god of matter). (Naturally, of course, we are also indebted here to C. G. Jung, but in this dream, it is important as we have here to do with the visitation of a woman.)

In the beginning of the dream, one only sees a tower which seems to refer to Jung's tower. I do not know whether or not there is a "north tower" in Bollingen, but the image of Philemon, Jung's "inner advisor" came immediately to mind. Marie-Louise von Franz taught me that we receive help through our dreams. It has slowly become an uncanny reality that, through dreams and active imagination, help can come to us. Synchronicity shows time and again that spirit and matter are secretly connected. Matter also has a divine soul, and there is still a lot to dig out and discover in this fertile ground.

My sadness today comes from my inability to more accurately express my deeply felt gratitude. My encounter with Marie-Louise von Franz changed my life; it gave my life a new direction. And although I am coming a bit late with my letter, Dr. Kennedy, this gratitude I do want to express to you.

With my best regards,
Françoise Selhofer

The Puer and the Patron

DARYL SHARP

Marie-Louise von Franz saved my life. It's that simple, and that complicated.

I didn't meet her in person until 1976, but already in 1970 her landmark book, *The Problem of the Puer Aeternus,* had opened my eyes to my personal psychology. Well, that's not entirely true; better say she prepared me for what was coming, which is to say that I could appreciate intellectually, with my thinking function, her analysis of the mother-bound man, but I did not truly see its relevance to me—from a feeling standpoint, that is—until I was on my knees three years later. Then her words pierced my heart. Her cogent comments on men who sounded suspiciously like me, devastating as they were to my image of myself, offered an implicit alternative to killing myself.

Needless to say, I took the alternative: I went into analysis. I was in England at the time, and my analyst was Dr. Anthony Stevens, a great admirer of von Franz. He helped me to my feet and on his recommendation—and that of the late Irene Champernowne—I was accepted for training at the Zürich Institute. I limped into Zürich in the fall of 1974. Marie-Louise von Franz was my beacon, but alas, she was already fully booked. I shopped around and found another analyst, the late Dr. Richard Pope, who was more than adequate for the likes of me, but that is another story.

As it happened, I then fell in with a shadow companion. Fraser Boa, a charismatic fellow larger than life, had also been accepted as a trainee and was looking for someone to share a house. Fraser had been a teacher for many years before he landed a job as assistant producer on the film *Murder on the Orient Express.* He was also Canadian, from London, Ontario, and he too had run out of steam, reached the end of his tether, and so on. Our dismal state was echoed by others in training, which is to say, we were all there because we had run afoul of our own psychology.

Fraser and I rented a house in the nearby village of Egg. In German, this place-name is pronounced "Eck," but of course eggs are ubiquitous symbols of new life, which heartened us both. His sister, Marion Woodman, soon joined us. She was a frumpy housewife then, just as neurotic as the rest of us.

Fraser became a close friend of mine, our relationship enhanced by the fact that Dr. von Franz was his analyst. Somehow he had wangled it. And thank goodness, because every time he came back from a session with her, we chewed over what she had said for hours. We found separate living spaces after six months, but the analytic sharing went on. I was continually in awe of Fraser's accounts of von Franz's understanding of his dreams. He would tell her a dream and stammer a few associations. She would come back with a full-blown interpretation of what the unconscious was saying to compensate his conscious attitude.

Well, my own analyst took quite a different approach toward me and my material, bless him, but what I heard from Fraser was at least complementary, and at best an analysis with von Franz, albeit vicarious. Fraser died in 1992 without ever knowing how envious I was when he began to refer to Dr. von Franz as "Marlus," the name by which she was known to intimates.

Marie-Louise von Franz was at that time a frequent lecturer at the Institute on dreams, fairy tales, and the symbolic importance of alchemy. At the very first lecture of hers I attended, I was fascinated almost as much by her dirty fingernails as by what she said. She was a handsome woman of fifty-eight, in the prime of life. She had a brilliant smile and was appropriately dressed. So what about those fingernails? I did not realize then that my dominant sensation function obliged me to focus on such outer details. Not to mention the fact that my attitude at that time was sadly blinkered, limited to persona perceptions.

Fraser enlightened me. "Marlus loves gardening," he said. "She was probably planting bulbs or weeding before she came, or maybe she just forgot to wash. Whatever. And so what? What you see isn't the sum total of what you get." Oh yeah? This was news to me but typical of what I learned from Fraser, an intuitive for whom time was flexible and boiling an egg was a hero's journey.

During my four years in Zürich, I read everything von Franz had published. Her fairy-tale interpretations took my breath away. Some of her lectures had been transcribed and were available from the Institute in mimeographed form. Several were published in the mid-seventies by James Hillman's publishing house, Spring: *The Interpretation of Fairy Tales, The Feminine in Fairy Tales, Shadow and Evil in Fairy Tales, Individuation in Fairy Tales.* I found these and others particularly valuable in amplifying the meaning of images that turned up nightly in my dreams. I devoured them and lamented the fact that they were not indexed. But not for long.

Before I went to pieces, I had been a freelance editor, and so I set about creating indexes for these books, as well as for my first love, *Puer Aeternus.* I photocopied my painstaking work and sold it to other students and past graduates. Eventually Spring bought the rights to these indexes and incorporated them in subsequent printings. The benefit to me was twofold: I absorbed von Franz's attitude toward the unconscious and I was able to pay my tuition fees.

I had analytic sessions with Dr. von Franz on two occasions, about a year apart. She lived and practiced in Küsnacht, in an unpretentious little house on the side of a hill overlooking the Lake of Zürich—15 Lindenbergstrasse. Her housemate was the late Barbara Hannah, whose biographical portrait, *Jung: His Life and Work,* published in 1976, is still among the best. I had heard the story that they lived together because Jung had decreed it on account of Miss Hannah's failing health. In spite of Miss Hannah's reputation for being cantankerous, I saw only affection between the two.

I remember her consulting room: simply furnished with a table and straight-backed chair, two comfortable armchairs face-to-face, and overflowing bookshelves. It was the same room she finally died in, which I was invited to view twenty years later, just before the memorial service. The only difference I saw was the addition of a single bed and flowers everywhere, giving it the appearance of a shrine. I also recall that she never billed me for those two analytic hours.

In 1976, when it came time for my propaedeuticum, those nerve-wracking mid-term exams at the Institute, I chose Dr. von Franz to test me on the psychological interpretation of fairy tales. I hadn't met her personally yet, though I dare say she knew something of me from Fraser's dreams. It was an oral exam. I was given twenty minutes alone to read the synopsis of a fairy tale. Then I was questioned by my idol, the Expert. In spite of having immersed myself in her work, I didn't do well. I sweated, I coughed, I stuttered; in short, I froze, completely complexed. I could not answer the simplest of questions.

After some twenty minutes, Dr. von Franz sat back and eyed me. "You are truly a mess," she said. "You are either a stupid ninny and shouldn't be here at all, or you have talents as yet undiscovered." On a grading from 1 (tops) to 5 (abysmal), a 3 was a bare pass, which is what she gave me. I crept out of that room feeling very grateful indeed, for it meant that I could then move on to the candidate stage and start taking clients of my own.

Two years later she examined me again. In the interim I had spent less time frolicking on the Niederdorf, Zürich's nightlife district, and more on why I was where I was. I had reread von Franz's books and I was intimate with Jung's Collected Works. I was as primed for my diploma exam on fairy tales as any horse is for the Kentucky Derby.

I was given a tale from the Grimm collection, "The Crystal Ball," and six hours in which to write a psychological interpretation. I had not read it before, but the motifs were familiar: crystal, eagle, whale, castle, forest, giants, magical hat, wishing, sword, etc., and, wouldn't you know it, an egg within which was the treasure "hard to attain." I wrote my head off and finished in time. The independent examiner refused a mark, saying, "He must have cheated." Von Franz gave me a 1 and penciled a terse note: "He knows his stuff."

In 1978, at the age of forty-two, I returned to Toronto as a certified Jungian analyst. Fraser had been back for a year, and Marion Woodman joined us in 1979. Thanks to the groundwork by laypersons who had founded the C. G. Jung Foundation of Ontario back in 1970, we three analysts, the first in Ontario, all had thriving practices. Still, I was restless. I had so much energy I thought I might explode. Theoretically it's possible. $E = mc^2$. If you have no place to put your energy it could build up inside until poof!—a burst of flame and at the speed of light you're toast.

For some time I had been trying to interest publishers in my diploma thesis on Franz Kafka, *The Secret Raven: Conflict and Transformation.* I had high hopes. The one hundredth anniversary of his birth was coming up, and then the sixtieth anniversary of his death. But there were no takers. I was frustrated. And then Marion and Fraser encouraged me to publish it myself. "Why not?" they said. "You have the tools."

Well, that was true. I knew what was involved in making and marketing a book. Yes, I thought, why not! Only I did not fancy being a one-shot vanity press, so I invited manuscripts from other analysts. Marion immediately offered her own thesis on obesity and anorexia, *The Owl Was a Baker's Daughter.* Fraser helped me design a logo. Then, on a sunny day in May of 1980, I plucked up my courage and called Dr. von Franz at her home in Küsnacht, not forgetting the six-hour time difference.

"Mr. Sharp?" she said. "In Canada? Oh, how are you? I have just come in from the garden. It is a wonderful spring for tulips, don't you think?"

I readily agreed, though I barely knew a tulip from a sunflower.

"Dr. von Franz," I said. "I am starting a publishing house and I'm interested in some of your unpublished seminars. I'm thinking of *Redemption Motifs in Fairy Tales, On Divination and Synchronicity,* and *Alchemy: An Introduction to the Symbolism and the Psychology.* I have mimeographed copies." She said she was very pleased to be asked. What is more, she graciously agreed to be honorary patron of Inner City Books. Those three books of hers, published in 1980, have sold over 60,000 copies to date, not counting foreign editions in ten languages.

In 1983, Fraser got a bee in his own bonnet. "I have an idea," he said. "You can make books; I know how to make films. I will film Marlus on camera interpreting dreams. Hey! What about it?"

"Not likely," I scoffed. "No analyst has ever done that, and she won't either."

My skepticism was ill-founded. Marlus agreed to Fraser's project, on condition that the dreams she was to interpret were told on film by the dreamers themselves, not by actors. "Without real dreams told by the actual dreamers," she said, "there is no integrity."

Fraser then started Windrose Films. He found people willing to recount their dreams on camera. He took these to von Franz and he filmed her interpreting them. The man I had known and loved as a scatter-brained intuitive got all the details right. The result was a stunning ten-hour film series, *The Way of the Dream.* It had its world premier, sponsored by Centerpoint in Cambridge, Massachusetts, in 1985. Since then it has had many showings around the world.

Time passed. I published more books. Fraser went on to film a six-hour series with Joseph Campbell, *This Business of the Gods.* He bought a computer and, with a little help from me on desktop publishing, he turned it and *The Way of the Dream* into books (both still available from Shambhala Publications in Boston).

Fraser's death in 1992 was a mighty blow. Von Franz sent a huge bouquet to the church. I mourned his loss, as much as any Enkidu would his Gilgamesh, but I continued to do what was right in front of me. Every six months, I sent von Franz a statement of her sales and a check. She once told me that I was the only publisher who ever paid her royalties without being sent a letter from her lawyer!

Periodically I wrote to von Franz asking if she had other manuscripts that Inner City might publish. My persistence was rewarded in 1996 when she offered *Archetypal Patterns in Fairy Tales* and reprint rights to *C. G. Jung: His Myth in Our Time.* And just six months before she died, she gave Inner City another hitherto unpublished Zürich seminar, *The Cat: A Tale of Feminine Redemption.* These were soon followed, posthumously, by new editions of *The Problem of the Puer Aeternus* (2000) and

Aurora Consurgens (2000). It is appropriate that Inner City's one hundredth title, published in 2002, was her *Animus and Anima in Fairy Tales.*

On the morning of February 17, 1998, I awoke to find a message on my answering machine from Chuck Schwartz, an old friend and expatriate Canadian, also an analyst, living in Devon, England. "Von Franz has died," I heard. "I thought you'd like to know." Dear Chuck. He had referred me to Anthony Stevens when I was *in extremis* so long ago. During our time in Zürich, he and I and Fraser and Marion were known as the "Canadian Mafia." Years later, when von Franz's beloved bulldog died of old age, it was Chuck who gifted her with a new pup on her birthday.

There was a similar message via e-mail from Bob Hinshaw, another friend and analyst, publisher of Daimon Books: "Sad news from Zürich. Marlus died early this morning. She has been ailing for quite some time and this was surely her deliverance."

I reeled. Oh no. I thought she would live forever. When I had recovered from this fantasy, I phoned friends and posted notices on the Internet. The response was immediate: heartfelt laments for her passing, commiserations to me. More than one correspondent noted yet another passing of the old guard, those who had worked personally with Jung.

The farewell service was scheduled to be held in the Reform Church of Küsnacht on February 26. I am averse to travel, especially to trips across multiple time zones, and so for a few days, I resisted the idea of being there. But in the end I could not not go; she was my patron, after all, and the inner urge to publicly honor our association was just too great. And what a joyful occasion it turned out to be: a simple service with three heartfelt valedictory addresses and a Schubert concert, followed by a sumptuous buffet and a seemingly endless supply of Swiss wine, all provided for in advance by von Franz herself. About six hundred of us mingled for hours, consoling each other, greeting old friends and making new ones.

In the midst of all this, I had a sudden realization. This dearly departed old woman, a self-professed thinking type who had often publicly confessed her difficulty with her inferior feeling function—to the extent of having to memorize collective expressions of sympathy, congratulations on weddings, etc.—had done *this* for *us*. Well, if that does not betoken an integration of opposites, I don't know what does. Thank you, Marlus, I thought, for your *sotto voce* example of the *coniunctio*.

So there it is. The worldwide Jungian community had lost a great lady. I had lost a cherished patron. But the spirit of Marie-Louise von Franz lives on—in her books, in those she worked with analytically, and in the many thousands of others who have been helped or influenced by her writings. Her legacy will surely be that she appreciated Jung's message and did her utmost to further it. And more, for she was not a mindless devotee of Jung. She made her own mark, put her own inimitable stamp both on Jungian psychology and on those she taught.

Personally, I feel privileged and fortunate indeed to be in a position to keep alive the work and spirit of Marie-Louise von Franz, to the benefit of everyone who strives to become psychologically conscious.

Listen to Your Dreams

NICHOLAS SPICER

Dear Dr. Kennedy,

Thank you for your invitation to contribute to the Festschrift for Marie-Louise von Franz, to whom so many owe so much and who is deservedly remembered with love and affection.

I have written a very short memoir of some events during my time training with her. Though there will be many contributions, I hope that my memories of my very dear teacher and analyst will be only a small wave in the great sea of warmth and affection which I expect the Festschrift to engender.

With sincere good wishes in this enterprise,

Yours,
Nicholas Spicer

Dr. von Franz interviewed me for an hour. When I left, she said, "After I have a dream about it, I shall let you know whether I can be your analyst." Even before she gave me her decision—indeed, even if her decision, or her dream's decision had been "no"—I knew I had arrived at home.

I told Dr. von Franz this dream.

> *I had found a young woman in a prison camp and helped to release her. On our journey, we found ourselves in a dark wood.*

I looked up as I said this. Dante filled the space between us. She smiled; no need to say anything.

> *In this wood, the young woman was in her own country, her own power. She embraced me and said, "I reward you for my release with the gift of a word of magic power, a secret word."*

Dr. von Franz leaned forward. We shared an interest in language. (I treasure a Japanese dictionary she gave me.) "What was the word?" I had a choice to make—and I made it. I told her the word. She got up and handed me the Greek and the Latin dictionaries. She took the more obscure languages, Egyptian hieroglyphic was one. There we sat, with five dictionaries on our knees. Then she said, "Excuse me, was that the end of the dream?" "Not quite," I said.

> *I asked the young woman, "If this word is secret, can I tell the dream to my analyst?" "Oh, yes," said the magical girl. "She will just think it's the kind of word she can look up in dictionaries!"*

And, she might have added, burst out laughing when the unconscious played its revealing tricks. My analysis with Marie-Louise was profound, challenging, and companionable. But what I remember most and best was how much of it was fun!

One day, I arrived for my hour and found Dr. von Franz with her leg in plaster. "What happened?" I asked. "Listen to your dreams," she said. "Yesterday I dreamed that I was a shepherd of snails—a snail-herd." (I wondered, am I one of those snails? One of the slow creatures in her care?) She said that, as she was getting dressed, she thought about the dream, of course, and thought that it was a reminder not to drive forward projects that have their own pace. She had a book to proofread, lectures to prepare, many things to do. She decided that she would drive them forward for just a week or two, and she would then put her feet up and let them go at their own pace, at snails' pace. On her way down stairs, she fell and hurt her ankle. Putting her feet up was imposed by the unconscious immediately! Better listen to one's dreams.

I was delighted by her letters. I had written to tell her I must cancel an appointment since I had to sell my house in England. She replied:

> Dear Mr. Spicer,
>
> Sorry you have to sell your house. But we are all wandering beggars in this world. I wrote you down for Mai 2nd at 3 p.m. O.K.?

During my analysis, I was studying Chomsky's linguistics and thought that there was a connection between his structural and transformational grammar and collective unconscious/archetypal structures. We talked about this on a few occasions. She disagreed. One day, long after my analysis with her was over, I received a letter from Dr. von Franz:

Dear Mr. Spicer,

About Chomsky, I now think you were right.

Both of these letters were signed "cordially yours." And cordially—in my heart—I carry her still; not a day passes, hardly an analytical hour passes without something from Marie-Louise von Franz enlivening my work and life—and thus the lives of many others. I had a dream about her today. With her example, I keep my letter short.

Ars longa; vita brevis.

Pleasure Being in Jung's Pocket

J. MARVIN SPIEGELMAN

I first met Dr. von Franz in the spring of 1953, when she came to Los Angeles to lecture. There was no Jungian society then, and I was not even a member of the Analytical Psychology Club, but since I had earned my doctorate in psychology in 1952 and had been in analysis (with Dr. Max Zeller) since the fall of 1950, I was permitted to attend. I had previously been present for the visits of several Zürich analysts such as Dr. Rivkah Schaerf, Ms. Barbara Hannah, Dr. Jolande Jacobi, and subsequently, Dr. C. A. Meier. For a young man (I was twenty-four when I started analysis), studying at a very rational and academic university, these visitors brought a powerful breath of cultured European spirit, deepened by Jungian psychology. This gave solace and inspiration to my parched soul, which had managed to meet the outer requirements of living but was thirsty inside.

I must say that Dr. von Franz was exceptional, even when compared to these very special visitors. She was brilliant, filled with information, just as intellectual as any of my professors, but oh, so much more substantial than any teacher I had yet encountered. I had the opportunity of having a private session with her and well recall that when I went to see her, I was trembling with the *numinosum* surrounding this treasured meeting. To my amazement, she trembled too, but neither of us said anything about it. She had a cigar box for the cash payment, which I thought odd but appropriate to her lack of pretension. She began, to my delighted astonishment, by telling me a dream that she had had the previous night, which was about ancient animals wandering in the Los Angeles area. I told her that she had indeed intuited a fact about my native city. The La Brea tar pits, in a park across the way from where I lived from age ten to age eighteen, had been filled with the bones and even bodies of many of these ancient creatures. As an adolescent, I went there to meditate at least once or twice a week and was subsequently to visit again, when I was twenty-seven and ready to get married. At that later time, the "ghost" of my grandfather appeared and directed me to walk to a nearby temple (unknown to me), where I encountered a rabbi, looking very much like my grandfather. I subsequently learned that this man had met my bride's rabbinical grandfather when the former, serving as chief rabbi of the German army during World War I, visited various towns on the border to see how their needs could be best served. Rabbi Sonderling was very impressed, he told us, that my bride's grandfather asked only that they be allowed to observe the Sabbath. These coincidences, later understood as synchronicities, were wonderfully appropriate for us, particularly for someone who subsequently performed our marriage ceremony. I report this personal experience here to indicate that my initial encounter with Dr. von Franz, as well as all later connections, were especially significant ones, either as to time or place or both, both synchronistic and filled with meaningful content.

Dr. von Franz lectured in Los Angeles on the *puer aeternus,* among other things, most brilliantly. In our private session, she interpreted my dreams with precision, directness, and depth of knowledge, as well as managing to connect with me personally and archetypally. I had hoped to work with her one day while training in Zürich. This longed-for possibility was delayed a bit. I completed my clinical training, married that same year, and was then called into the U.S. Army (this was at the end of the Korean war), despite my previous two-year stint during World War II in the merchant marine. This time, however, I served as a psychologist at a large hospital and clinic, again for two years. At the conclusion of this tour of duty (a "good" arising out of an initially perceived "evil"), I was awarded financial help (the GI bill) to attend the C. G. Jung Institute in Zürich.

I had hoped to work analytically with both Dr. von Franz and Dr. C. A. Meier, having previously arranged to see the latter. I discovered that they did not work well together, so I felt compelled to put off individual contact with Dr. von Franz until completing the propaedeuticum. I was compensated for this loss by being able to attend every one of her lectures, on fairy tales in particular. As is known to "all the world," Dr. von Franz's courses were marvels of information, insight, creativity, and depth. I had never in my life had a teacher who so combined knowledge with depth. Those seminars subsequently became the books she is so well known for, but thanks to a devoted class member, we were privileged to be able to purchase mimeographed copies, which I took back to America with me when I graduated in 1959.

When I completed the propaedeuticum, I happily approached Dr. von Franz for control work and initially this went very well. After a time, however, conflict arose. I think this was basically because I was unable to contain the differences between my training analyst, C. A. Meier and my control analyst. With pain and sorrow, I was compelled to stop working with her for a time. Some months later, I wrote to her, expressing my regret at having had to stop the control work and hoping that our relationship would not be damaged thereby. She wrote back a wonderful letter, thanking me for taking the trouble and risk of writing to her. She herself had been disturbed by our conflict and did not know how to repair the breach. Furthermore, she was very grateful that I had done this. Well, one can imagine how moved I was by this eros response from a most esteemed teacher, one that I had previously experienced superficially as "tough." Our subsequent connection went quite well indeed.

A few years later, when I returned for a stay in Zürich, I had arranged for a session with her. The night before, I attended a party at which, alas, I had a little too much wine. Conversation ensued in which I had said that I regretted that Dr. von Franz was "too much in Jung's pocket." My remark was both stupid and envious. A pupil of hers was there, however, and immediately telephoned her about what I had said. When I arrived the next day for the interview, Dr. von Franz was not to be found. After a time, I returned to my hotel and found a note stating that she would not be able to see me. Sadly, I contacted her again, but the damage was done. Several letters were exchanged between us, in which she expressed her pleasure at "being in Jung's pocket," and we both were able to laugh about it.

This somewhat stormy aspect of our relationship was to change a few years later when Dr. von Franz came to Los Angeles once again to speak at a conference. By then, I had resigned from my local Jungian society (only to resume membership some fourteen years later). I had again asked to see her, and this time she replied very graciously indeed. She invited me to have dinner with her at her hotel at the beach and was glad to have the conference pay the bill! We had a wonderful evening, in which she understood very well my reasons for resigning from the society. She endeared herself even more fully to me by saying that the individual is so much more important than professional societies, which often betray individuation at the first opportunity. In short, she supported me fully. Following that meeting, I had several powerful dreams, two of which portrayed the Self in both a personal and transpersonal way, while another one presented Dr. von Franz as deeply supportive of my writing. In this dream, she assured me that my work did indeed have significance beyond "writing for the desk drawer," as she was often fond of saying. As a matter of fact, all nineteen of my books (authored, co-authored, and edited) have been published since then.

Following that magical and fulfilling evening, there was occasional correspondence between us over a number of years, most importantly when I was facing a period in my life in which I lived with fear from a perceived outer threat. Again Dr. von Franz was both supportive and helpful. When that fear was relieved, I wrote to her that I had had a most powerful experience, feeling angels singing the praises of God within me. I told her that up until that time, I had always wondered why there were a whole group of angels whose only function was to praise God. Was God, then, like some sort of Mafia chieftain who needed endless adulation, despite (or because of?) displaying obvious darkness? That experience of being "delivered from evil" and knowing that those very angels were singing in my own soul solved that question for me. It is not that God (the Self) needs or does not need that praise; rather, there are autonomous forces in the psyche that proclaim that praise and express gratitude when the soul experiences deliverance. It is just so. And I would now spontaneously add: thank God!

It is my final personal experience with Dr. von Franz that truly caps this lifelong connection with that outstanding personality. In 1995, at the time of the IAAP Congress, I had the great honor and pleasure of seeing both of my important Jungian teachers in Zürich, C. A. Meier and M.-L. von Franz, not long before they both died. Dr. von Franz had responded to my earlier letter announcing my coming and invited me to visit her at her home in Bollingen. Friends had advised me that she continued to be far from well and that I should expect to spend no more than a few minutes with her. I was glad to have any time at all, sensing that this would be the last occasion that I would have a chance to see her face to face. My wife joined me in taking the train out to Bollingen, and we then gradually made our way up to her mountain retreat. About halfway up, when we asked directions, we were told we were on the right path. Some few hundred yards from the top, my wife chose to wait for me, sitting on a comfortable bench with a nice view. I continued on, found Dr. von Franz's house, and knocked, for a moment anxiously remembering that unhappy event in the past when she failed to appear (following the party). Her companion answered the door, however, and immediately ushered me into Marlus's presence (we had been on a first-name basis for some time, actually). Dr. von Franz was almost crippled now, but still in fairly decent spirits. After the usual preliminaries, she suddenly asked about my "knight." I was astonished. I had sent her a copy of my first book, *The Tree of Life: Tales in Individuation (Psychomythology)*, some twenty years earlier. It was a fictional presentation of ten different stories of individuation in men and women from different nations, religions, and ethnicities, all of whom meet at the Tree of Life. The lead character of that book and its two sequels was a knight. This archetypal image had been central in my own life process from early childhood onward. Dr. von Franz's only comment when she received the book, long ago, was to wonder if it should not have been exposed to the world. I was never clear as to why. Was it meant "for the desk drawer," as she was fond of saying, or was it too personal? I do not know. Now, twenty years later, she told me how much she appreciated that tale and that her own animus had also presented himself powerfully as a knight. Our conversation then grew more emotional and intimate, and when she leaned forward for me to kiss her, I was not surprised. It was a true culmination of our eros connection, which, I think, was powerfully constellated at our very first meeting, almost a half century earlier.

After this shared moment, Dr. von Franz told me a number of her recent dreams, all quite impressive. One that I feel can be told here was that the Self appeared and announced that she indeed had been a great scholar. After telling this dream, Dr. von Franz said that there are many aspects of the Self, and she was grateful for manifesting some of them, but others had not been realized. This was said in a very matter-of-fact way, without regret or doubt. I affirmed that her work was a great gift to all of us and I was sure that it would be even more appreciated in the years to come. She responded that this was perhaps so, but she, like Jung, was not terribly optimistic about either the fate of Jungian psychology or even our civilization. She also said that she was very ready to leave life now and was hoping for the best for others. She added that she could still appreciate how the Self was continuing to appear for her, particularly in her solitude in her garden and when she gazed out over the world below.

Instead of the expected ten minutes, I was with her for more than an hour and a half and left in a heightened state of feeling. I knew that I had been privileged to share a long-term relationship with a most outstanding individual. I was weeping when I came back to where my wife had been waiting for me, and she patiently accompanied me back to the train station in silence. Only on the ride back to Zürich was I able to relate the experience to her. She embraced me, too.

Jungian psychology was fortunate to have so many gifted "first generation" people. Those of us in the second generation can only express our appreciation and continue onward in the service of the psyche and of individuation. In a changing and uncertain world, we can surely do so by helping our pupils and analysands to do the same. For special and unwavering support in this worthwhile endeavor of the soul, I am especially pleased to thank Dr. Marie-Louise von Franz.

I am aware that there is currently a move within the broader field of Jungian psychology to disparage what some see as the idealization of Jung, in particular, and some of his immediate followers, among whom the most gifted, perhaps, was Dr. von Franz. I am also aware that much of what I have written here may be so dismissed by this same chorus. While I am painfully aware of shadow issues (and know of them quite well in Jung, von Franz, and myself), I want to suggest that such a reductive move may also be simply the need for some people to get rid of the masters in order to find their own way. In so doing, one might then merely be repeating a variant of Freud's Oedipus complex without having transcended or outgrown it.

Another possibility that comes to mind arises from the East. Gurus there often have pictures of their teachers and teachers' teachers behind them as they present themselves to the public. That sense of continuity of tradition (instead of revolution) is also a very beautiful image for some of us to treasure. It is this image that gives me sustenance as I approach my own final years. I thank Dr. von Franz for her devotional nature, which provides us with an example of this other way, one adding a much-needed feminine perspective to the old myth. Perhaps I may note that on the outer wall of a bookcase in my consulting room, just opposite my chair, and out of sight of the analysand, there sits, at the top, a picture of my ancient and honored grandfather (who lived from 1854 to 1951). Below him is a picture of Jung, meditatively sitting at the seaside. A small photo of von Franz rests just above his head to the left. Below that pair of photos is an antique map of Zürich, reminding me of my extraordinarily rich years of study at the Institute in the late 1950s. At the bottom is an ancient imaginal map of Jerusalem. In this way, I too honor my spiritual ancestors and teachers. I am glad to have them all present when I am devotionally engaged in the work of the psyche.

Some Images of Dr. von Franz

MURRAY STEIN

It is an honor to be invited to contribute a short article to a Festschrift commemorating Dr. von Franz. As for so many others, her lectures and writings were deeply influential in my training as a Jungian analyst. I will never forget the first time I heard Dr. von Franz lecture. This happened during my first year of training, in early 1970. The lecture took place in the evening and was held in a hall outside the Institute, to accommodate the large audience. As it turned out, this was the first in her famous *puer aeternus* series. For me, it was a numinous experience. I thought God was speaking. She seemed to know everything. In an amazing fashion and without a text, she ranged over history West and East, mythology, philosophy, anthropology, and a host of other specialized areas. Never in my previous academic training had I heard such far-reaching and profound reflections. When I told this to my analyst the next day, he only smiled. I did not realize at the time what a big reputation Dr. von Franz had. After that, we got down to the business of applying some of her insights on the *puer* to my own life, which was not such a comfortable experience.

Later, while still in training, I had the pleasure of editing her book on creation myths for Spring Publications. She was the most objective author I have ever worked with as an editor. No detail was too small for her careful consideration, but one never sensed a personal investment in the outcome of discussions, only a serious psychological attitude toward the work.

One of the features of great personalities like those of Dr. Jung and Dr. von Franz is that their presence and influence continues to move us as strongly as ever after they pass away. Many of my analysands over the years have dreamed of Dr. Jung, for instance, and invariably these dreams have had important symbolic meaning. Synchronicity also seems to strike in the vicinity of such psychologically important figures. I will give an example, this one involving Dr. von Franz.

On the day I received the invitation to contribute to the Festschrift for Dr. von Franz in the mail, I also received by email a dream from a friend, Don McNair. He has no connection to the Psychological Club and of course knew nothing about the Festschrift in preparation. I opened the email first, but being pressed for time I glanced at it quickly, only noting that he said that he had had a dream the night before in which Dr. von Franz appeared. As I read through the Festschrift invitation, I saw that donors were asked to contribute accounts, including synchronistic events or other relevant unconscious constellations related to her. There is also an interest, the announcement said, in learning from dreams *how the unconscious perceives her.* Astonished, I went back into my computer and read Don's dream more carefully. Here is the extraordinary dream as he wrote it down:

> *I have come to Zürich to visit Dr. Marie-Louise von Franz. As I walk along a street or in a park among many trees, I look down and see a bas-relief image of a woman under a thin film of red clay dust. I realize that it is an obsidian sarcophagus and think to myself, "There's a mummy in it." To the right of it there is a large mollusk shell made of pure gold. It reminds me of those beautiful "turkey wing" shells I've found on the coast of South Carolina except that it is a long diamond shape rather than*

wing-shaped. It is about a foot long and is covered with embossed designs, quite beautiful. It "buzzes" because of a rapid fluttering of wings, and I realize there is a creature in it that is "more than a butterfly." I gently open the shell and see the creature. It has a face with humanlike features.

I arrive at Dr. von Franz's house with the shell in my hand. She comes out on a sunporch and greets me very warmly. She is petite and attractive, no glasses, with dark blonde hair tinged with gray. She is wearing a gray-brown pantsuit. She appears to be about seventy or seventy-five years old. I am holding the butterfly cupped in my hands over the center of my chest. I open my hands and show it to her. She tells me the name of the butterfly creature, though on waking I cannot remember it. She invites me to dinner. Somehow the plans change to preparing a banquet for an elderly man, Jung-like but not Dr. Jung. I start working on a dish for the banquet. I am mixing ground meat and bread crumbs in a large silver bowl with my hands. I form it into large meatballs 2 inches in diameter. I look around and see lots of people milling about to my left.

Murray Stein shows up with a mug of beer in his left hand. The mug is round on the bottom and square on top with the handle at a corner, giving the top a diamond shape. It is clear glass. I say, "Let's go buy our guest a gift." Murray says, "Let me finish this beer." I look in a large room to the left, which is filled with tables full of stacks of Swiss chocolate and lots of people, mostly women, shopping. I say, "There's nothing appropriate there." I think about the collective, "harassed and helpless, like sheep without a shepherd."

Murray and I meet up with Dr. von Franz on the porch again. She is on her way to give an impromptu lecture, in a hall where the old man has already arrived. She has a folder of notes and tells us she doesn't know what she will choose to talk about. Then she says, "Don will give me an idea. He is really bubbly and he will also challenge me on my thoughts." Then Murray goes ahead of me, shopping, and I set out to meet him.

Of course, this dream has a lot of personal meaning for the dreamer, who has long been a serious student of Dr. von Franz's writings and has seen her on film, but I believe the fact of this synchronicity and the archetypal symbols in the dream lend it a more general meaning as well, one from which many people can benefit. He told me as well that while he has dreamed many times of Dr. Jung this is his first remembered dream of Dr. von Franz, which adds forcefully to the impact of its synchronicity.

This synchronicity consists not only in the meaningful coincidence between my receiving the Festschrift invitation by mail and the dream's occurrence to Don and its subsequent arrival in my computer, but also in the conjoint theme of celebration. We have here a conjunction of two occasions of celebration. On the one hand, there is the celebration of Dr. von Franz with the Festschrift, and on the other hand there is the celebration in the dream of the "Jung-like" old man (who himself also surely represents a union of the opposites—young and old!). To me this says, in a brief and clearly encoded way, that an important *coniunctio oppositorum* has come into play. In this event, Wisdom and Wholeness are being raised up for honor and consciousness. What could be more needed in our time of darkness and wanton one-sidedness? What could be more deserving of celebration?

There is also the striking suggestion that in the dream image of the creature who is "more than a butterfly" and has a human face a new, or perhaps better said, a re-newed aspect of the collective unconscious is approaching human consciousness. This figure is reminiscent of other mythological animals with human faces, theriomorphic representations of the gods. I would interpret this as an augury for the new millennium: a new archetypal image and value is emerging into consciousness. Naturally Dr. von Franz, with her vast store of knowledge, can name the creature! No doubt we will hear more about it in the years to come. It has to do with the new god image that is emerging in this aeon.

The dream's presentation of Dr. von Franz shows her in brown earth tones with a warm and feeling demeanor toward the dreamer. She is also intellectually creative and playful. To me, her spirit appears to be well and vibrant, in the afterlife as she was in this life, and clearly she is participating in the psychological process that is unfolding in our time. Even though she stands outside of time, she also participates in it. This is the meaning of her noted age (she is in her seventies) in the dream account.

Certainly making a present to her in the form of this Festschrift is also celebrating the life and ongoing historical presence of Dr. Jung, to whom she was so deeply dedicated. Beyond even that, it is celebrating the psychological values (the "gold") to which both are eternally committed.

Music in Dreams

HILDEMARIE STREICH

September 28, 2002

Dear Dr. Kennedy,

Enclosed please find an abridged English translation of my research work on the theme of music in dreams, which, inspired by your letter, I would like to dedicate to Dr. Marie-Louise von Franz.

The dedication of this work to her has a special reason. In 1965, I met Dr. von Franz for the first time at her home in Küsnacht where she had invited me for a visit. I had just completed a five-year training and control analysis as part of the educational program in analytical psychology in Berlin. At the recommendation of my training analyst, I reported the results of my research work on the theme of music in dreams to Dr. von Franz, a theme which, at that time, was in its earliest pioneer phase.[1] To my great joy and relief Dr. von Franz was genuinely enthusiastic and thought—as did my training analyst—that this work, along with the interface between analytical psychology, psychological diagnostics, music, the science of music, and music therapy—was a constellation that C. G. Jung had long awaited. She then recommended to the C. G. Jung Institute in Zürich that I give lectures and courses. And thus between the years 1967 and 1978 I lectured many times. For the initial impulse to all of this, I wish to thank Dr. Marie-Louise von Franz.

During the time of my lecture series in Zürich I had—much to my great benefit—the occasion to go to lectures of Dr. von Franz and to cultivate relationships with Cornelia Brunner, Jolande Jacobi, Franz Ricklin, C. A. Meier, Alfred Ribi, James Kirsch, and others, all of whom I wish to thank for the valuable material they gave me on music in dreams.

In the beginning, above all, was that inspiring encounter with Marie-Louise von Franz, who I thereafter visited whenever I was in Zürich. She told me many of her dreams and was glad to exchange her ideas about them with me.

As I was about to give my first lecture in English, I had a dream in which Dr. von Franz said to me: "Just give your lectures in English freely. Your English is quite good. Spoken freely, they will come across the best." The dream encouraged me. The next day, I told the dream to my audience and then held my lecture freely. Without this dream I would never have taken the risk, as my English was anything but perfect. My audience, nevertheless, was gracious and grateful.

Although I could report so much of what Dr. von Franz and I spoke about in our conversations, I hope the following contribution will suffice.

With warm greetings,
Hildemarie Streich

Contents of dreams that involve music themes are not limited to the practical field of music with its rich variety of musical instruments and their vast range of expression. We also find hidden in the unconscious depths of the human psyche evidence of archaic musical concepts and structures whose very origin was an important issue in ancient and medieval thought. Music often appears in dreams as a therapeutic agent of the psyche. So whenever music is used for its harmonically balancing, leveling, stimulating, or calming effects, the unconscious of modern men and women reaches back to the ancient therapeutic experiences of humankind that were mediated via music. Music reaches from the depths of the psyche up into consciousness, from within outward, and serves as a cathartic healing agent adapted to the problems and the personal needs of the individual, often initiating new forms of inner development.

The Meaning of Music in Ancient Times

The words *music* and *harmony* shared the same meaning in ancient times. Since the dawning of human thought, music has been considered to be a quality of both the cosmic and divine worlds, belonging as well to the realm of matter with its organic and inorganic elements and to the psychic and psychosomatic worlds.

In Greek mythology, Harmonia was worshipped as the goddess who unites opposing forces. A daughter of Ares (god of war) and Aphrodite (goddess of love), she represented the harmonic forces responsible for musical order in the world. Etymologically, the word *harmonia* comes from the Greek in which the syllable *ar* or *har* means the uniting of opposites in a fruitful and dynamic whole. Thus "true music"—understood as harmony—can only be found in uniting the organic, the psychic, and the cosmic or heavenly realms, integrating their inherent opposites in a holistic totality whose different qualities manifest themselves in four main aspects:

Musica coelestis or *divina*	the music or harmony of the heavens
Musica mundana	music or harmony of the spheres
Musica humana	psychosomatic music, harmony
Musica instrumentalis	instrumental and vocal music[2]

In the view of the ancients, the whole of creation with its deepest realm meets in a structured, unified, and whole world that does not know of a separation of the individual realms or aspects. These dimensions complete, overlap, and complement one another. They can be compared to the rungs of Jacob's ladder connecting heaven and earth. The teachings of the ancients interpret Jacob's ladder as the tree of life or the Sephirot tree.

Jacob's Ladder of Music

In medieval traditions concerning Jacob's dream, the ladder between heaven and earth is sometimes thought to possess four great rungs which can be seen as analogies of the four great aspects of music. Here the rungs are considered to be:

> four worlds, one upon the other, which are not separated according to our conception of time and space, but permeate each other in the here and now. The World of God overlaps the World of Ideas which overlaps the World of Invisible Form not yet materialized, and this in turn overlaps the World of Matter.[3]

The ancient conception of music is apparently similar to the conception of the four rungs of Jacob's ladder representing four realms or worlds permeating and completing one another so that by their cooperation the integral whole comes into consciousness. Each part can only be understood if seen as one part of a larger whole. Only a quartet of all the four aspects of music is able to give us the true *musica* or *harmonia.*

According to ancient teachings, the ladder to heaven which appeared in Jacob's dream has become an earthly perceptible reality (and a conscious-immanent reality) in Christ as the incarnation of the Logos, the creative sound at the very creation of the world. In his colloquy with Nathaniel, Jesus implicitly refers to Jacob's ladder: "Verily, verily, I say to you, hereafter ye will see heaven open and the angels of God ascending and descending upon the Son of Man" (St. John 1:51, Gen. 28:12). Christ is here seen as the ladder to heaven, as the reconciliation of opposites, as the mediator between above and below, as the living, healing energy, possessor of the keys to hell, triumphant over death (Rev. 1:18). With this in mind, we are able to understand St. Jerome speaking of *Christus Summus Musicus,* that is, Christ as the universal musician in whom, as in Jacob's ladder, heaven meets earth, time, and eternity.

The following presentation of present-day musical dreams will show us that experiencing music as an entirety is not only a phenomenon of days long past, but rather a psychic reality waiting to be individually recognized and realized in the lives of modern people.

Present-day Dreams

The musical content found in the dreams of contemporary people is well related to the ancient concept of music as harmony. The deepest parts of our psyche still harbor a knowledge of music as a whole, as a unifying, harmonizing, and purging force seemingly no longer recognized or understood by rational thought. Accordingly, dreams with images of disharmony, of musical destruction, or of blockages tend to occur when one is unaware of disturbances in the harmonic order of the psychic and psychosomatic forces. Their task is to show these disturbances so that they can be recognized and remedied, thus offering the dreamer a chance to regain lost harmony. Musical motifs may take the form of a musical mandala, a symbol of the center, a goal to be achieved, or the unity of opposites. And they do this either in order to point out possibilities of order and harmony hitherto unknown yet now to be realized, or in order to serve as a temporary compensation for a condition of distress and disorientation.

A distinct group of music-related dreams can be seen to occur as a prelude to the very beginnings of a new phase in the dreamer's development. One might conclude that here music serves as a herald presaging changes to come. There are dreams that use musical imagery focusing on instruments or musical occurrences, and these may come at any time whatsoever. Closer examination of the music motif may be essential in the interpretation of such dreams. Dreams, however, do not always place the music motif in a central position. It can also be found in an unobtrusive and modest position in the background. Nevertheless, it may be well worth while to heed even the most minor occurrence of music motifs or references. To a much higher degree than at first assumed, their analysis may lead to enriching the conscious mind with new knowledge that, clad in seemingly insignificant attire, may be all too easily passed over unawares.

We will now proceed to the presentation of a small selection of dreams with music motifs that have an initiating character opening new possibilities of insight, development, healing, or growth. They are taken from the unpublished series of lectures titled "Music in Dreams" given at the C. G. Jung Institute in Zürich.

Examples of Music-related Dreams

The Music Tree

The following dream is from a thirty-nine-year-old teacher, a woman who was a German Protestant but whose religious heritage included French Catholics as well as Jews. At the time of the dream, she was trying to find some way to unite these differing religious traditions within her own individual personality.

> *I am in a church like the church in Birnau, the very famous baroque pilgrimage church on Lake Constance with marvelous frescos on the ceiling. I am standing up on the gallery. Strangely, this gallery is like the huge and broad bough of a tree which grows from the depths of the earth and climbs high into the blue sky, past the clouds and beyond, into the heavens. Standing quite at ease on a strong branch of this tree-gallery, I look up to the ceiling above and see a host of angels busily playing music. But there is no fresco painted on the ceiling as in Birnau, and there is no stone, but rather there is something like a musical heaven so close that I can almost touch it. Everything is most real and alive. The music rendered is of an extraordinary beauty, joyous and profound, and*

it serves to link heaven and earth. Moreover, the church's nave below is not made of stone but of farmland that looks like the fresh-scented, fertile soil of spring which seems to be absorbing the current of heavenly music pouring forth from above in order to return it later in a transformed variety of fruits, flowers, and grains.

This dream of the tree linking heaven and earth by means of music and extending right down to the root of all things does not remind us so much of Jacob's ladder or the tree of life but more of St. Jerome's description of Christ as the universal supreme musician in whom all aspects of music and harmony, chord and discord, are united. The dream image gave the dreamer both deeper insight into an inner experience of the essential possibilities in the relationship of spirit and matter, of above and below, reason and emotion, or Protestant-Catholic-Jewish ancestors, and of heaven and earth. This dream also inspired her profoundly in her work and proved to be a fruitful catalyst enriching her future life.

The Broken Cello

A thirty-seven-year-old social worker, who played no instrument (certainly not the cello here), sought psychoanalytic treatment for her severe depression. At the beginning of her therapy, she related the following dream:

My cello is broken and out of joint. I cannot play it anymore. The strings are broken, and the resonant chamber is damaged. I am supposed to take it to a violin maker. Someone says to me, "It will take a long time, but given patience and precision work, your cello will be sound again."

The musical instrument here is essentially used as a comprehensive visual image of the dreamer's back trouble and her disturbed state of mind much in need of healing. The shape of the cello renders the idea of the woman's bodily form as a kind of protomusical instrument. But as for this woman, the instrument is not intact and cannot fulfill its vocation of sounding its unique voice and finding its place in the greater living, breathing orchestra of humankind. It is out of joint, says the dream; it cannot sound because the strings are broken and the resonant chamber damaged. We should note here that the English word *sound* also means healthy, intact, stable, reliable, and so forth.

And indeed, the main course of the dreamer's desolation was her dissociation from herself and her environment. Certain instances in her biography had led to the woman losing her backing on various levels. A parental background of a despotic father and a compulsive mother led to considerable suffering as a child and the loss of her initial trust, which in turn broke the strings linking her with our transcendental background, that is, she had lost her *religio.* In consequence, she was no longer able to respond when called to do so. Cutting her connections, she grew increasingly lonely. And out of touch, she grew ever more out of tune. With no strings intact, the instrument was no longer sound. Visiting the violin maker is the only way to make it sound again. Thus a way is offered to overcome the chaos and destruction from which she suffers in a gradual process of healing.

The dream is helpful in four ways. First, it unambiguously states what is wrong. Second it states a clear demand to seek help. Third, it offers an encouraging hope for recovery. And fourth, it advises patience and diligence for such a protracted undertaking.

Visual dream images of damaged musical instruments can impressively indicate the kind of distress from which a person is suffering and the causes for that condition and offer a suitable remedy. In such contexts we find images of splits, tears, partial or complete destruction, negligence, soiling, and so forth. Not always, however, is the chance for healing indicated nor a phase of consciously facing the problem initiated.

In the course of this woman's analysis, the image of the cello together with other music imagery kept emerging, commenting on the gradual process of healing as well as on the hindrances that occurred. At a later stage in her development, the patient dreamed that she had a viola da gamba, a small instrument rather like a cello, and she was supposed to take lessons. This dream marked the beginning of yet another new phase coinciding with her changing jobs and renting a small flat. It also led to obtaining a real viola da gamba and beginning music lessons. As for her inner life, she had grown to be a somewhat sounder person, a little more at home with herself; contact with her own inner life had been made. She now had to learn how to play the instrument "of herself," that is, to find her own voice. Little by little, she then resumed contact with the world around her. In this phase, her dreams showed images of her making music together with others and of the joys and sorrows and difficulties that go with it.

The Black Man's Song

The following dream comes from a twenty-six-year-old American man of Jewish origin suffering from an inferiority complex. He had committed a criminal offense, was ashamed of his race, professed atheism, and, in his own view, was an utterly unmusical person. In his dream, he takes a walk with a black man who is singing a long song about his life and its problems. The song is also a religious one expressing a yearning for the return home. The song is called "Home to Moses, Home to Christ, Home to God." Deeply moved by the black man's song, the dreamer tells him that he is his friend. On waking up, the song remains with him and accompanies him all through the day.

This dream initiated a new attitude toward the dreamer's life as well as toward his race and the dark brother in his own soul. In a most impressive way, the dream complements the dreamer's conscious atheist attitude and indicates a longing to return to his roots, to the home offered in the religious experiences of his forefathers. Up until then, this wish had been repressed and therefore unappreciated and unfulfilled.

Musical Structures

The following dream came from a seventy-seven-year-old psychiatrist who neither read nor played music. Up until the time of the dream, he had appreciated music solely as a "language of feelings." He dreamt:

I see a large sheet of music, and on this sheet of music is drafted a most profound system entailing the very roots of music and the psyche. Overjoyed, I look at this sheet whose music I can both see and hear resonating in geometric-mathematical structures such as I have never experienced or been conscious of before. There is a lot more to grasp than I am capable of comprehending. I wake up wondering how can I find access to these archaic structures of music that are also the basic structures of the psyche?

For this dream, I would like to thank James Kirsch, M.D., Jungian analyst and founder of the C. G. Jung Institute in Los Angeles. Born in Berlin, James Kirsch emigrated from Nazi Germany to London and from there later to the United States. On the occasion of the Eranos Conferences in Ascona, Switzerland, Dr. Kirsch and his wife discussed the meaning of music in their dreams with me, and on following visits to Europe they brought with them numerous music-related dreams from their clients and their training analysts for interpretation. Their contributions greatly enriched my collection of musical dreams. The following dream, told by a sixty-eight-year-old American author, is one of their contributions.

The Dockworker's Dream

On a New York waterfront dock at night, a high-spirited union meeting cum celebration is taking place. Dockworkers—blacks and whites, fathers and sons—are present. Then suddenly, in the foreground, one of the black leaders begins to play beautiful, deeply moving jazz on his brilliantly polished trumpet. I immediately hear another trumpet responding further away and closer to the water's edge, and this one is played by a prominent white dockworker. And as the music floats back and forth between these two men, I realize that they are engaged in a dialogue: they are actually talking in a loving, good-natured fashion. I am deeply stirred by this duet. Suddenly two more trumpets join them, played by their sons. And the colloquy floats back and forth in vibrant jazz. Then the black musician in the foreground lifts his trumpet to the black, starless sky, and I see the notes issuing from his horn and planting themselves in the blackness of the night. The phrase flashes through my mind: "written on the wind in gold." It is a thrilling dream.

In a musical fashion, this dream initiates a new phase in the dreamer's inner development in respect to the harmonic and highly dynamic jazz ensemble composition of the opposites formerly experienced as being in bitter combat. We find these opposites expressed in the blacks and whites playing their trumpets in a wonderful and mutually complementary manner of music making. Thus, the dreamer was shown a peaceful solution to the most urgent problem of racial discrimination as well as the equally pressing question of how to achieve a productive cooperation of conscious and unconscious as well as the forces of light and darkness within.

Another set of opposites can be seen in the different generations, an issue that was acutely felt by the dreamer. In his outer life, he was grappling with issues in his relationships both to his parents and to his children, whereas in his inner life interests and needs appropriate to his age frequently and vehemently collided with urges and drives belonging to a younger and rather adolescent stage equally alive in him.

Then there is the musical relation between the colors black, white, and gold. In their symbolic aspect they can be seen as representations of the stages through which our psyche passes ever and anew in its development. From time immemorial, black (for instance, the *nigredo*) has been considered to represent the dark, unprocessed, and often chaotic and initial stages of all things emerging; white (the *albedo*) as the cathartic phase of purgation and clarification; and gold (*citrinitas, rubedo*) as the phase wherein we see the dawning of new perception and of an individually novel approach to life.

Finally the dream shows yet another way of communing, which is of a more religious kind: the musical communication of man with what is above him, planting his music into the nocturnal darkness of the divine presence.

Like a musical sketch of the next phase to come, the dream preludes the tasks and themes that the dreamer will now have to elaborate in his life with patience and perseverance.

Dreams of Professional Musicians

Musical dreams of professional musicians tend to take a professional character. Sometimes they are musical nightmares concerning the loss of sheet music or musical instruments. They may also be admonishing the dreamer in times of stress or when one is on the verge of losing one's emotional, "musical" balance. The following two dreams are taken from a dream series covering more than forty years given to me by a sixty-seven-year-old musician who had never undergone any form of psychoanalysis before. Yet in his life he had been frequently impressed by musical dreams that helped and inspired him, and he had taken to recording them for further reflection.

Johann Sebastian Bach

"When I was thirty-five years old, I was writing a book on musical ornamentation. Before I could hand in the manuscript to the publishers, it got destroyed in a bomb attack. About this time I had the following dream:

> *I am walking along by myself when I suddenly notice a companion by my side. When I see his friendly broad countenance and his pink coat with its characteristic silver buttons, it dawns on me that this is Johann Sebastian Bach, just as I had known him from the pastel drawing in the collection of Carl Philipp Emanuel Bach (in the collection at Thuringia in the upper valley of the Rhine). It was but his ghost, yet quite real and friendly in the fashion of Thuringians. I was overawed. We kept walking in silence while I tried to make up my mind about what would be the proper way of addressing him: organist in Weimar, concertmaster in Köthen, choirmaster in Leipzig, and, ah, yes, royal Polish composer* (Hofkompositeur) *at the Dresden court. At last I plucked up my courage and said:* 'Herr Hofkompositeur . . . *about this ornament in your English Suite in D minor. May I ask you how you used it? You see, I am rather at a loss how to get it right, and am really so glad to have*

> *this chance to ask you.' To my infinite amazement, and with a marked Thuringian-Saxon accent, Johann Sebastian simply answers: 'Ah, well, actually I am not sure myself. Sometimes it is like this, sometimes like that,' and then he walked off."*

Talking to Wolfgang Amadeus Mozart

"About five or so years later, when I was about forty years old, I once dreamt that I was going for a walk in Vienna.

> *I found myself in the street called* 'Auf der Weiden.' *Suddenly there right next to me was Mozart. I was taken aback, and overjoyed. I could feel a flux of communication between us, yet tried to think of the proper way to address this beloved and incomparable master. The director of the royal orchestra was Salieri, while Mozart was known as* Hofkompositeur *(court, or royal, composer). I noticed that Mozart was reading my thoughts and was himself amused. And so I said to him: 'Look,* Herr Hofkompositeur, *look here. This is where you used to live.' There was a plaque on the house saying* Schwarzspanienhaus *(Black Spanish House). (The actual house had long been demolished, and—as I remembered on waking up—it was Beethoven and not Mozart who used to live there.) The plaque was shaped like an old-fashioned weather vane and said in bronze letters: 'Former House of Wolfgang Amadeus Mozart. The Mozart Society. Open from 10 A.M. to 12 P.M.' Almost overcome by the fact that he had lived in this house, I say:* 'Herr Hofkompositeur, *here, in this very house, you used to live.' To my utter surprise, Mozart answers with a marked local accent:* 'An Scharrn hab' I da g'wohnt, dass war ja im Haus nebenan!' *('What a lot of rubbish that I lived there, it was in the house next door'). Eagerly I reply that one ought to inform the Mozart Society of their mistake. But Mozart says:* 'Ah was . . . , 's Mobiliar is eh nit echt, und's is ja eh wurscht, wo s' mich verehr'n, in dem oder in dem Haus' *('Ah so what, the furniture isn't genuine anyway, and I couldn't care less whether they honor me in this house or that'). After this amusing reaction, Mozart's spirit disappeared."*

Both of his composer dreams greatly helped and inspired the musician, for they encouraged him to strive for an optimum in the synthesis of a formal academic approach to music coupled with free artistic interpretation. His performance thus gained an unusual liveliness and transparency—drawn right from the source one might say—which then won him international acclaim.

Dreams on Death and Dying

In some dreams, music seems to play the role of the conductor of the soul in helping the soul enter into life after death. In instances like these, the music heard is of an indescribable beauty and leaves the dreamer feeling much comforted and ascertained of timeless forces that exist beyond death. Thus, some of these dreams render an intense experience of music as a messenger of realities invisible to us. Then there are other dreams in which doors open that lead into a hitherto unknown land.

Heavenly Music

In a dream shortly before his death, an eighty-six-year-old man, wise with age but fatally ill, heard "wonderful celestial music of indescribable beauty which convinced him deeply of there being some great benevolence surrounding, embracing, and supporting the universe." Music serves here as a messenger bearing tidings of a force that transcends empirical knowledge and the human capacity for understanding so that, for the sake of more subtle experiences, our senses of perception adapt and perceive those invisible realities of inner and outer worlds.

Music, Word, and Light

The inner kinship of sound, word, and light is one of the earliest experiences of our psyche. The dream of a contemporary woman shows the enduring relevance of such an experience. In her dream, music, word, and light worked together, heralding her impending death while opening doors to a hitherto secluded world. In the dream, her late husband plays the role of the bearer of the word and the conductor of the soul. The day before her death, this fifty-nine-year-old woman dreamed that she heard exquisite music of such an overpowering beauty that it exceeded the powers of description. As the music resounded, a large door opened, allowing a powerful current of light to pour in. And in this light stood her husband, who recently passed away. He then stepped toward her with a radiant smile and said: "I have not come for you today, but I will come tomorrow." And indeed, the next day she passed away peacefully with a remarkably joyous smile.

Conclusion

Both in the dreams during our lifetime as well as in dreams dreamt on the threshold of death, music may appear as the "conductor" of the psyche. In the first case, music opens the doors of our mind, leading to new stages of inner growth. In the latter, music leads the way into an existence after death, spanning the gulf between life and death. This is obviously quite in accordance with the ancient meaning of music as harmony, as the force which—against all odds—achieves the connection of apparently incompatible contradictions into an integral whole. Thus music-related dreams can be seen in context with the four great aspects of music and harmony that were discussed at the beginning, aspects that possess no fixed parameters but overlap and permeate each other.

Most of the music motifs in dreams make use of the rich and almost inexhaustible store of imagery supplied by practical music. When we take a closer look at this element in the world of matter, we find psychic and cosmic-divine musical forces intertwined with practical music making that need to be recognized and permitted to gain influence in our lives. By pointing out either harmonic possibilities or disturbances of the harmonic order, musical motifs in dreams refer to music in its ancient meaning as harmony and reveal a deep need for compensation within the psyche. In times of disunion, dispersal, discord, disorientation, destruction, and horror, the healing forces within the psyche seek images representing the integral whole. Disconnection from these images does a great deal of harm. Regaining a living connection to them can help remedy such ailments. Here, as in other cases we have seen, music may serve as a kind of therapeutic agent of the psyche, providing catharsis to disparate conditions and initiating and conducting new phases of development.

NOTES

1. Hildemarie Streich, "Musik im Traum," in *Wiener Beiträge zur Musiktherapie, Band 3: Theorie und Klinische Praxis,* Dorothee Storz and Dorothea Oberegelsbacher, eds. (Wien: Edition Prasesen, 2001), pp. 73–98.
2. The latter includes the diametrically opposed orders and structures complementing one another in the organic and inorganic realm on earth.
3. A. Peter, *Zohar-Studien I–IV* (Berlin: unpublished manuscript, 1943).

My "Encounter" with Dr. Marie-Louise von Franz

VRENI SUTER

Just about four years ago today, I "met" Dr. von Franz. I had first heard of her in my analysis, in my work on dreams, and in my own unconscious, and then I became acquainted with—and learned to appreciate very much—her books. When I heard that a Festschrift in honor of Dr. von Franz was going to be written, I wanted to make some sort of contribution. Although I never personally met Dr. von Franz, I felt in an inexplicable manner close to her and thought that I would very much enjoy involving myself in some way in her honor.

It often seemed to me as though I was touched by her spirit in such a way that I could feel her warmth, her humor, and her wisdom. She accompanied me as an inner friend, and I held inner conversations with her, asked her questions—what she would do?—and so forth. My encounters with her were something that happened to me and from which I was touched. And then I met her in a dream.

I knew that Dr. von Franz always asked her own unconscious or listened to its reactions when she wanted to write or undertake something, and thus I wanted to do the same. The unconscious, I hoped, would answer me as to whether or not I should make a contribution and, if so, how or what my contribution should be. The night after I had heard about the Festschrift, I had the following dream.

> *February 16, 2002. I am lying in bed and to my right is a second bed in which Dr. von Franz is also lying. She says to me: "When the green frog comes, then everything will come into order." Then she becomes increasingly agitated and tries to explain it to me. She searches for the German word that would express what she is trying to say but cannot find it. Then she says in English: "Duplic completion." As soon as these words are spoken, she becomes even more agitated and says that "one never has too little money, for instance," and then added in a rather uncanny manner that "the devil notices and can do nothing more." She was in an intensely agitated state because she wanted to say something but did not know how. Then I took my hand from under the covers and reached out to her. I awoke with my heart racing.*

After this dream, everything was somehow different than it had ever been before. First, because von Franz's strategy really does function: one can ask the unconscious a question and one then may receive an answer. I had just experienced this myself. In no other way could I have believed such a thing could happen. I was truly shocked.

Second, which turned everything upside down, was that the dream did not express something vague, uncertain, or otherwise harmless enabling me to comfortably maintain my peace of mind. Instead, I totally lost my inner repose, for I found myself confronted with an important and urgent message that directly challenged me and could not be annulled or ignored. And what is more, what was the meaning of the green frog, or "duplic completion," or a condition where everything is in order in such a way that evil loses its power? And what is the nature of the relationship between the frog, "duplic completion," and the devil? These questions have occupied me intensely from then on.

I knew that Dr. von Franz loved frogs. And that unlike Jung (who sat by the lake and played at digging out his waterworks), she preferred to sit and watch the goings-on of the frogs in her pond.[1] From a psychological perspective, she shows how the frog is associated with reincarnation and resurrection as well as with love-magic, sexuality, and the mood of springtime with its brimming abundance of nature.[2] In the dream, it is a green frog that should come. Dr. von Franz notes that the color green points to life, procreation, and resurrection. And, as she goes on to explain, the frog in particular in dreams represents an unconscious impulse that has a decisive tendency to become conscious. There are impulses that are reluctant to become conscious, she notes; one must in a way make an effort to lift them into consciousness. But there are other impulses that approach consciousness with a powerful energetic gradient; they practically force their unconscious perception of their existence upon us. The frog represents just such an impulse, an impulse that refuses to be dismissed. (One thinks, for example, of the urgency of the frog prince.)

As Dr. von Franz says in my dream, the approach of the green frog—this unconscious urge toward renewal and rebirth—serves to bring everything into order. And she attempts to explain this state of order, so difficult to describe, with the expression "duplic completion."

The word *duplic* is not found in my dictionary but rather similar words such as *duplicate* or *double,* which mean a correspondence, a doubling, an exact replication, or two things that are exactly the same. *Completion,* of course, means to complete, to finish, to achieve closure, to conclude, to fulfill. The frog then catalyzes something similar to a doubling of a conclusion, in essence a twofold form of completion. But how am I to understand how something that is fulfilled and complete can become even more complete, fulfilled, or perfected? Or is she referring to different dimensions?

Dr. von Franz explains that a doubling of motives generally refers to something that is approaching the threshold of consciousness.[3] When a person dreams of two identical dogs or identical people, then it would mean that this content is emerging up out of the unconscious and approaching the threshold of consciousness. As it comes close to this threshold, it then splits or divides into two. At the threshold of consciousness a doubling phenomenon can occur indicating that that which we call time is an archetypal image that is not yet fully conscious for us. We do not yet know what time really is, and it may be here that the moment has come in which the archetype of time is approaching the threshold of consciousness. Von Franz notes that, as far as she knows, the concept of a twofold order is found everywhere. She, like Jung, names one aspect "acausal orderedness" (which is timeless) and the other "synchronicity," synchronistic events appearing then in linear time.[4]

This material, along with the urgency and agitation of Dr. von Franz's communication to me in the dream, is a clear indication that something is standing on the threshold of consciousness. But . . . what is it?

The assertion from Dr. von Franz in my dream that "the devil . . . can do nothing more" indicates that this content—which is making itself acutely noticeable—must be dealing with the problem of evil. But how then should evil be conquered in a world where it blatantly rules and against which I feel more than helpless? Or, concretely asked, how am I supposed to be able to deal with it?

Jung says that evil has become a determining factor in reality and cannot be done away with by simply changing its name.[5] We have to learn how to cope with it because it wants to live with us. There are situations, however (as Dr. von Franz describes), where it is best just to get out of the way of evil. She mentions the example of Buddha, who simply was not there when he was stricken with the attack of twenty thousand demons. They were left with the disappointment of pointlessly wielding their weapons in front of an empty throne. The Buddha's stance is an example of an introverted approach to avoid a direct confrontation with evil and not to allow oneself to be involved in emotionality and affects but rather to withdraw into the emptiness of the Self.[6] In *The Interpretation of Fairy Tales,* Dr. von Franz expresses the same attitude when she writes that there are situations in which one has to fully give up what one wants, and in this manner one slips out from under the danger; one simply is no longer there and thus nothing can go wrong. When one is confronted with a hopelessly wrong situation, one must simply risk the jump into nonexistence. And from there one can survive.[7]

I carried these thoughts about with me but found no conceivable connection between the green frog, the "duplic completion," and the ensuing powerlessness of evil. And I found no conceivable or concrete connection to me. How does something so difficult have anything to do with me? Isn't it simply a mystery that is impossible for me to unravel? On the other hand, the dream held fast, and I was unable to forget or ignore it. It was here to stay and would not leave me in peace.

Compelled by an irresistible urge, I drove to Bollingen and went to Dr. von Franz's tower hoping to find the answer to this mystery. I thought that maybe somehow her spirit would inspire me, or maybe the frogs in the pond would be forthcoming with some answer . . . anything. And then: there stood the tower, lonely and abandoned. I could not spot a single frog in the pond. There was simply nothing there other than a squirrel snuffing about and mosquitoes who took me for their hot lunch. The loneliness and emptiness made me sad, and no secrets were revealed.

Disappointed and ashamed of the illusion that I was seeking something when in fact I actually had no idea what it was, I left the tower and turned back. On my way, I discovered a little path crossing the fields and decided to walk along it. How can I have been so silly and hoped for something like a miracle? Pensive and irritated with myself, I plodded forward. Everything around me was so quiet and abandoned that even a swarm of flies buzzing up from fresh cow dung made me jump back. And then I saw him. Farther down below, working away at a block of salt, stood a large black bull. I slowly proceeded in order to figure out how my path could best pass around him. But as I looked around, I saw the situation was hopeless. I had somehow landed inside his paddock. He looked up, thoughtfully inspected me, and then returned to his salt, which was apparently more interesting . . . looked up again, then returned to his activity. I slowly realized that there was nothing else for me to do than retreat. It was a long way back, and in the end I had to cross a threefold barbed-wire fence in order to get out of danger.

I then stopped at a gap in the hedge that grew along the bull's paddock and looked back. There he was again. He now stood just where I had been standing a short time ago and stared in the direction of my retreat. Although his massive strength and vitality were so much greater than mine, he was certainly no devil. Nevertheless, I was more than glad not to be there anymore. And then on the evening of the same day I also met the frog. It hopped in front of my car on the road, paused, then squatted. It showed no further intention to move, and I had no other choice than to carefully drive around it.

After the experiences of this day, I felt increasingly affected and concretely struck by these events that simply would not let themselves be ignored. My understanding of the world was considerably shaken. I no longer knew which reality was real. I had the impression that the outer world depicted the inner world of my questions and reflections. Or it was as though outer things would behave as symbols of my inner life. Jung's question arose in me: What is more real—the one that is mirrored or the mirror that is used?[8] The very basis of my point of view was suddenly and unexpectedly altered. It was a shock. Never before was it so clearly set before my eyes that outer things could be symbols, or that which we name psyche and matter—seen either from the outside or from within—actually represent one and the same reality.[9]

From the point of view of analytical psychology, these experiences have to do with synchronistic events. Jung's concept of synchronicity denotes a meaningful coincidence of inner and outer events in time without the two events being causally dependent on one another.[10] This meaningful coincidence in my case was, on the one hand, my queries and thoughts that I was carrying around with me and, on the other, my encounter with the bull and then the frog.[11] That the appearance of these animals in time and space before me was caused by my thoughts can be excluded with certainty. At this moment—when my perception of the world and my understanding of things is so intensely challenged—another possible conception of the world becomes apparent in which the inner world and the outer world no longer appear to be absolutely divided but, in a rather inexplicable manner, are interwoven and overlapping. One has a hint of another point of view, another dimension, and also of what Jung meant when he spoke about the *unus mundus,* the one world, and what might have been the dimension or the point of view Dr. von Franz referred to in my dream when she said "duplic completion."

Jung said that we cannot visually conceive of this world; it extends fully beyond our conscious ability to comprehend. We can only conclude or surmise that somewhere there is such a reality—we could call it a psychophysical reality—that sporadically manifests in synchronistic events.[12] Dr. von Franz elaborates on this by saying that such phenomena affect the individual like messages out of the primordial matrix of the unconscious, and they can only be really understood by the individual. The mystery of their singular experience lies in the mirroring of both realities, the one in the other.

Through my dream and the search for the meaning of this important message, and the investigation of its mystery, I was drawn deeper and deeper into something strange, something that I could not grasp. Just as the frog actually emerged and crossed my path in the real world, so I was led in the outer world to understand what it means to find oneself in a hopelessly false situation, to retreat and "no longer be there." However, the puzzle was by no means solved nor the mystery revealed. On the contrary, they were extended by the experience of a notion of the ungraspable, of a world in which the opposites of inner and outer, and of good and evil, constitute aspects or points of view of the same unknown reality, and even a hint at what "duplic completion" could possibly mean.

I will continue to carry this mystery around with me and reflect on it, for I must occupy myself with it. And here Jung gives me support when he says:

> It is important that we have a secret and that we have a notion of that which is unknowable. It fills our lives with something impersonal and numinous. Whoever has not experienced this has missed something important. One must experience that one lives in a world that is in a certain respect full of mystery, that things will happen and be experienced which remain inexplicable, and that our lives are not restricted to those experiences which occur within our own expectations. The unexpected and unheard of belong in this world. Only then is life complete.[13]

As von Franz emphasizes, a conscious content like the frog (a cold-blooded animal at home in the water) should be left in its element and not disturbed by an eager desire to understand. She writes that if one notices that an unconscious fantasy is beginning to emerge from within, it is wise not to interpret it too soon. Do not tell it that you know what it is and do not force it into consciousness. Just let it simply live in that you leave it halfway in the dark. Carry it around with you and observe where it goes and where it is heading toward. Much later you will look back and ask what you were doing the whole time and realize that you got close to a strange fantasy that then led you to an unexpected goal.[14]

What had actually begun in innocence, namely, the idea that I might be able to contribute something in honor and gratitude to Dr. von Franz, developed in an unexpected manner. It confronted me with problems, questions, mysteries, events, and apprehensions that I could not have dreamt of, as one so easily (and mistakenly) says. My "encounters" with Dr. von Franz are actually encounters with the world of the unconscious and the creative, a living matrix of all things. And I reach out to this world, so the dream, as a sign of acceptance and in readiness to perceive and grapple with its messages.

NOTES

1. Suzanne Wagner, "Ein Gespräch mit Marie-Louise von Franz," *Jungiana,* Reihe A, Band 11, p. 31.
2. M.-L. von Franz, *On Dreams and Death* (Chicago: Open Court, 1998), pp. 44ff in the German edition; and *The Feminine in Fairy Tales* (Boston: Shambhala, 1993), pp. 27ff.
3. Again, the threshold of consciousness associated with the frog.
4. M.-L. von Franz, *Wissen aus der Tiefe (On Divination and Synchronicity),* p. 107.
5. C. G. Jung, *Memories, Dreams, Reflections* (New York: Pantheon Books, 1963), p. 329.
6. M.-L. von Franz, *Shadow and Evil in Fairy Tales* (Boston: Shambhala, 1995), p. 268.
7. M.-L. von Franz, *Psychologische Märcheninterpretation (The Interpretation of Fairy Tales),* p. 179.
8. C. G. Jung, "Psychotherapists or the Clergy" (1932), in *Collected Works,* vol. 11 (Princeton, N.J.: Princeton University Press, 1969), par. 500.
9. M.-L. von Franz, *Archetypal Dimensions of the Psyche* (Boston: Shambhala, 1997), p. 366 in the German edition.
10. Ibid.

11. The author uses the word *synchronicity* to mean two relatively coinciding events that correspond in meaning but which have no causal connection. This reflects the more popular usage of the term which refers to the principles of acausal orderedness and the *unus mundus.* Jung and von Franz define synchronicity as a special instance of the *unus mundus* in which—in a singular moment in time—a conjunction of psyche and matter appears as a creative act, demonstrating a spontaneous manifestation of inner and outer realities that coincide in their meaning. M.-L.von Franz, *Number and Time* (Evanston, Ill.: Northwestern University Press, 1974), pp. 6ff, 11f.
12. M.-L. von Franz, *Wissen aus der Tiefe (On Divination and Synchronicity),* p. 127.
13. C. G. Jung, *Memories, Dreams, Reflections* (New York: Random House, 1963), p. 358.
14. M.-L. von Franz, *The Interpretation of Fairy Tales* (Boston: Shambhala, 1996), pp. 98ff in the German edition.

Becoming the Woman You Are Supposed to Be

DELORES TAYLOR-LAUGHLIN

Many years before I ventured to Zürich to see Marie-Louise von Franz, I had a series of dreams that took place ten days before Christmas in the year of 1966. The dreams were of an older woman who would come to me with five great lessons filled with knowledge to teach me how I could and should become the woman I was supposed to be, a woman in my own world and time.

On the first night, we traveled to different places so she could show me what it was I was to learn. Then she told me she would be coming for ten sequential nights, spending two nights on each of the five lessons. I remember asking her, "Are you sure you are supposed to be coming to me? I think you may be making a big mistake." She just looked at me and laughed. The dreams were beautiful, but because of my own insecurities, they frightened me. They seemed like they were too much of a responsibility, and I already had enough of that in my life, at least that was my excuse for my actions.

Regardless of my efforts to try and stop the dreams, each night they would come. Every night they were different with the older woman continuing to guide me. (As I think back on it now, I believe deep down I did want the dreams, because they showed such richness of wisdom and love, but at the same time I feared them. I know now that my unconscious had to be heard and nothing was going to stop it.) The dreams went on for nine nights.

Then on the tenth and last night, Christmas Eve, I was determined and decided I had had enough. (I think this last dream was going to be too much for me to handle. Everything was already way over my head.) So, I stayed up all night; that way I couldn't possibly have any more dreams. Right? Well, I was succeeded in staying awake through the night by keeping myself very busy. Then as dawn came, I thought to myself, "I'm sure I'm safe now," and I sat down with a cup of hot tea. No need to say more . . . I had the last dream. Again, it was unbelievably beautiful. The older woman was transformed into Christ, standing luminescent on top of this majestic mountain. I was in a state of utterness, of wonderment. What does this all mean? What am I supposed to do? How? Why? Even as I write it now, I can't find the words to express what was going on inside of me. It was unbelievable.

I tell you this because it wasn't until I made my first trip to Zürich, alone in a foreign country, that I realized what the dreams were all about. I told Marie-Louise the dreams, and I remember her laughing and saying, "That had to stop you." I realized that even though I had actually been born on September 27, 1932, in the small town of Winner, South Dakota, it was as though I was really for the first time born *inside.*

During the following seven days that I spent with Marie-Louise, as I had done previously in my dreams with the older woman, I realized the earlier dreams were absolutely necessary. They enabled me to accept what was happening to me, while alone, here in Zürich. I no longer was afraid. I had been given the confidence to face my unconscious, and I knew I had the responsibility of growing up inside and finding out just who I was and where I was going with my life. Because like everyone, I had made so many mistakes and was hurting so very bad inside, I had to do something. I also knew I couldn't stay awake my whole life, as I had tried to do on that Christmas Eve in 1966, to hide from whatever it was I was running away from. I had tried that before and knew it wouldn't work this time either.

Marie-Louise von Franz made my understanding and belief of all of this possible. She was, for me, a great example of inner strength, of love and caring, of wisdom, of patience, of acceptance, of what one is capable of inside and out, and most of all, belief of what we all have inside, both the good and the bad, with the knowledge and wisdom to accept it all and ourselves for what and who we are and to realize we have to work to make it better for ourselves and thereby better for those around us, particularly for our loved ones. She took the fear of the unconscious away for me and made it real.

I think the thing I most appreciated about her, which for me was a tremendous help in facing all that we all have to face, was her sense of humor. She had a way of getting into those tight hidden corners of the unconscious that we all keep trying to push down deeper and deeper, but end up dragging them up while laughing our heads off and holding our sides from the pain, which only happened when working with her.

She was a very wise woman and a true woman in the deepest sense, and I loved her for that and for sharing it with me so that maybe someday I could also learn it and share it with others and let them know the who, what, where, and why of that magnificent woman . . . Marie-Louise von Franz.

Thank you, Marie-Louise von Franz.

Sisters and Brothers in the Spirit

CARL R. WALKER

Dear Dr. Kennedy:

Enclosed is my dedication to the memory of Dr. von Franz. I hope it meets with your approval. She continues to be a constant inspiration to me as I work on a manuscript with the help and guidance of the Self that she helped me to discover.

Even a title for my work in progress, "The Age of the Illusionment," came to me in the middle of the night as the result of a kind of revelation in which she and my self seemed to have a part. I didn't mention these things in the dedication at the risk of seeming too sentimental, but as you said in your letter, "our hearts know, not the others." I have expressed my feelings and emotions and hope I have stopped short of writing something hagiographic.

Warm regards,
Carl R. Walker

I first became aware of the work of Dr. Marie-Louise von Franz in 1976 when a friend gave me a copy of her book, *C. G. Jung: His Myth in Our Time,* as a present for my fifty-third birthday. I had been reading and collecting Jung's books since the 1950s, beginning with *Symbols of Transformation* and *Psychological Types.* Having spent many hours relentlessly pouring over these complex works, to discover the lucid and down-to-earth prose of Dr. von Franz after struggling through the gold mine of Jung's great opus was like suddenly finding diamonds in profusion, little points of light that led to an understanding of what depth psychology was all about. From that moment on, I knew that I had found a guide, someone I could depend on and trust on my long journey in search of self-knowledge, and she never let me down.

In 1950, at the age of twenty-seven, I left my birthplace in a small town in Vermont to attend school in New York City. As luck would have it, I found a place to live in a rooming house for young students, across the street from St. Paul's Roman Catholic Church, headquarters of the Paulist fathers whose work was concerned with bringing converts to the faith. Our landlady was a winsome Irish lady, a member of St. Paul's parish who soon had us attending mass every Sunday. This proved to be a new experience for me since Religion was hardly ever mentioned by anyone in my family, and I grew up without any knowledge of spirituality and no exposure to creeds, dogmas, or rites of any kind.

It turned out that my newfound friends were involved with something called, at that time, existential Roman Catholicism, and we were soon reading Jacques Maritain's major work, *The Degrees of Knowledge,* along with books by Paul Claudel, Gabriel Marcel, as well as the vagaries of St. Thomas Aquinas and his *Summa Theologica* and the philosophy of G. F. W. Hegel.

In the meantime, our group of young men were beginning to find the life of a convert to the church a bit of an encumbrance when it came time for what we looked upon as "good clean fun." We managed to stay out of mischief for a couple of years until the day we discovered that we were living in something called "the age of anxiety" and that the new experience was to be found as members of the Ramakrishna Vivekanada Society, whose headquarters were not far from the campus of Columbia University where some of our friends were students. There we discovered the Bhagavad Gita and the Upanishads and became friends with two of the swamis in residence at the center who were engaged in translating some of the ancient Indian texts into English.

I soon discovered that the treasurer of the society was a well-known German Freudian analyst named Eilhard von Domarus, and since it was considered fashionable at the time to have something called an anxiety neurosis, I decided to become a patient of his and underwent a two-year analysis with him. Although I worked very hard and wrote down and discussed hundreds of dreams, I never felt that I benefited much from the experience. However, all was not lost because I did learn about the work of C. G. Jung since he and von Domarus had known one another in Germany before the war. It was thanks to him that I found Jung's book on psychological types, which opened up a whole new world for me, something that became a lifelong preoccupation with Jung's work. I had a strong feeling that the unfinished business of my bout with Freudian analysis would one day be taken care of.

After eleven years in New York, I had completed my formal education and had an opportunity to move to Connecticut where, in addition to a job, there was a very active Jung group. I continued to be troubled by a lack of self-knowledge, something I felt could be rectified by a successful depth analysis, but the details of the process were still shrouded in darkness. A few days before I was to leave New York, I remember standing by myself in the middle of my half-empty flat and suddenly uttering aloud a sort of prayer, to nobody in particular, that I would one day undergo some sort of apotheosis before my life on earth was over. I was not even sure of the meaning of the word nor of the fact that my request might be considered an act of hubris. But some lares and penates must have been lurking near my hearth because, from that day on, unseen forces seemed to insist that I not forget my heartfelt entreaty. The next week, at the age of thirty-eight, I left New York for a new life in New England.

My decision to move to Connecticut proved to be a wise one and teaching at a university there provided access to a great library as well as a group of people who were sympathetic to the work of both Professor Jung and Dr. von Franz. In the early 1970s, I acquired volume 11 of Jung's *Collected Works, Psychology and Religion,* which included the Terry Lectures that had originally been published for the foundation by Yale University Press in 1938. This book reawakened the interest in religious studies that had begun in 1952 in New York, and which continues to be a pressing preoccupation of mine to this day.

As time passed, I discovered that coming to terms with spirituality was something I would have to address, but exactly how it would happen and when was totally beyond my comprehension. In retrospect, I am convinced that without the books of Marie-Louise von Franz as my inspiration and a growing familiarity with Dr. Jung's great opus, I would never have found my way to spiritual enlightenment.

Nine years of hard work passed quickly by and in 1970, at the age of forty-seven, I received an offer of a position from a small school in Maine that would prove to be the most important move I would ever make.

As I approached my late forties, I gradually became aware of the fact that in spite of a successful career and many good friends, something important was still missing from my life and for the first time in many years I felt the need for another try at analysis. Once settled in my new job, I decided to see whether I could find a list of Jungian analysts in the United States and was surprised to find such a list in the college library. At the time I decided to move to Maine, I was not aware that the small town of Brunswick had a very active Jung group, and I was pleased to find that the chairman was a professor of religious studies who held weekly meetings in his conference room. Serendipity, or perhaps those same lares and penates from long ago, seemed to be dogging my footsteps, and sure enough I found the person for whom I was looking. Furthermore, he had retired and was living just a few miles away in the tiny town of Readfield, and his name was Heinz Westman.

After a long and successful career as analyst and writer in Germany, England, and New York, Dr. Westman was working on what was to be his final literary effort, a book called *The Structure of Biblical Myth: The Ontogenesis of the Psyche.* In his youth, he had been analyzed by Dr. Jung, along with a group of young men from Germany, and in 1923 he had decided to become an analyst after reading Jung's newly published *Psychological Types.*

I decided to write Dr. Westman a note and ask him whether he would accept me as a patient; he replied that he was busy working on his manuscript and had retired because of rather poor health. He added that if I would write him a letter and let him know why I thought he might help me, he would consider and let me know. I mailed the letter with little hope that I would be lucky enough to be accepted and endured a week of acute apprehension as I waited. One week later, I was delighted to find that he would welcome me at the beginning of the fall semester and had given me two hours a week until the following summer. My visits continued for the next three years and changed my life completely.

The analysis began with instructions to place a pad and pen beside my bed and carefully record any dreams that occurred during the night. I hoped I might be fortunate and have a series of interesting dreams such as I had read about in Jung's books, but alas, much to my initial disappointment and regret, no such dreams appeared. As a result of an unfortunate and wretched childhood, during which I was deprived of any affection or warmth, I entered adult life with no trace of self-esteem and a totally unconscious inflation of my ego as a miserable attempt at compensation.

My hard work in the middle of the night brought forth a long series of what seemed to me dreary and forlorn dreams, utterly sad and cheerless. I seemed always to be lost in desolate old buildings, empty and abandoned, in which I was trying to find my way. I moved aimlessly, climbing about on high beams across great empty spaces in what seemed to be a hopeless quest for deliverance from something that had no name. Dr. Westman wisely refrained from alleviating or explaining the significance of these dreams and always listened carefully with deep feeling and great concern, offering me his fiat to continue my journey and persevere.

Nevertheless, my visits were by no means depressing in any way, for we discussed at great length the work on his book, and I was allowed unlimited access to his great library. I ended up with a weekly private tutorial in the humanities and comparative religion by a patient and devoted friend.

Along the way, during my three years of analysis with Dr. Westman, I encountered many ghosts who made themselves known in diverse ways. There was an illusive shadow who appeared in occasional nightmares, the result of my destructive inflated ego, and later, a cold, negative anima figure because of early experiences with a wicked stepmother. And the dreams that were concerned with my endless struggle to find a way out of my labyrinth continued unabated.

The end of my sixth semester in analysis was coming to a close, and one day I learned that failing health and the pressure of seeing his book into print were forcing Dr. Westman to terminate our meetings. He assured me that he would keep in touch and that I should call him if I felt the need of a bit of encouragement. About two months later, I awoke one morning with a new and wonderful feeling of joy and self-esteem which took me completely by surprise. I spent two or three hours in a kind of reverie and finally managed to write Heinz a short note telling him as nearly as I could about my experience. He answered quickly to say, "What you are writing about yourself was a long time in the coming. To the degree you accepted yourself, you came down to earth, i.e., to your Self."

I now felt I could safely leave the security and reassurance of my weekly visits and made the last entry in my journal, which I quote verbatim:

> Spring, 1983: Dr. Westman would not let me "worship" anything. He kept urging me to be myself. All the trappings of "culture," "theology," "philosophy," etc., are not the way "it" happens. The free-flow from the unconscious just happens if we withdraw the "projections" but it doesn't come unless we constellate a "field" by seeking self-knowledge. The round, the idea of completeness (alchemy), is a fact but it doesn't save the world. Only Christ within us is the answer because of the Incarnation and the Resurrection.

Now, anyone who has undergone a thoroughgoing depth analysis by an analytical psychologist knows how difficult it is to recognize a projection, then isolate it and come to an awareness that the very thing we find irritating in a neighbor is a fault that exists in ourselves. It was at this point in what was to be my post-analytical period that I experienced the first instance of what I will call synchronicity in a budding relationship with Dr. von Franz.

One day not long after I was on my own, having suffered from the realization that withdrawing a particularly nasty projection by no means meant that it had been banished and sent into limbo, I decided to take a walk and visit my favorite bookstore. After an hour or so, as I was getting ready to leave, I noticed a small book in a green dust jacket with the title, *Projection and Recollection in Jungian Psychology,* and the name of the author in very small print, von Franz. I quickly took the book and found a chair in a corner and opened it to the page that listed the contents. I remembered how much I had enjoyed her book on Jung and now proceeded to find once more a beautifully organized outline of all the things I needed to know about projections; I heaved a sigh of relief and started to read. The next thing I knew, an hour had passed; the bookstore was closing, so I quickly paid for the book and left.

During the next few days, I read and reread all about projections and once again was struck by finding the same delightful insights presented in a no-nonsense style and her charming use of colloquial English made reading about very complex things a pleasure. I began to watch for the works of Marie-Louise von Franz as they became available in English and now have her entire opus, including *Muhammad Ibn Umail's Hall Ar-Rumuz* and *The Cat.* Before I leave my adventure with projections and recollections, I would like to add that it was here that I first learned about the golden ass of Apuleius and the related material about the Self. A few years later, I was fortunate to find Dr. von Franz's book by that title, without which I would never have come to know and establish a relationship with my self.

My next experience with the books of Dr. von Franz came a few months later, and once more it happened as a result of serendipity. In spite of my having been exposed to so many wonderful insights during my analysis, I was finding it difficult to come to terms with the necessity of taking action and addressing lingering problems in the light of what

I had learned. Once more, quite by chance, I found another work by Marie-Louise von Franz in a bookstore called *The Problem of the Puer Aeternus,* which provided me with some concepts and a vocabulary that described something called "the provisional life," an image I still find useful to this day, not only as it applies to myself but as a description of the behavior of untold numbers of males in public life all over the world today.

The early 1990s were a difficult time for me; I was trying to make peace with the fact that old age was now a reality and it was high time to think about the future in terms of a few, rather than many, years. I felt compelled to share with others the fruits of a lifetime devoted to a widening of my consciousness, as Jung had suggested that we do, but something was still missing. Somewhere there lurked some still-unfinished business, but I was at a loss to think what it might be.

In the early spring of 1995, I began to have a strong impulse to write, and in early May, I had what to me was a "big dream."

> *I was sitting in a large warm room in semidarkness. A tall male was standing over me and I felt totally at peace. He did not speak but I sensed that he wanted to tell me something important. Suddenly I saw an image of a beautiful calico cat in full color, and she looked at me intently for a few seconds and I awoke with a feeling of contentment and peace.*

The next morning I awoke at two A.M. with a strong impulse to write Dr. von Franz a letter and tell her how much her work had helped me to make peace with what seemed to be an ongoing process of individuation. I mentioned the fact that I was looking forward to finding a copy of her book, *The Golden Ass of Apuleius,* and that I was still having trouble dealing with that stubborn inflation of my ego. I also mentioned an interesting book that I thought she might enjoy and offered to send her a copy. Dawn was breaking as I finished writing, and I fell into a deep sleep in which I had the following dream:

> *I was in an unfamiliar setting in a foreign country, and it seemed I was about to meet Dr. von Franz. I entered a rather large room where she*

seemed to be, along with a few others. In the center was a sort of miniature cone-shaped stone mountain about twelve feet high. There were small tubes or pipes with odd fittings running up and down the sides which were full of pure crystal-clear water that had a special significance for me. Dr. von Franz seemed to be there while I enjoyed the experience. I moved to a sort of covered porch, open to a lovely landscape where there was a large flying machine, not an aircraft but a kind of portable device for exploring the countryside. A blonde man, about forty-five years old, who also seemed to be an aspect of Dr. von Franz in some way, was working around the machine and was experimenting with a smaller version that would be easier to manage. I also met a friend of Dr. von Franz, a younger woman with reddish hair. I awoke with a delightful feeling of freshness and very positive feelings.

(P.S. I always have to be very careful of flying too high; a recent reading from the I Ching brought hexagram no. 34 with four changes, 9 in the first place, 9 in the third place, and 6 in the fifth and sixth places. Perhaps the dream is showing me a way where flying too high can be managed without disaster.)

I decided to attach the dream and the postscript to the letter and mailed them off to Switzerland.

On May 25, 1995, I received a little note from Marie-Louise von Franz in answer to my rather long and windy letter:

25th May, '95

Dear Mr. Walker,

Your letter touched me. As from a brother in the Spirit. I don't know the book of Maccoby. Could you send me a copy? Tell me how much I owe you. I am too ill to dictate long letters, but I will react.

With my warmest good wishes,
sign. Marie-Louise von Franz

In her own succinct and inimitable way, she gave me a compliment I will always remember, and I know that her warmest good wishes are with me still.

Over the next two years, I received ten little notes from Dr. von Franz, the final one on April 21, 1997. In the meantime, I continued to collect her books, and on July 31, 1997, I found the revised edition of *The Golden Ass of Apuleius: The Liberation of the Feminine in Man.* I hasten to confess that it took me at least three months to read and study this book, and I had a feeling that what had been known to me as concepts gleaned from a continuous study over some forty-five years in the field of Jung's psychology were now being broken like eggs by this woman. She seemed intent on giving me a chance finally to make an omelet that would provide a kind of spiritual nourishment for my soul.

At last I was able to understand who it was that awakened me in the middle of the night and replaced my dreams with revelations. Thanks to our beloved Marie-Louise, it finally dawned on me that although I heard no voice nor did I see an image, He was none other than my self. I was now able to accept a vocation and dedicate the rest of my life to His service.

In closing I would like to quote a few sentences from the last page of *The Golden Ass of Apuleius* (p. 230) that spoke directly to me:

> It takes a strong consciousness, which is flexible and modest enough, to be able to accept what the unconscious—the gods—has to say to us, and to realize the will of the gods, of the god who manifests himself to us, and to put us into his service, without forgetting the individual limits of our human nature.
>
> . . . .
>
> It is up to us to pay attention and to allow the development of that which within us seeks to fulfill itself.
>
> . . . .
>
> I hope that these attempts at a psychological interpretation, which are often only tentative suggestions, have conveyed to the reader the following: that this novel of Apuleius is a highly important "document humain" which one can even put next to Goethe's *Faust.* . . . It leads into the deep-

est problems of Western man and points symbolically to developments which today we still have not realized in consciousness.

If I may say so, I feel very strongly that our author has seen to it through her book that certainly some of us can now understand these developments beyond any reasonable doubt.

Coda

Our heroine mentioned on page 89 of her book, *The Golden Ass of Apuleius,* that one can say the incarnation of the feminine principle in a woman is still on the program for the coming centuries and is beginning to become urgent today. As a result of my own personal experience I can say that through her life's work, Dr. von Franz was living proof that a daughter of Sophia had indeed incarnated in the body of a woman. How else could she have shown me, a man, the way to a realization of my self as the supreme principle?

Respectfully submitted,
Carl R. Walker

A Stone and a Dress

SATOMI YOSHIDA

A little stone sits on my desk. It strongly reminds me of the person who gave it to me in 1987 and her room, which it originally belonged to. I had taken analysis from her for several months and was soon going back to Japan. She knew that I had been uncomfortable in my country and still felt uneasy. She took a half-cut volcanic stone from the window ledge and handed it to me. She said, "You are a very introverted person. You may not look so nice outside but you have beautiful things inside just as this stone has crystal part in it." I clearly remember the voice when Dr. Marie-Louise von Franz said this.

The stone has been encouraging me ever since. It is 500 grams in weight, 10 centimeters in diameter, and fits into the palm of my hand. It is the shape of a half of an avocado pear without its stone. The uncut surface is rough and gray, covered with beige spots. The stone is smoothly cut, and I can see that the globe stone within has an empty part in its core, covered with the crystal part tinged with pale blue and many tiny spots of rainbow brightness. And there is a bit of sooty part, too. The stone reminds me of both stillness and dynamics. I associate it with crystallization, rainbow-colored light, a vessel, a sphere, the earth, Nature, and the self. I grappled with the theme of the self, Jung's key concept, on my master's thesis. I think I need much more wrestling with this theme from now on.

I wonder how many times Dr. von Franz made me change dramatically and deeply. It was an autumn day in 1986 when I visited her for the first time. It was no easy task for me. I was so nervous. I could not speak German and was not good at English at all. She must have had great difficulty in having a conversation with me. That was my first trip abroad, and I had never even met a Westerner in my small town in Japan. I was very surprised to see a Swiss man sneeze on the street on my first day in Zürich and felt strange because I had rarely seen a "live" Westerner.

At that time, I had severe problems and had lost my self-confidence and felt very pessimistic about the future. I felt alone. I wasn't able to establish good relationships with my parents and friends. Every human relationship tired me out, and I had no energy left to go to high school normally. The counseling and psychotherapy I took didn't do any good. I was deeply ashamed and hurt. I didn't like what I was at all. I could do nothing but blame myself. I was very shy and timid but necessity drove me to take a step in coming to Switzerland alone to see Dr. von Franz. I had read her books, *C. G. Jung: His Myth in Our Time, The Problem of the Puer Aeternus, The Feminine in Fairy Tales,* and *Shadow and Evil in Fairy Tales,* and also *Man and His Symbols,* in Japanese, and I had great respect for her. Those books had already influenced me. The idea that caught me was that the unconscious is tremendously influential and it has both good and evil power. The way of her dealing with the unconscious was so interesting as well as persuasive. I felt as though she was discussing my problems. I was very grateful to know that she was able to see me. But at the same time, I was worried about whether it would work.

I had known through her works that Dr. von Franz was a very intelligent and resourceful person and full of insights. Having a person-to-person relationship to her made me find other aspects of her personality. I don't think I have to write about how kind and how warmhearted Dr. von Franz was. Everyone familiar with her must know very well. She cared about not only my psychological situation but also traveling and living expenses. I could hardly believe my ears when she, the authority, Dr. von Franz, offered me a very inexpensive analysis fee!

The first session with her delighted me, and I found myself hopping down the hill on the way home. I think I had been frozen in horror by my frightening experiences, and I began melting on that day, for I felt that she understood my problem, the terrible pressure I felt from people around me in Japanese society. I was in tears with joy, and Dr. von Franz also seemed to be moved to tears hearing me describe my own experiences. I can clearly recall her words, "I was moved," in a soft, low-key voice. That was quite a moment. She even hugged me tightly! I didn't know how to react, but I was overwhelmed by happiness. She told me that there was nothing wrong with me, but I was just too complicated. She advised me that I should be freer and wilder, as a little child or an animal. "Don't be afraid. Be free. Don't doubt. Be a child. Don't study too much, Satomi." That was not easy at all, though. She told me to go to the zoo and see how animals act. I visited one in Zürich, but I was half in doubt about whether it worked. Her charming dog, by the way, always came to me and sat down by my chair, often on my feet, during the sessions. He, or she, had an Italian name, Laura (I'm not sure if the spelling is correct). I liked the dog very much. Laura's leisurely movement and his smell relaxed me.

I visited Zürich from Japan to see Dr. von Franz twice and could take two series of analyses from her. We talked a lot about my dreams once a week on the first visit, and once every two weeks on the second visit, for several months each stay. I was very lucky. It was in 1993 when I met her for the last time; I was going back to visit her for one day. Zürich and Küsnacht had become very special places for me. I was very fond of the path and the scenery there and the little pears in the box I bought in front of the beautiful farmhouse on the way home from her place. I met many kindhearted people during my stay. The sound of the tram and the church bells lingered in my ear for a while after I came home from Zürich.

She once told me that love and sadness always go together. When I received notice of her demise, I was very shocked and sank in grief. I regretted not having written letters to her for a while. I was very sorry and sad that I didn't notice her critical condition and could do nothing when her hour had come. Not a prayer. Not a word to express my gratitude. . . .

But my sad days didn't last long. Dr. von Franz appeared in a dream unexpectedly:

> *I come to attend Dr. von Franz's funeral. I am overwhelmed with grief. When I enter the room, there she is in high spirits! She is taking a black feminine one-piece dress out of her coffin, which looks like a case of a musical instrument. She is alive and very well. What is more, she looks very cheerful and even younger! I am struck dumb with astonishment. Dr. von Franz wears the black lace dress gracefully, and she is walking with light steps. She takes my hand into her own, and we are going out.*

In this dream, she looked full of life and very cheerful. It made me feel relieved and very happy from the bottom of my heart. The black dress doesn't seem to be one for mourning but just one of fashionable clothes. In reality, I had never seen her like that. She was always in dark suits and looked like she didn't care much about dressing up. The great scholar might have been in a more surrealistic world. She was often in cheerful mood, but sometimes looked tired and not in good health. In this dream, she looked perfectly well and moved so gracefully.

Dr. von Franz gave me the stone in the beginning of our relationship and left me that dream, image of the black feminine one-piece dress and being in good spirits, when she met her end. I don't know how to express my gratitude. It is thanks to her that I have nice people I can trust now. Needless to say, I miss Dr. von Franz very much, and I wish I could ask her advice as to whether I'm still on the right track. Even now, I sometimes wonder whether my introverted nature causes problems in my life when I feel small. Problems and emotional conflicts are likely to continue to occur at every stage of life. The stone and the dress will keep giving me important messages from now on as I grow.

After Dr. von Franz passed away, I met a man and got married. That's one of the surprising changes for me. Does it have something to do with the dream of the dress?

Marie-Louise von Franz and Shakespeare's *Hamlet*

JOSÉ ZAVALA

In October or November 1971, I went to an analytical hour with Marie-Louise von Franz. In the course of that hour, I told her one of my dreams in which the motif of Shakespeare's *Hamlet* occurred. She did not ask me for associations but rather began directly to discuss the dream. "Hamlet is the one who cannot kill the illegitimate lover of his mother, thus he cannot love the anima who then commits suicide. Hamlet remains a failure not because he was a coward, but because he is exaggeratedly correct." For a short moment, she was silent and reflective. Again she began to speak and added that "what I wrote about in *Puer Aeternus* is the surface of the mother complex. Hamlet is the abysmal and darkest depths."

It never failed to astound me how often Marie-Louise von Franz could explain, elucidate, and capture an entire life process with such a brevity of words in so short a time. Words that were simple and natural, but they penetrated the depths and so often hit the mark.

I noted down what she said about Hamlet shortly after the hour but took little notice afterward. A while later, as I was leafing through C. G. Jung's *Zarathustra Seminar* for very different reasons, it came back to me as I read Jung's comment about the conversation between Zarathustra and the dwarf. Here he says:

> This passage is great language. . . . These monumental short words of wisdom come from the intestines of the world. They are like the words of Lao Tse, or Pythagoras, or Heraclitus—short and pregnant with meaning.[1]

Marie-Louise von Franz always spoke to me with simple, yet pregnant words when it had to do with the objective experience of psychic contents. They were words that not only harbored striking wisdom but were also vibrating with vigor, a vigor that was never eccentric but out of which I could draw the very substance of life. This strength was a product of her deeply and innermost consciously lived experience of psychic reality which she bore to the extreme. Marie-Louise von Franz was not simply content to approach and delineate human psychic reality with pure scientific reasoning; she also experienced it and lived it. Out of this human, thoroughly lived experience emanated her resounding golden laughter, which she never lost even in the face of her own death.

The scientific dealings with her became real experience because of the wisdom that was always filled with eros. It is this synthesis that was of such precious value when one was with Marie-Louise von Franz. But that was the honor of those who actually had the chance of working with her. The rest of the world knows only her intellectual work, namely her books, in which one perceives but a shimmer of her real and unique being. That which personally touches me the most is the deep respect I always feel when I think of the awe and the religiosity with which Marie-Louise von Franz grappled with the contents of the unconscious. I can only join Hamlet in saying:

> The rest is silence.

NOTE

1. C. G. Jung, *Nietzsche's Zarathustra: Notes on the Seminar Given in 1934–1939*, vol. 2, James L. Jarrett, ed. (Princeton, N.J.: Princeton University Press, 1988), p. 1272.

The Trout

IDA REGINA ZOCCOLI

Des Menschen Seele
gleicht dem Wasser.
Vom Himmel kommt es,
Zum Himmel steigt es
Und wieder nieder
Zur Erde muss es,
Ewig wechselnd.

W. Goethe, "Gesang der Geister über den Wassern"

During Marie-Louise von Franz's funeral service, so as to respect her deathbed desire, Schubert's quintet, "The Trout," was played. The sonata's allegro, andantino, and scherzo describe the life cycle of the trout, which spends its days leaping joyfully in the river. I wish to remember Marie-Louise through this last desire of hers, in other words, for her hidden, intimate, Zen aspect, which Silesius transmits to us from Chuang Tzu: "I am conscious of the joy of the fish in the river through my own joy as I stroll along the river banks."

Both von Franz's writing and her lectures are the reflection of her psychic experience, and therefore through them we come to discover not a series of abstract ideas but the continual flux of her most intimate psyche related to daily life.

When she states that hers was a very simple life, we have to agree with her, since life is simply a harmonic unfolding of one's individuality. "My biography," she states, "is revealed in my writings." That is because what she wrote—and to a large extent they are the lectures delivered at the Jung Institute—always corresponded to her life experience of that specific moment. Such was my experience during the twenty-one years of analysis with von Franz. She was my teacher, but above all, my analyst. A true analyst is a guide who makes one's daily life meaningful, trying to get through to one's very essence, never trying to indoctrinate his or her listener. This is exactly what she so generously did during her lectures at the Jung Institute, where she had quite different duties to carry out. Certainly every aspect about her was a lesson, depending, of course, on the extent to which my psyche managed to assimilate her teachings and apply them to my daily life.

On one occasion, enthusiastic about a dream she had, she exclaimed, openheartedly, "to be . . . the most important thing is to be," and continued, "Yes, the real problem is not what we do, but what we are," and then she added, contemplative, "*bien difficile.*"

Our relationship through analysis began in one of the halls of the Eranos conferences. In those days, Eranos was still a holy of holies which one could enter only if well-presented by one of the conference masters; I therefore remember how trembling and timorous I was when I approached her, getting up from my seat and going toward that woman—in one of her gray suits—sitting quietly in the "professors' corner." Although "Hephaestus" was the only word she uttered, it clearly expressed the myth which, according to her, I inspired.

For that very reason, I immediately asked her if I could begin analysis with her. I used to drive alone the 642 kilometers from Florence to Küsnacht but was never late for an appointment, and, what is more important, I never had an accident, a delay, or breakdown. In recent years, improvements have been made to the highway but previously it was by no means easy to drive over the St. Gotthard Pass. Consequently, I chose the longer but less dangerous St. Bernardino Pass and still have fond memories of its charming scenery.

On Sunday mornings when I absentmindedly set out on my journey back to Italy, I used to drive to the Rappersville side of the lake, stopping for a moment in front of Jung's house so as to call him to mind; likewise, I would stop in front of the Bollingen Tower; and then I had a further pause higher up in the woods, where on several occasions people stopped to ask me if I needed help. I must have made a strange impression, immobile and apparently idle on those narrow little roads. It is place that encourages meditation; so when we did analysis at Küsnacht, I chose to end my day's activity in front of her holiday house, her tower, where she had me as a guest in the summer.

Jung had let her build a tower at Bollingen like the one he owned on the lakeside, but it was to be built high up in the woods and to be different from his, which, as everyone knows, he had built with his own hands and which was a round tower.

When you enter this square room, dark owing to its small windows and sparsely furnished, apart from the fireplace you see nothing but a large stone sink with a fountain in the middle of it. That was how Marie-Louise wanted it: water and fire and land and sky. She said she used to sit there in the evenings, waiting for nightfall. I never asked for explanations about her choices: I was privileged enough to be able to discover them. Until a few years ago, on the field behind the tower there were her ducks, which paddled in the fountain; she smiled fondly when she mentioned them. In the early years, I underwent analysis holding the paw of a female bulldog, her bitch Laura, who lay at my feet and wanted that close contact. "She's Petrarch's Laura," she observed, laughing.

How often we used to laugh, smile, and joke together! It was part of our love of life. In my presence, she was always spontaneous and smiling. We shared an ironical and derisive attitude toward life's difficulties; I wish to reveal this unknown side of her though I am reluctant to admit certain aspects of her personality, for fear of disclosing a professional secret. However, it seems to me that official biographies overstress the fact that she was a highly cultured, rational woman and a "thinking mind." My impression was somewhat different. To tell the truth, when her illness became a real burden, we often ended our meetings, half-joking and half-sarcastic, singing an old French popular song: "*tout va très bien, Madame la Marquise, tout va très bien, tout va très bien. . . .*"

One of my painful memories is of when she talked openly about her Parkinson's disease. I explained that during my career as a neuropsychiatrist I had seen miracles performed through various operations. "Some attempt must be made. . . ." Nevertheless, one day she explained, "An eminent specialist has examined me, he's the world authority in this field." While I was feeling optimistic and thinking, "these Swiss doctors are the avant-garde in the field of medicine," she continued: "His exact words were: 'Miss von Franz, there is nothing we can do for your Parkinson's.'" To tell the truth, no specialist had examined her, but the fact had been revealed to her in a dream. That conversation took place years ago, and in more recent years she used to say, almost regretfully, "Parkinson's usually lasts for seven or eight years, mine has gone on for eighteen. . . ." In spite of the suffering which she must have had to bear, her illness was a giant that she was able to come to grips with. She managed to transcend it. Lord knows how often I was unable to distinguish reality from dreams in her accounts, and even now I'm unable to separate one from the other. The same can be said for my own life. Fortunately, life offers us a positive side which we can all share in enjoying!

Let's go back to talking about her and of the psyche's most secret aspects, so as to *scrivere più per extenso* (every now and then, she used this funny, imprecise Italian, perhaps because it was easier to remember!). In her last letter to me, she encouraged all of us to study hard, not only for personal satisfaction but above all to spread Jung's teachings.

Let's go back to her cherished Zen aspect and continue to stroll up and down the riverbanks, let's listen and participate in the joy of the trout leaping joyfully in the water. *Che più?* (What could be more perfect?)

PART EIGHT

Published Works in English

Books

Alchemical Active Imagination. Boston: Shambhala, 1997. © Stiftung für Jung'sche Psychologie and Emmanuel Kennedy. First published by Spring Publications, Irving, Texas, 1979.

Alchemy: An Introduction to the Symbolism and the Psychology. Toronto: Inner City Books, 1980. © Stiftung für Jung'sche Psychologie and Emmanuel Kennedy.

Animus and Anima in Fairy Tales. Toronto: Inner City Books, 2002. © Stiftung für Jung'sche Psychologie and Emmanuel Kennedy.

Archetypal Dimensions of the Psyche. Boston: Shambhala, 1997, and Einsiedeln: Daimon Verlag, 1994. © Daimon Verlag, Einsiedeln. Contents:

- "Highlights of the Historical Dimension of Analysis" (1977)
- "Antichrist or Merlin? A Problem Inherited from the Middle Ages" (1980)
- "The Transformed Berserker: The Union of Psychic Opposites" (1985)
- "The Unknown Visitor in Fairy Tales and Dreams" (1974)
- "The Bremen Town Musicians from the Point of View of Depth Psychology" (1970)

"The Cosmic Man as Image of the Goal of the Individuation Process and Human Development" (1970)
"The Self-Affirmation of Man and Woman: A General Problematic Illustrated by Fairy Tales" (1975)
"In the Black Woman's Castle: Interpretation of a Fairy Tale" (1969)
"The Discovery of Meaning in the Individuation Process" (1971)
"Individuation and Social Relationship in Jungian Psychology" (1975)
"Nike and the Waters of Styx" (1985)
"The Individuation Process" (1968)
"Jung's Discovery of the Self" (1949)

Archetypal Patterns in Fairy Tales. Toronto: Inner City Books, 1997. © Stiftung für Jung'sche Psychologie and Emmanuel Kennedy.

Aurora Consurgens: On the Problem of Opposites in Alchemy. Toronto: Inner City Books, 2000. © Stiftung für Jung'sche Psychologie and Emmanuel Kennedy. First published by Pantheon Books / Bollingen Foundation, New York, 1962. A companion work to C. G. Jung's *Mysterium Coniunctionis.*

C. G. Jung: His Myth in Our Time. Toronto: Inner City Books, 1998. © Stiftung für Jung'sche Psychologie and Emmanuel Kennedy. First published by the C. G. Jung Foundation, New York, 1975.

Creation Myths. Boston: Shambhala, 1972. © Stiftung für Jung'sche Psychologie and Emmanuel Kennedy. Republished in 1995.

Dreams. Boston: Shambhala, 1991. © Daimon Verlag, Einsiedeln. Contents:
"The Hidden Source of Self-Knowledge" (1973)
"How C. G. Jung Lived with His Dreams" (1972)
"The Dream of Socrates" (1950)
"The Dreams of Themistocles and Hannibal" (1980)

"The Dream of Monica, Mother of Saint Augustine" (date unknown, prior to 1991)
"The Dreams of the Mother of Saint Bernard of Clairvaux and the Mother of Saint Dominic" (date unknown, prior to 1991)
"The Dream of Descartes" (1952/1968)

Individuation in Fairy Tales. Boston: Shambhala, 1977. © Stiftung für Jung'sche Psychologie and Emmanuel Kennedy.

Jung's Typology. With James Hillman. New York: Spring Publications, 1971. © James Hillman/Stiftung für Jung'sche Psychologie and Emmanuel Kennedy. Republished in 1995.

Light from the Darkness: The Paintings of Peter Birkhäuser. Basel: Birkhäuser Verlag, 1980. © Birkhäuser Verlag Basel.

Muhammad Ibn Umail's Hall Ar-Rumuz: Clearing of Enigmas—Historical Introduction and Psychological Comment. Switzerland: Fotorotar, 1999. © Theodor Abt.

Number and Time: Reflections Leading toward a Unification of Depth Psychology and Physics. Evanston, Ill.: Northwestern University Press, 1974. © Stiftung für Jung'sche Psychologie and Emmanuel Kennedy.

On Divination and Synchronicity: The Psychology of Meaningful Chance. Toronto: Inner City Books, 1980. © Stiftung für Jung'sche Psychologie and Emmanuel Kennedy.

On Dreams and Death. 2nd edition. LaSalle, Ill.: Open Court, 1998. © Stiftung für Jung'sche Psychologie and Emmanuel Kennedy. Originally published by Shambhala, 1986.

Projection and Recollection in Jungian Psychology: Reflections of the Soul. LaSalle, Ill.: Open Court, 1980. © Stiftung für Jung'sche Psychologie and Emmanuel Kennedy.

Psyche and Matter. Boston: Shambhala, 1992. © Daimon Verlag, Einsiedeln. Contents:

"Matter and Psyche from the Point of View of the Psychology of C. G. Jung" (1970)
"Symbols of the *Unus Mundus*" (1963)
"Time: Rhythm and Repose" (1978)
"The Psychological Experience of Time" (1978)
"Psyche and Matter in Alchemy and Modern Sciences" (1975)
"Some Historical Aspects of C. G. Jung's Synchronicity Hypothesis" (1985)
"The Synchronicity Principle of C. G. Jung" (1979)
"A Contribution to the Discussion of C. G. Jung's Synchronicity Hypothesis" (1983)
"Some Reflections on Synchronicity" (1984)
"Meaning and Order" (1981)
"Time and Synchronicity in Analytical Psychology" (1966)
"Concerning Meeting Points and Differences between Psychology and Physics" (1981)

Psychotherapy. Boston: Shambhala, 1993. © Daimon Verlag, Einsiedeln. Contents:

"Self-Realization in the Individual Therapy of C. G. Jung" (1977)
"The Inferior Function" (1971)
"Active Imagination in the Psychology of C. G. Jung" (1957)
"On Active Imagination" (1978)
"The Religious Dimension of Analysis" (1983)
"The Religious or Magical Attitude toward the Unconscious" (1993)
"Some Aspects of the Transference" (1973)
"Projection" (1980)
"Profession and Vocation" (1978)
"On Group Psychology" (1973)
"Drugs in the View of C. G. Jung" (1974)
"The Religious Background of the *Puer Aeternus* Problem" (1962)

Shadow and Evil in Fairy Tales. Boston: Shambhala, 1995. © Stiftung für Jung'sche Psychologie and Emmanuel Kennedy. First published by Spring Publications, New York, 1977.

The Cat: A Tale of Feminine Redemption. Toronto: Inner City Books, 1999. © Stiftung für Jung'sche Psychologie and Emmanuel Kennedy.

The Feminine in Fairy Tales. Boston: Shambhala, 1993. © Stiftung für Jung'sche Psychologie and Emmanuel Kennedy. First published by Spring Publications, New York, 1972.

The Golden Ass of Apuleius: The Liberation of the Feminine in Man. Boston: Shambhala, 1992. © Stiftung für Jung'sche Psychologie and Emmanuel Kennedy. First published by Spring Publications, Irving, Texas, 1970.

The Grail Legend. With Emma Jung. New York: G. P. Putnam's Sons/C. G. Jung Foundation, 1970.

The Interpretation of Fairy Tales. Boston: Shambhala, 1996. © Stiftung für Jung'sche Psychologie and Emmanuel Kennedy. First published by Spring Publications, New York, 1970.

The Passion of Perpetua: A Psychological Interpretation of Her Visions. Toronto: Inner City Books, 2004. © Stiftung für Jung'sche Psychologie and Emmanuel Kennedy. First published by Spring Publications, Irving, Texas, 1980.

The Problem of the Puer Aeternus. Toronto: Inner City Books, 2000. © Stiftung für Jung'sche Psychologie and Emmanuel Kennedy. First published by Spring Publications, New York, 1970.

The Psychological Meaning of Redemption Motifs in Fairy Tales. Toronto: Inner City Books, 1980. © Stiftung für Jung'sche Psychologie and Emmanuel Kennedy.

The Way of the Dream. Boston: Shambhala, 1994. © Fraser Boa. Contents:

Descent into Dreamland
Charting the Unconscious
The Structure of Dreams
The Living Symbol
The Ladder to Heaven
The Forgotten Language
Our Shadow Knows
The Devouring Mother
Slaying the Dragon
Looking Through the Moon
The Inner Bride
Hell Has No Mirrors
The Hanged Man
The Tyrant
Flying Through Roofs
The Inner Guide
Liberation of the Heart
Liberation of Relationship
Dreams of a Lifetime
The Maker of Dreams

Time, Rhythm and Repose. London: Thames and Hudson, 1978. © Stiftung für Jung'sche Psychologie and Emmanuel Kennedy.

IN PREPARATION:

The Visions of Niklaus von Flüe. Einsiedeln: Daimon Verlag. © Stiftung für Jung'sche Psychologie and Emmanuel Kennedy.

Articles, Interviews, and Forewords

"A Conversation with Marie-Louise von Franz" with Susan Wagner, in *Psychological Perspectives: A Journal of Global Consciousness Integrating Psyche, Soul and Nature,* "An Homage to Marie-Louise von Franz—Concentrate the Heart," no. 38, Winter 1998–1999, pp. 12–39.

The interview was conducted in 1977 as part of a film project produced by the C. G. Jung Institute of Los Angeles. Parts of this interview can be seen in the documentary film *Matter of Heart* (1985). The entire interview is available on video as part of the series *Remembering Jung* and is distributed by the bookstore of the C. G. Jung Institute of Los Angeles.

"Analytical Psychology and Literary Criticism," in *New Library History,* vol. 21, no. 1, Autumn 1980–1981 (Charlottesville, Va.: University of Virginia).

"Archetypes Surrounding Death," in *Quadrant,* Summer 1979 (New York: C. G. Jung Foundation for Analytical Psychology), pp. 5–24.

"A Woman's Way: A Conversation with Marie-Louise von Franz," with Donna Spencer and Ernest Lawrence Rossi, in *Psychological Perspectives: A Journal of Global Consciousness Integrating Psyche, Soul and Nature,* no. 22, Spring-Summer (Los Angeles: C. G. Jung Institute, 1990), pp. 102–121.

"C. G. Jung and the Problems of Our Times," in *Quadrant,* Fall 1969 (New York: C. G. Jung Foundation for Analytical Psychology), pp. 4–12.

"C. G. Jung's Library," in *Spring* (New York: C. G. Jung Foundation, 1970).

"Consciousness, Power and Sacrifice," in *Psychological Perspectives: A Journal of Global Consciousness Integrating Psyche, Soul and Nature,* vol. 18, no. 2, Fall (Los Angeles: C. G. Jung Institute, 1987), pp. 375–385.

"Conversations on *Aion;*" in B. Hannah, and M.-L. von Franz, *Lectures on Jung's* Aion (Wilmette, Ill.: Chiron Publications, 2004), pp. 125–206. © Stiftung für Jung'sche Psychologie and Emmanuel Kennedy.

"Conversations with Marie-Louise von Franz at Seventy: Too Close to a Divine Secret?" with Ernest Lawrence Rossi, in *Psychological Perspectives: A Journal of Global Consciousness Integrating Psyche, Soul and Nature,* vol. 17, no. 2, Fall (Los Angeles: C. G. Jung Institute, 1986), pp. 375–385.

"Daimons and the Inner Companion," in *Parabola, The Magazine of Myth and Tradition,* vol. 6, no. 4 (Denville, N.J.: Society for the Study of Myth and Tradition, 1982), pp. 36–44.

"Forever Jung: A Conversation with Marie-Louise von Franz," with Jonathan Cott, in *Rolling Stone Magazine,* no. 461, November 21, 1985. Also published in Jonathan Cott, *Visions and Voices* (New York: Doubleday, 1995).

"Foreword," in Barbara Hannah, *Encounters with the Soul: Active Imagination as Developed by C. G. Jung* (Wilmette, Ill.: Chiron Publications, 2001).

"Foreword," in Siegmund Hurwitz, *Lilith—The First Eve: Historical and Psychological Aspects of the Dark Feminine* (Einsiedeln: Daimon Verlag, 1992).

"Introduction," C. G. Jung, *The Zofingen Lectures,* William McGuire, ed., and Jan von Heurck, trans. (Princeton, N.J.: Princeton University Press and London: Routledge and Kegan Paul, 1983), pp. xxi–xxv.

"Introduction," E. A. Bennet, *Meetings with Jung: Conversations Recorded during the Years 1946–1961* (Einsiedeln: Daimon Verlag, 1985), pp. 9–11.

"Jung and Society," in *In the Wake of Jung: A Selection from* Harvest, Molly Tuby, ed. (London: Conventure, 1983), pp. 25–40.

"Love, War and Transformation: An Interview with Charlene Sieg," in *Psychological Perspectives: A Journal of Global Consciousness Integrating Psyche, Soul and Nature,* no. 2, Spring-Summer (Los Angeles: C. G. Jung Institute, 1991), pp. 54–63.

"Meaning and Order," in *Quadrant,* Summer (New York: C. G. Jung Foundation for Analytical Psychology, 1981), pp. 4–22.

"On Love, Maturity and Happiness: An Interview with Marie-Louise von Franz," by Joan Juliet Buck, in *Vogue,* November 1986, pp. 206–216.

"Peter Birkhäuser: A Modern Artist Who Strikes a New Path," in *Spring* (New York: C. G. Jung Foundation, 1964), pp. 33–46.

"Saint Exupéry's Little Prince," in *Harvest* 2 (London: Analytical Psychology Club, 1955), pp. 74–102.

"The Geography of the Soul: An Interview with Marie-Louise von Franz," in *In Touch,* Summer (Nashua, N.H.: Centerpoint, 1993).

Also published in *Jungian Directions,* Winter-Spring (Vancouver: C. G. Jung Society, 1994), pp. 2–5.

"What Happens When We Interpret Dreams?" in L. C. Mahdi, ed., *Betwixt and Between: Patterns of Masculine and Feminine Initiation* (LaSalle, Ill.: Open Court, 1987), pp. 434–438.

MARIE-LOUISE VON FRANZ'S FINAL LECTURE:

"C. G. Jungs Rehabilitation der Gefühlsfunktion in unserer Zivilisation" ["Jung's Rehabilitation of the Feeling Function in Our Contemporary Civilization"], published in J. F. Zavala, G. Ruska, and R. Monzo, eds., *Beiträge zur Jung'schen Pyschologie: Festschrift zum 75. Geburtstag von Marie-Louise von Franz* [Contributions to Jungian Psychology: Festschrift for the 75th Birthday of Marie-Louise von Franz] (Valencia: Victor Orenga, Editores, S.L., 1980). Not translated into English.

Films with Marie-Louise von Franz

1982

"Marie-Louise von Franz. Bollingen, September 1982"
Produced by Françoise Selhofer.

A transcription of the text appears in *Jungiana,* Verlag Stiftung für Jung'sche Psychologie, Reihe A, Band 2, Zürich, 1989, pp. 15–33.

The text of the film was originally in German but is now available in English, French, and Spanish. In this film, Marie-Louise von Franz speaks about her life, her encounter and collaboration with C. G. Jung, her understanding of Jung's psychology, and her own work. She answers questions on dream interpretation, creativity, synchronicity, alchemy, and some of the burning problems of our times. The film can be ordered at Fotorotar AG, CH-Egg, Zürich, Switzerland (ISBN 3-87089-375-3). © Stiftung für Jung'sche Psychologie.

1987

"Die Visionen des Niklaus von Flüe. Eine Interpretation von Marie-Louise von Franz" ("The Visions of Niklaus von Flüe: An Interpretation by Marie-Louise von Franz")

Produced by Televisione della Svizzera Italiana under the direction of Guido Ferrari.

The text of the film is printed in *Jungiana*, Verlag Stiftung für Jung'sche Psychologie, Reihe A, Band 9, Zürich, 2000, pp. 11–41.

The film can be ordered at Fotorotar AG, CH-Egg Zürich, Switzerland (ISBN 3-908116-94-5).

1988

"The Wisdom of the Dream"

A video interview with Marie-Louise von Franz broadcast on a Channel 4 Television series in London. See also S. Segaller and M. Berger, *Jung—The Wisdom of the Dream* (Boston: Shambhala, 1989).

1988

"The Way of the Dream"

Produced by Frazer Boa and Windrose Film Productions, Toronto, Canada.

Featuring interpretations of dreams gathered by Fraser Boa from ordinary men and women on the street and interpreted by Marie-Louise von Franz. The film can be ordered at Windrose Films LTD, c/o G. Chalmers Adams, 1255 Yonge Street, Suite 100, Toronto, M4T 1W6, Canada. The film transcript was published in F. Boa, *The Way of the Dream: Conversations on Jungian Dream Interpretation with Marie-Louise von Franz* (Boston: Shambhala, 1994).

Marie-Louise von Franz left numerous unpublished lectures, papers, and major works related to alchemy, mythology, fairy tales, dreams, active imagination, synchronicity, and other subjects. The heirs of the literary estate of Marie-Louise von Franz, the Stiftung für Jung'sche Psychologie, and Emmanuel Kennedy are presently in the process of publishing these works, the first volume being *Animus and Anima in Fairy Tales.*

Made in the USA
Las Vegas, NV
23 October 2026

56345759R00371